PRAISE F

"Julie Peters has given us a work on sexual trauma that is at once sweeping yet intimate. On every page there is the vibrant energy of intellectual curiosity as well as the searing truth of lived experience. In her book, she challenges us to not just be readers, but also witnesses to her journey. It's at times painful, often humorous, always illuminating. Anyone who has been touched by trauma knows that there's a resonance that lives on long after in the body and mind. But in her near-experience book, Peters also shows us the resilience and radiance."

—Ian Kerner, PhD, sex therapist, and *New York Times* best-selling author of *She Comes First*

"Wow. Beautiful. Kudos. This book is such a compassionate, nuanced look at an incredibly complex, deeply-entrenched set of flawed societal norms and patriarchal beliefs about power, sex, punishment, and entitlement. And most importantly, some great advice on healing; helping survivors and society in general."

—Paul Gilmartin, host of the *Mental Illness Happy Hour* podcast

"It is a rare and wondrous thing to read a book that seems to see into the most secret and private corners of your life, your body—that seems, in fact, to have been there for a long time, waiting to provide you with what you had not known you'd desperately needed. Julie Peters has written such a book. With unwavering honesty, penetrating insight, warmth, humor, and aplomb, she lays out strategies for a tangible, nourishing, and vitally ferocious self-love. The book is written from the perspective of a survivor of sexual assault (and what a tremendous and generous gift it is for those who have shared the experience), but the practical and practicable wisdoms here are for everyone. The reader feels variously transported to a therapist's office, a research facility that studies modes of gentleness, a night spent talking over wine with a dear and learned friend, and into the center of a circle in which a witch mixes her healing potions and sings her wild incantations. I hope that (particularly straight, cisgendered) men will join me in reading this book—both for the insight into the lives of the women (and other-gendered folks) who surround us, with whom we are intimate or not, with whom we share space, and for the revelations it offers into our own lives, our own fraught relationships with pleasure, food, addiction, sex, our bodies. As Tony Kushner writes in *Angels in America*, 'The Great Work Begins.' Julie Peters provides us a map."

—Jeremy Radin, poet, author of *Slow Dance with Sasquatch* and *Dear Sal*

"Julie Peters' new book *Want: 8 Steps to Recovering Desire, Passion, and Pleasure After Sexual Assault* provides women who have experienced sexual assault with a roadmap toward healing their shame and rekindling their desire. What's unique about this book is that the sexual assault that the author shares about so vulnerably happened when she was an adult, with a 'best friend' whose advances she had been rejecting for months. Peters takes readers on her own personal journey from trauma to reconnecting with her body, emotions, and eventually her own desire and sexuality. While the book is well thought out and researched, it is Peter's no-nonsense, tell it like it is, personal narrative that is both refreshing and so relatable to many women's experiences. Add this book to your bookshelf!"

—Xanet Pailet, Sex & Intimacy Educator and Coach, author of the best-selling book, *Living an Orgasmic Life: Heal Yourself and Awaken Your Pleasure*

"This book paves the way forward to newer, better sex and relationships for sexual assault survivors. Julie Peters weaves personal experience and research to bring us readers deep into the psychology and physiology of sexual desire post-assault. This book empowers survivors to go beyond the limiting 'healing' narrative our culture imposes and to reclaim sex as a source of pleasure and joy moving forward. It's full of practical strategies for a better sex life—strategies that take into account survivors' histories and challenges."

—Katie Simon, writer whose work has appeared in *The New York Times*, *Medium*, *The Washington Post*, and more

"This is a potent, provocative, multi-sided look at deep and painful issues between the genders. Julie's depth of knowledge in this work is illustrated by her ability to know when to engage difficult edges and when to hold people to account, as well as when to bring levity, breathe, and remind of us of our shared humanity. Her profound courage as a rape survivor to share so deeply is matched by the wisdom of her nuanced exploration of violation pattern in broader society. She is able to do so with an utterly non-shaming and compassionate voice that also consistently includes and thoughtfully considers the victimization of men, transgendered, and non-gender binary people. Her voice is just the kind of eldership that is so needed in the complexity of gender identity, power, and violence issues."

—David Hatfield, M.A., M.Ed., process facilitator and consultant, Canadian coordinator for International Men's Day, founder of Manology: Exploring 21st Century Masculinity.

"Julie skillfully weaves together science, history, and feminist and trauma theory with her own sexual assault and healing. She offers practical trauma-informed tools for the reader to support their own safe embodiment and writes in an honest, funny, and hopeful way about the struggle to make sense of the world and our lives and how to thrive in the aftermath of trauma. Her heartfelt writing reaches out to the reader, like a friend who bears witness to your most vulnerable moments while mirroring them back in her own. I think that this book is a must for anyone wanting to understand their own journey after trauma and needing the support of a wise, compassionate, and well-informed presence along the way."

—Nicole Marcia, MA, trauma-informed yoga therapist

"Reading *Want*, I found myself exhaling deeply every few pages. Peters sets out to do what many survivors wonder, at one point or another, if we're capable of doing: she seeks to heal from her assault by understanding it from every direction. From within the body. From fields upon fields of research. From turning toward the wound as opposed to away from it, all the while remaining transparent about how she's learning right alongside us. In the same candid and warm tone you'd expect from sitting down to drinks with your best friend, Peters shares frankly and sincerely as she moves through each new learning, be it clinical, physiological, or societal, holding it up to the light to see where it might fit best in the very real, intricate mess of moving beyond the harm that's done to us."

—Kelsey Savage, writer and sex educator

"Despite sexual violation being an enragingly common story, Julie manages to pull out her own unique narrative, and, in true yogic tradition, seeks unity with self to self, self to others, and others to self. Simply astounding."

—Monique Desroches, trauma-informed somatic therapist

"Julie Peters brings pleasure to life after sexual assault through vulnerable stories, supportive tools, and social critiques. This blend of thoughtful work will support folx in their healing and their growth. I am so into a world where we encourage more understanding of our complex humanness, and Julie allows us to breathe with her and try together. Powerful, vivid, and profound; Julie welcomes you to yourself."

—Tanille Geib, sexual health educator

"Julie has eloquently navigated the fine balance of trauma and triumph. She articulates perfectly an application for healing, infusing a gentle, knowledgeable language with a lightness that is hard to achieve in this subject. Her blend of earnest personal sharing and well-researched material drew me in and left me enthusiastically turning page after page and nodding my head in solidarity. This book gave me permission to go deeper into my own experiences by being delighted and eager to use her techniques and practices of self-acceptance and care. Practical, playful, and poignant, Julie's perspective reads so clearly and genuinely I truly feel this book is a must for any survivor or ally wanting to deepen their journey of healing."

—Lola Frost, international burlesque artist, exotic dancer, and instructor; co-owner of the Vancouver Burlesque Company.

"An educational approach to regaining your power, *Want* talks honestly about the realities of sexual assault and how to take control over your pleasure and your life in its wake. *Want* is a restorative text, offering readers a hand, a shoulder, and a toolkit. Peters is a wise, warm, and compassionate companion through the most challenging of experiences. *Want* is a place of sharing, a place of grace, and a clearing in the woods; it is as personally tailored to its readers as any book can be. *Want* will put you first and is a tremendous resource for coping with assault."

—Erin Kirsh, award-winning poet published in *Geist, Qwerty, The Malahat Review,* and others

Want

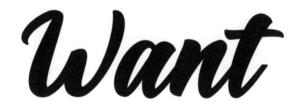

Want

8 steps to recovering desire, passion, and

pleasure after sexual assault.

JULIE PETERS

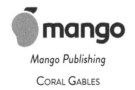

Mango Publishing

Coral Gables

Published by Mango Publishing Group, a division of Mango Media Inc.

Cover and Layout Design: Jermaine Lau

For permission requests, please contact the publisher at:

Mango Publishing Group
2850 Douglas Road, 2nd Floor
Coral Gables, FL 33134 USA
info@mango.bz

For special orders, quantity sales, course adoptions and corporate sales, please email the publisher at sales@mango.bz. For trade and wholesale sales, please contact Ingram Publisher Services at customer.service@ingramcontent.com or +1.800.509.4887.

Want: 8 Steps to Recovering Desire, Passion, and Pleasure after Sexual Assault

Library of Congress Cataloging
ISBN: (p) 978-1-63353-964-8 (e) 978-1-63353-965-5

Library of Congress Control Number: 2019935689

BISAC category code: HEA042000 HEALTH & FITNESS / Sexuality

Printed in the United States of America

This book is dedicated to you, the reader, in honor of all that you've survived.

CONTENTS

SURVIVE

What I remember most is what happened after.

I'm sitting in my car, staring out the windshield. It's raining, and it's late, maybe three or four in the morning. The wipers are on, but the car is not. I watch them spread the rain across the windshield (badly on the right side, that wiper has been broken for years). I listen to the rhythmic *squee* for a while, staring, not quite able to turn the car on and drive myself home. My thoughts don't seem to want to take an order. I'm not physically hurt, I'm fine. I'm fine. I think I'm fine. But I left my best friend's house at three or four in the morning in the rain because I needed to get the hell out of there. And now I'm sitting here across from his apartment, listening to a broken windshield wiper, not getting the hell out.

I don't know how long I sat there before I finally figured out I could turn the car on and go home. Sometimes I try to remember, really get the details in order, sort out what happened, go back to the beginning and think it through till the end, but it's difficult, like trying to get ants to walk in a straight line. It gets mixed up with other memories— the other times he'd tried to touch me when I didn't want him to. Or when he pushed me into his room and locked the door behind him. Or trying to leave earlier that same night, sitting on the stairs, my coat half on, him pleading with me to stay, me making him promise nothing would happen. I remember enough, anyway.

When a bad thing happens, you have to survive twice. First, you have to survive the thing itself. You have to be physically alive after the thing has happened. That's certainly key to the whole process. But then you have to survive again, to get through the consequences of the thing that didn't kill you. You have to figure out how to be a person in a world where your trust in people or your faith in what you think the world is has been shattered. Survival is a gift, but not always the kind you want. Sometimes it's like the worst of grandma's Christmas sweaters, because still existing after a terrible thing happened is confusing and painful and sometimes itchy and definitely comes back every Christmas.

If something like this has ever happened to you, congratulations! If you're reading this, you are a survivor. But then, of course, there's everything after. You have to cope. Then you have to forgive yourself for whatever devastation the coping caused in your life. You have to survive your own survival.

How to Use This Book

I don't know what will help you in your healing journey, but I can certainly share what has helped me. I don't want to preach at you or give you a bunch of advice you don't want to take. So I've separated out my suggestions for some things you can try into these handy little boxes. You're welcome to try the suggestions in these boxes anytime you like or ignore them altogether. It's your choice.

SURVIVING THE MOMENT

I hate thinking about what happened to me. I still feel shame burning the back of my throat when I think about how long it took me to realize that what happened was a violation. I wish I'd resisted more, fought, run away. The guy wasn't even that much stronger than me—he was one of those nerdy beanpole types who wouldn't raise a hand (but knew how to whittle your self-esteem down to a husk). I wish I'd been able to sit with my feelings and trust my gut and tell that guy to die in a fire. I apologized to *him* when I told him we couldn't see each other anymore. I didn't understand why I felt so repulsed by this nice guy who had violated me. It was confusing. It felt like my fault. Sometimes it still does. Maybe it was. I don't know.

Writing this book is hard, partly because of how certain I am that you, as you read my story, will judge me for being so stupid and weak. When I sat down to start writing this chapter in the bright new coffee shop in my neighborhood with the sleek counters and gourmet glass coffee bean smelling dome thingies, I opened my computer and promptly burst into tears. The barista very sweetly came by to wipe the table and quietly ask, "You okay, honey?"

It's just that I don't know that I have the right to tell this story when so many more horrible violent traumas have happened to so many others. Do I even have the right to my own reaction? Do I deserve to heal from something that someone else may not have found so devastating? How can I claim to know anything about healing when I was so stupid in the first place? (I did not say any of this to the barista. To the barista, I smiled effusively and told her yes and thank you for asking.)

Honestly, I don't know the answers to these questions. If you want to judge me for what happened, there's not a damn thing I can do about that. But one thing I do know is that I am far from the only woman to experience one of these creepy nonconsensual sexual experiences that may not have been especially physically violent but that broke something in me anyway. Every woman I know has experienced some level of sexual violation. I know a few of the guys have, too, along with many transgender and nonbinary individuals. Some of us were groped as children and didn't know what it meant at the time. Some of us have woken up with a date, a friend, or an ex-boyfriend already inside us. Some of us were too drunk to really know what we were consenting to or said yes when we really meant no. Some of us have been verbally abused and manipulated into doing things we didn't want to do. We've been stalked, catcalled, followed home, and felt up at work. Some of us were abducted by strangers and raped in an alley at gunpoint, that happens too. But a lot of our experiences happened at the hands of someone we trusted. However gently we were violated, we were still violated. It changed us for the rest of our lives.

TEND AND BEFRIEND

I'm sure I'm not the only survivor who suspected that the fact that we complied with what was happening meant we caused the assault in some way, that we have no right to be angry, or that it was our fault. Well, let me clear that one up once and for all: honey, it was *not your fault* (nor mine, either). And I'm not just saying that: it's science!

When we're stressed, we react with what's called the fight-or-flight response. When faced with a predator, our bodies flood with stress hormones like adrenaline and norepinephrine and our blood rushes out of our sexual and digestive organs and heads to the limbs, where we can throw some 'bows or get the F out of the way. As it turns out, though, this type of stress response has mostly only been studied in male animals. Females—that is, mammals with vaginas—were often left out of the research on stress, along with a whole lot of other things that have been studied in labs, too. Guess why? Yup, it's periods! Female animals tend to have periods, so the hormone fluctuations make our bodies harder to study in clinical trials of anything. Thanks for including only half the population, medical science!

In 2000, Dr. Shelley Taylor et al. published a paper on a type of stress response that seems to affect female animals (humans, rats, sheep, and some primates) disproportionately.[1] Taylor doesn't get into the specifics for how this might affect a transgender individual, but the gender variation in stress responses does seem to be related to hormonal patterns (as opposed to specifically one's genitals, though pregnancy plays a role). The paper does, however, clarify that it's not a completely consistent variation across gender lines. We should always be careful when we point to strong differences between the sexes from an evolutionary standpoint. It's easy enough to be biased, even in scientific research, and, in general, all humans are more similar than they are different. Nevertheless, Taylor's theory makes a lot of confusing things suddenly start to make sense. In addition to fight-or-flight, female animals can generally display a whole other stress response called "tend and befriend."

The idea is that female animals are less likely to survive by fighting or fleeing. They may be smaller and/or slower than their attackers, but they also might be pregnant or carrying helpless young. So rather than a rush of adrenaline, some of us get a squirt of oxytocin, a bonding hormone, instead. Oxytocin tends to be inhibited by testosterone and boosted by estrogen, so tend and befriend disproportionately affects women, girls,

1   Taylor, Shelley E., Laura Cousino Klein, Brian P. Lewis, Tara L. Gruenewald, Regan A. R. Gurung, and John A. Updegraff. "Biobehavioral Responses to Stress in Females: Tend-and-Befriend, Not Fight-or-Flight." *Psychological Review* 2000, Vol. 107, No. 3, 411–429, University of California, Los Angeles.

and other people with female-like hormonal patterns. The "tend" part makes sure we don't abandon our babies when shit goes down, and the "befriend" part helps us find allies to protect us when we know we can't protect ourselves. Surely a huge part of why naked humans with their soft nails and rounded teeth have made it this far is because we know how to rely on each other.

Female animals will often turn to each other in times of stress and try to develop networks to protect one another. This is pretty cool, especially considering how our culture tends to pit women against each other in competition (see: any reality TV show), but consider what can happen when someone you already see as an ally attacks you. Your first response may not be to fight and scream. Your instincts might urge you to connect instead—to placate. Appeal. Please. Try to calm him down. Shut up and give him whatever he wants so that he doesn't kill you. Sound familiar?

For a long time, I believed I had lost my power. Then I believed that asshole *stole* my power. But maybe neither is true. Maybe my power didn't go anywhere. Power doesn't always look like standing up, screaming, or running away. Maybe it's powerful that I let what was happening play itself out until the moment when I could safely slip out without causing a scene or further aggravating his anger. I always saw it as a weakness that I dissociated and went passive while it was happening, but perhaps it was a very old and actually quite effective survival instinct called tend and befriend that allowed me to get the hell out of there—still alive.

We live in a culture that tends to value men and masculine qualities more than women and feminine qualities. We are used to seeing medicine and evolution through the male gaze, and perhaps we see power that way, too. We need our male and female superheroes to be strong, and most of them can also literally fly—they've got fight or flight on lockdown. We tend to assign a wage to labor that is physical or intellectual, but emotional labor like caring for children, cleaning the house, and making plans for the family generally goes unpaid or underpaid. We don't respect "chick flicks" that depict female characters in the process of learning to connect. We restrict films that show sex and award Oscars to whichever films have the most disturbing violence. We don't mind pretty frilly things on super thin fashion models but get very uncomfortable with men who want to wear flowy garments or bright colors. Our culture has a problem with honoring and respecting the feminine, whether it comes in a male or female body. So perhaps you and I are conditioned to see tend and befriend as less powerful than fight or flight, even though it is just as powerful. You know how I know that? Because we survived.

I think tend and befriend might help explain a lot of our confusion around sexual violence. If part of our stress-response wiring is to placate and please, it makes sense that some perpetrators might actually think we are consenting, even if we manage to get a "no" out of our mouths at some point during the experience. I know (at least) one woman who avoided having sex with someone by bargaining for a blow job instead. She didn't exactly come out ahead (pun intended), but the girl survived. We get through these experiences and avoid more explicit violence by pretending it's okay with us.

When we speak up later and say we didn't want to do what we did, these perpetrators might be surprised because they were looking for and expecting a yes, and placating seemed close enough. No wonder we're all so lost about what consent means.

I suspect many of us are using this strategy more than we know, not only in sexual situations, but also at home, with our families, with our partners, and even in boardrooms. We know we should probably lean in and talk back and get mad when men interrupt to mansplain back to us what we were just saying, but we often don't because in a really old place in our tiny little reptilian brains, we know we should be nice because we don't want to get murdered.

As irrational as this might sound—and, guys, believe me, I know most of you are not out here trying to murder anyone—a lot of women have a very deep fear of our intimate male others, whether this comes from experience, generational violence handed down to us from our great-grandparents, or the ambient information we get from our news and entertainment. Men's roles are generally limited in our blockbuster films to savior/protector or villain/rapist, so a lot of us have these simplistic roles stuck in our unconscious minds. We never want to consciously believe our loved ones would hurt us, but the truth is, they do—a lot. An overwhelming amount of rape and nonconsensual sex happens with the men we know and trust. Over half of all the murders of women in the US are at the hands of a current or former male partner.[2] Congratulations on your recent nuptials! You just gained a life partner, the opportunity to share your Netflix subscription, and a significant increase in your chances of death!

Of course, sexual violence, trauma, and survival responses don't only happen to women at the hands of men. If anything, we are conditioned to expect women to be victims and to silence men who experience violation. The truth is, all humans have the capacity to be violent and the capacity to be afraid. It's not only men and women who have to figure out how to survive each other. We live in a world where certain groups have been oppressed and treated with violence by other groups, both historically and currently. Being a person of color, transgender, visibly gay, differently abled, or even just being a smaller-sized man could be reasons to have a range of survival responses ready to go in your pocket. Tend and befriend might be one of them. What if we considered this response normal, effective, and even powerful? We play nice with our attackers and our oppressors because we are trying to survive. It's not enough and it doesn't have to be the end of the story, but there can be no healing if we don't survive to fight (or flee or befriend) another day.

---

2   Donaghue, Erin. "More than half of the women slain in 2017 were killed by family or partners, study finds." CBS News, Nov 27, 2018. https://www.cbsnews.com/news/more-than-half-of-women-slain-in-2017-were-killed-by-family-intimate-partners-study-finds/

Seeing Your Survival as Powerful

Consider a bad experience you've had. This could be a traumatic experience if you feel comfortable going there, but if you prefer, practice with something milder, like going through a breakup, losing a job, moving to a new city, or having an argument with a friend (as long as you don't consider these too traumatic!).

⊕   What did you do? Think about the actions that you took to get through the initial experience and/or the aftermath.

⊕   Pause to consider that whatever happened, however messy it was, whatever regrets you might have about it, and no matter how long it took, you made powerful choices because you survived.

⊕   Consider the possibility that these actions you took are not reasons to see yourself as disempowered but are exactly the opposite: reasons to believe that you are powerful, that you do have the power to survive and to continue to take your healing into your own hands.

⊕   Take a few moments with a journal and write down each of the things you did phrased like this: "I ___, and I survived."

TRAUMA AND THE BRAIN

Trauma is a strange animal. It's not always big and dramatic; sometimes it's small and subtle. The definition of trauma has shifted and widened in recent years. Traumatic stress tends to be triggered by witnessing or experiencing actual or threatened violence, according to the International Society for Traumatic Stress Studies.[3] What "violence" means isn't as clear as we might think, either: the World Health Organization defines violence as "the intentional use of physical force or power, threatened or actual, against oneself, another person, or against a group or community, that either results in or has a high likelihood of resulting in injury, death, psychological harm, maldevelopment, or deprivation."[4] Violence can be physical or psychological, and can manifest as injury, threat, or even neglect. Some people are traumatized indirectly or vicariously when a loved one is going through something. For some people, emotional losses like divorce or custody battles aren't necessarily marked by violence but are traumatic anyway. This can make trauma a little hard to spot and a lot more common than most of us think.

Traumatic stress or PTSD also doesn't necessarily follow any of these kinds of experiences. If a plane were to crash leaving a number of survivors, only some of them would be traumatized. Some would have traumatic stress reactions that would resolve

---

3   "What is Traumatic Stress?" International Society for Traumatic Stress Studies webpage accessed Nov 2018. https://www.istss.org/public-resources/what-is-traumatic-stress.aspx
4   "Definition and Typology of Violence." Violence Prevention Alliance, World Health Organization. Nov 2018 http://www.istss.org/public-resources/what-is-traumatic-stress.aspx

in a few weeks, others would have the longer-lasting and more serious post-traumatic stress disorder (PTSD), and still others would be just fine. The classic symptoms of traumatic stress include trouble sleeping, mood swings, nightmares, an enhanced startle response, anxiety, depression, and social withdrawal. It's common for trauma survivors to have a hard time remembering the traumatic event itself, despite the sudden unbidden flashbacks that happen for some of us. Trauma is triggered by an external event, but ultimately it's something that happens inside of us.

Trauma shuts down our ability to see the world as safe and predictable. Kids who grow up in an unpredictable environment can have a tough time figuring out how the world is supposed to work in the first place. Being traumatized as an adult can mean losing some of our most precious illusions about the world, like that we're safe most of the time, that people are trustworthy, or that God is on our side. These comforting perceptions aren't exact truths about the world, but they are handy: it's hard to relax when the sky could fall at any moment. I mean—it could. Reading the news makes you feel like the sky is falling right now. The sky is falling for real people all over the world all the time. The world is not only immoral, it's barely comprehensible. Even physicists don't totally understand the fundamental principles of how the universe was born and continues to be a thing. But you can't walk around feeling like you have absolutely no control over anything (even though—and I hate to break it to you—it's true!). You still need to get to work in the morning, you know?

Being sexually assaulted by my best friend was, to put it mildly, confusing. I denied it for a long time because I didn't want to face the scary realities it brought up. If my best friend had assaulted me, then how could I ever trust my instincts with men again? How could I trust anyone anymore? If my "no" didn't matter, then how could I ever stop anyone from doing whatever they wanted to my body? How do you walk around in the world without an intact "no"? The experience broke several core beliefs I didn't even know I had. In order to heal, I had to look at what had been broken, see if I could glue any of the pieces back together, throw some of them out, and start building a whole new worldview from scratch. This was not easy. I survived the assault, of course, but first, the sky had to fall.

LIBIDO AS LIFE FORCE

When you're stressed all the time, whether from trauma or for other reasons, your physical body doesn't function well. Stress hormones keep telling your body to evacuate the blood and energy in your organs and send it to the limbs so you can fight, run, or freeze. Your rational mind goes into hiding, and your fear brain takes over. Your intestines aren't able to manufacture your mood hormones properly, and your sexual organs shrink up inside of you like terrified raisins. You might get that tend-and-befriend oxytocin boost, which makes you want to cling to certain people or, I don't know, get into a relationship with some boring dude you don't really like because he seems safe and probably won't rape you. You almost certainly lose your desire for sex.

Yes, I said it! it's a thing. Loss of sexual desire is a normal reaction to being sexually assaulted. Surprising, right?

We are a culture that is obsessed with sex but that doesn't value libido. We love objectifying people and their body parts, usually in the service of selling something, but we don't often think about how libido drives us in our day-to-day lives. Libido isn't just about sex. Libido is about power, passion, intensity, connection, and the sort of life desire that makes you want to take risks and try new things. When St. Augustine first wrote about libido in 426 CE, he used the phrase *libido dominandi,* which means "will to power" or "dominating lust."[5] In Sanskrit, the word *iccha* means both desire and will, the representation of what we want and our ability to go for it.[6] *Iccha-shakti* is a phrase that's sometimes used to mean life force, and it's related to the energy of the goddess named Shakti, the feminine form of power. People who are genuinely connected to their own sexual energy tend to be powerful—and not in a power-over kind of way, but in the sense that they know who they are and what they want. They are not afraid to try things, to invent, to show up, to make a mess. That freaks us out, so we try to corral libido into the realm of sex alone, where we can contain it and put rules around it and close it away, preferably into heterosexual married middle-class bedrooms.

Feminist critic Audre Lorde writes about the erotic as a "power which rises from our deepest and nonrational knowledge," a power that is often cut off and silenced in an oppressive society.[7] This is an energy of being connected to ourselves, of being unafraid to feel our most intense emotions. Lorde finds this energy in herself within

> *the open and fearless underlining of my capacity for joy, in the way my body stretches to music and opens into response, harkening to its deepest rhythms so every level upon which I sense also opens to the erotically satisfying experience, whether it is dancing, building a bookcase, writing a poem, or examining an idea.*[8]

When we're connected to our erotic energy, we have access to our deepest desires and feelings. We're connected to our own flow, and we're not trying to stop ourselves from feeling anything. Some of us use sex as a strategy to shut down our feelings, but this isn't true libido, that's a craving that comes from a place that wants to avoid feeling. If we're having sex because we want power over someone or because we're trading for something else, like intimacy or security, we're paradoxically shutting down our own libido, our genuine connectedness to who we are and what we want. Sexual energy can be channeled into work, friendships, art, and, sure, building bookcases. Celibate monks and nuns can be deeply connected to this erotic drive and channel it into their spirituality. It's sexual energy that doesn't have to be about sex with another person.

---

5   Stack Pole, Gregory. "Peter Brown on Augustine on the Libido Dominandi." Into the Clarities, Feb 19, 2016. https://intotheclarities.com/2016/02/19/peter-brown-on-augustine-on-the-libido-dominandi/
6   Brooks, Douglas Renfrew. *The Secret of the Three Cities: An Introduction to Sakta Tantrism.* Chicago, University of Chicago Press (1990) 96.
7   Lorde, Audre. *Sister Outsider: Essays and Speeches.* Berkeley: Crossing Press (2007): 53–54.
8   Lorde, Audre. *Sister Outsider: Essays and Speeches.* Berkeley, Crossing Press (2007): 56.

After the assault, I lost this energy. It wasn't just that I didn't feel like having sex, but I also didn't really feel plugged into anything. I didn't have any joy. I felt that I was going through the motions of life, letting other people make my decisions for me. My erotic drive was shut down, pleasure was a great distance away, and I didn't have the motivation to change anything about my life. This was what I now think of as the fog of trauma. You don't usually even know you're in it until you wake up. It took me four years to wake up.

Our erotic energy lives in our deepest places, in our guts and in our genitals. I thought of this when the pop singer Cardi B was asked how she felt on the red carpet at the 2018 Grammy Awards, and she said in an excited singsong voice, "I feel it all! Butterflies in my stomach and vagina!"[9] Truly, what a delightful twist on an old adage. Our stomachs and vaginas are the deepest sources for our "yes" and "no" feelings, around sex of course, but also about which projects we want to take on, which people we feel safe around, how to stay close to our ethical convictions. These are the places where things feel right or wrong to us. These are physical and not always rational places—the stomach and vagina, sources of a very true wisdom for women (though I have no doubt men get this feeling, too, in their stomachs and testicles, perhaps).

As it turns out, vaginas have a "pulse" that is measurable in lab settings, which many women have noticed piping up from time to time. The vaginal pulse shows up in all kinds of situations, sexual and otherwise. Naomi Wolf discovered this vaginal beat in her research for her book *Vagina: A New Biography*; in the book, she interviews women who report feeling it in all sorts of places: while hiking next to a beautiful view, feeling the thrill of the racetrack, listening to music, and crossing the finish line at a marathon. I've been paying attention to this recently, and sure enough, it's right there: I get a little quiver most often when I come across a really good line of writing that rings true for me, or when I look over a really high balcony, or when I make out with boys. Wolf explains that the existence of this vaginal pulse suggests

> *that a woman's relationship to her own mind and body is erotic first; that her existential excitement at being alive and responsible to the world around her is erotic first; and that this eros comes before any erotic awakening triggered by an "other."*[10]

So Cardi B was onto something there—when we're connected, safe, and feeling, for lack of a better term, "right" about the world, we get butterflies drumming a beat in our vaginas. When trauma happens, whether it's sexual in nature or not, it taxes our sense of safety, the normal functioning of our brains and our organs. The beat goes quiet. We're cut off from our deepest sense of ourselves, our passion, creativity, love, and joy. It's like someone has killed the butterflies.

9   "Cardi B Says She Feels Butterflies in Her Stomach and Vagina At Grammys Red Carpet (Looped)" Jan 28, 2018. https://www.youtube.com/watch?v=GR4VnAu58UI
10   Wolf, Naomi. *Vagina: A New Biography*. New York, Ecco (2013): 278.

Meditation for Sexuality as Life Force Energy

One really sweet way to connect with your libido is to imagine it inside of your body and meditate with it. Here's how:

⊕ Set a timer for ten minutes for this meditation. It's completely fine to do it for a longer or shorter amount of time according to your comfort.

⊕ Lie down on your back with your knees bent and your feet on the floor. Let your feet widen a bit so your knees can fall into each other. Take a few deep breaths and let your belly relax as much as you can.

⊕ Place your hands on your low belly, or right over your genitals. Breathe deeply and imagine sending the breath to this place, low down into your soft belly, into the bowl of your pelvis, into your genitals. Try to relax everything. No resistance from the breath at all.

⊕ Notice how you feel. Does it feel easy to breathe into your belly, your pelvis, your genitals? Do you feel tension here? Does the tension move with your breath or stay stuck?

⊕ Try not to judge or worry about whatever is happening here. Do your best to be present and compassionate with whatever you're feeling in this area. Simply inviting the breath into this zone will help you reconnect to your libido energy. Stay with it.

⊕ Imagine that there is a specific kind of energy, this sexual energy, living deep in your pelvis. You might be able to feel something, but if not, imagine it. Maybe it has a color or looks like water or light.

⊕ Imagine the energy moving with your breath, and see if it can move into different areas of your body. Perhaps you can feel it move into your heart, your throat, or down your legs into your feet.

⊕ Keep breathing, gently imagining this energy moving through you until your timer goes off, though you're welcome to stay longer if you like.

⊕ When you are ready, you can gently roll to one side and then up to a seat. Then press your hands into the floor and imagine the earth taking any pain, fear, shame, or discomfort that's ready to be released from your body (and it's okay if it's not ready to go). Take a deep breath, shake out your hands, and see how your day may feel a little bit different.

WHAT TO DO WHEN A WOLF HAS PEED ON YOUR HOME

Tracey Lindberg's novel *Birdie* is about a young indigenous woman dealing with the consequences of sexual assault alongside the many generational traumas that attend growing up indigenous in Canada, a country that has colonized and oppressed indigenous people for a very long time. The narrative is woven through with scenes like this one:

> *When she looks back, that old young owl,*
> *She sees that*
> *her home, her tree, had become*
> *ravaged with wolf urine*
> *and twisted with heat.*
> *Curled and gnarled, she is unable to sleep there.*
> *She begins to travel at nights*
> *because she cannot sleep in her home.*
> *She doesn't know what*
> *She's lookin' for*
> *But she keeps goin' and goin'.*[11]

When I read this, I felt a hot light run through my heart, and yup, right down into my vagina. It describes so perfectly what it feels like to be sexually assaulted, to feel that someone has broken into your home, defiled it, and then didn't even stick around to see what would happen next.

Our first and only true homes are our bodies. There are no other true homes. But when we do not feel that our bodies truly belong to us, when we don't feel safe in them, how can we rest? How can we sleep at night or replenish our resources with our kitchen counters covered in wolf urine? So we flee, we run away from our ruined homes, we try to avoid our own bodies, to get away from the smell and the shame of the violation.

When we can't go home, we can't ever turn off the stressed-out sympathetic nervous system state to repair and recover. We don't want to stop and restore ourselves. It's too painful to slow down to rest and feel our feelings. Instead we distract ourselves with work and create more anxiety in our lives, so we have something to focus on that isn't the defilement at the center of our beings. We do not want to sit with our feelings because our feelings are very, very bad. We can't feel sexual when we don't feel safe. Neither can we digest. So what happens when we're traumatized, hypervigilant, and super stressed after a wolf peed all over our homes? Low sexual desire. And sometimes diarrhea.

In order to heal, we have to go home. We have to clean up all the wolf piss and figure out how to get the smell out. It's infuriating to have to clean up someone else's mess, but that's what we have to do. The act of the cleaning doesn't absolve the wolf. Rather, it's an act of love for your own home, your body. For me, the process of cleaning and recovery within my body was a more loving practice than I had ever experienced within myself before. My home is more mine than it's ever been.

This is challenging work, and we can't force ourselves to be ready for it. I think it took me so long partly because I didn't start out with a really strong sense of being at home in my body. Hitting puberty was confusing, not only because of all the hormones, but

11   Lindberg, Tracey. *Birdie*. New York, HarperCollins (2015): 230.

because of how my body was suddenly out there, being perceived as sexual, commented on, and grabbed. Becoming a sexual being came along with all kinds of scary stuff, like adult men catcalling my eleven-year-old body on the street, grabbing my ass in public places, or preying on high school girls to take them into the park to "practice" kissing. (Guys, I did this! I went into a park with a strange man and kissed him so I would learn to be better at kissing boys! Can you even believe I wasn't murdered? No one tell my mother.)

Growing up in a world that objectifies and preys on young women isn't exactly conducive to feeling secure about what belongs to you and what doesn't. My tend-and-befriend strategy up to that point had been pretty much to say yes to everything so I could seem cool and game and, you know, not get murdered, but I always thought I had a "no" I could use if I needed it, like an ace up my sleeve. But when I finally pulled the ace out, some asshole peed all over it anyway. My body was a place that had never been good, had never been whole, had never really been mine, and might as well have been soaked to the floorboards in wolf pee.

Body as Home

Journal with the following questions. Take as much time as you need; feel free to take one or two questions at a time and return to the others on a different day.

⊕   What is your relationship to your sexuality?

⊕   What is your relationship to your genitals? Do you touch them? Look at them? Feel the butterflies in them leading you to your "yes" and "no" responses?

⊕   How did your relationship to your sexual self change at puberty?

⊕   Where there any experiences or physical changes to your sexual self throughout your life that shifted your perception of your own sexuality?

⊕   Do you feel ownership over your body?

⊕   How do you respond when your body is sick or injured? Do you touch it? Medicate it? Feed it? Rest it? Share it with others? What others? Doctors? Lovers? No one?

⊕   Who has control over your body?

⊕   Does your body feel like home?

ADDICTION AS A SURVIVAL STRATEGY

So what do we do when home has been colonized by someone else's choices? How do we handle it when we can't face cleaning up someone else's territorial piss? Well, we get out that psychic Febreze, cover up the smell, deny everything, and figure out a way to keep goin' and goin'.

For a lot of us, this looks like addiction. Addiction doesn't always mean alcoholism or drug dependency, though of course it can. Addiction often means goin' and goin', it means doing whatever we can to avoid feeling our feelings. We drink, we smoke. We gamble. We shop. We exercise too much or work to exhaustion or stay in bed all day. We binge on TV. I had a *close* relationship with the show *Grey's Anatomy* during a stretch of my survival phase—and thankfully all fifteen seasons (and counting) are available on Netflix.

I remember how comforting it was to feel so strongly about these fictional characters, because it felt so much less complicated than being in my own mind, my own body, and my own relationships. Addictive behaviors like these can be a boon in a lot of ways because they can turn the volume down on the painful thing you somehow both can't remember and can't stop thinking about.

There's a lot of shame that comes along with addiction, but I think it's actually pretty amazing that human beings have the ability to find tools that help us dissociate or numb ourselves. Sometimes our own minds are absolutely unbearable, and we have this almost mystical ability to exit our bodies and exist on some other plane when the plane we're on sucks too much. It's an incredible tool for survival.

Of course, the tools we use to numb and dissociate also tend to have some pretty serious consequences, not the least of which is that these tools tend to self-perpetuate at the cost of absolutely everything else. After the assault, I was diagnosed with Generalized Anxiety Disorder, which sounds like a problem of modern life where you just feel anxious all the time for no particular reason—which is exactly what it is. One of the fun consequences of this disorder is that when I get anxious in general, just kind of anxious about life and the fact that I have a vulnerable set of guts, I pick up more work and take on more appointments, which also makes me feel anxious—but in a more *familiar* way: a way that I chose, that I have control over. Logical, right? It sort of works, but it pins my nervous system into a spin cycle that makes me feel—get this—generally anxious. It's a short-term solution that exacerbates a long-term problem.

When I do this, my reptilian brain—that is, the very old, primitive, survival-oriented part of my brain that is driven by fear, emotion, and the present moment—is in control. This is the oldest part of the brain structure, which I sometimes affectionately call "Lizard Brain." It connects directly to our nervous systems and is a basic structure that we share with reptiles. It is much louder and more powerful than my Wise Brain—the newer, more reason-oriented part of the brain including the neocortex, which takes into account the past, the future, and, you know, actual reality. Wise Brain needs things like good food, rest, and a general sense of safety to work properly. Lizard Brain avoids those things so we never have to be in a state where we might feel our feelings. I think it's vitally important to understand that while Lizard Brain might be messing up our lives in some pretty serious ways, it is also desperately trying to help us.

There's something for me about smoking cigarettes when I'm feeling really low. I once heard that we carry grief in our lungs, and that feels so true for me—it's like I want to fill a certain void with horrible toxic smoke when I'm in my lagoon of sadness. I remember going through a heartbroken phase where I would take my dog out, cigarette and lighter hidden carefully in one hand, and go to the farthest end of my neighborhood where I could be sure no one would notice me, peer around for any onlookers, sit down on the pavement in the rain, and light up, my dog looking at me like I was crazy. I'd puff away at my shameful habit, stoppering the tears with nicotine and tar, hiding from everyone, as pathetic as possible—and inevitably a neighbor would notice my dog (an implacably chipper Pomeranian mix) and cheerfully say hello, interrupting my high-drama reverie. Smoking seems to pull me down to earth, returning me to my heavy body, letting me settle fully into my feet. I'm also quite sure no one in my life would ever tell me to light up, so I can be 100 percent sure I'm making a choice about my body that is completely mine. It's terrible for me, and I usually regret it immediately, but for a moment, it makes me feel better.

It's not just the cigarettes, either. I've gotten drunk because the spins and then the next day's brutal hangover gave me something other than my feelings to focus on for a while. I've had a string of one-night stands with people I didn't really like because it made me feel powerful, like I was in control of my body, even if it didn't feel good. Even if it hurt. When the high wore off enough for Wise Brain to wake back up, I'd feel a bolt of shame, and that was all Lizard Brain needed to get back in charge and take me through the cycle all over again. I'd work on it, try to do better, fail, and then say, "Fuck it" and find some other way to avoid myself.

For me, the key to getting out of the cycle was targeting the shame. Lizard Brain is not my enemy. Lizard Brain is trying to help me survive. When I can see my addictive behaviors as the desperate attempts to avoid pain that they are, I can thank my Lizard Brain for helping to protect me and then try to figure out a way to address the pain, be brave, and face myself anyway. We need to understand that if we have addictive tendencies, that's because we are still trying to fucking survive, even if the thing we're surviving happened years ago. We have to see and appreciate and forgive that in order to move on.

Feeling Safer When You're Freaking Out

If you're able to notice yourself in an addictive behavior, in a panic, unable to sleep, feeling anxiety rising, or just coming out of a stressful or triggering situation (but you know you're physically safe), try these quick and simple grounding techniques that may help calm down Lizard Brain and bring Wise Brain back into the room:

⌗ Inhale deeply and slowly through your nose, and then exhale through pursed lips, like you're blowing a leaf slowly away from you. Do this five times, then switch: inhale through pursed lips like you are sipping through a straw, and then exhale through your nose.

⊕   Look around you and count how many red objects there are in the room. Then count how many green objects are in the room. Then count the blue.

⊕   Pick up an object in the room and describe it in as much detail as you can. What does it look like? What does it feel like? Does it have a smell? What about a taste? A sound?

⊕   Shake: some animals shake after they've escaped a predator, like they are shaking off the stress. Jump up and down, shake your hands, shake your head. Shake for a minute or two, then become still and see if you feel any better.

WHEN THE BUTTERFLIES CALL YOU HOME

The good news is, no one, not even your self-sabotaging habits, can completely kill the butterflies in your vagina (or testicles, or wherever they live). Sometimes it takes years or even decades to get through the survival phase, but eventually the body will rebel against our coping mechanisms in some way or another in an attempt to get us to face ourselves. The butterflies will stage a revolt.

A system that is constantly stressed is suffering, and it will make that suffering known. Denial is a subtle form of constant stress that taxes the immune system over time and can literally make us sick. Denial is not a great long-term strategy. I often think of those first four years after the trauma as a kind of sleepwalking, a total avoidance of my feelings, but it wasn't really that simple. My nervous system was fighting me all the way. I would have terrifying recurring dreams of being chased by a man I had to kill before he killed me, or about huge hulking killer whales swimming just beneath the surface of a deep body of water, about to rise up and consume me. I startled a lot, and while I never quite had a panic attack, it felt like my heart was always beating just a little too fast. I would get stress hives and long flus that would force me to lie down for weeks. I am a yoga teacher in my thirties who got pneumonia twice. Pneumonia! It was kind of embarrassing. I'm in the wellness industry, guys. My body would find some highly dramatic way to make me sit down and feel my feelings. I'd just have to lie there, ill on my couch, with the memories coming back and my stomach cramping, and cry.

There were two triggers that helped me start to clue in that maybe I should pay attention to all these physical reactions. The first was a pamphlet created by the poets Mindy Nettifee and Rachel McKibbens that was being passed around within a community with which I was involved. It had been discovered that one of our prominent male members was repeatedly raping young women in the community. Everyone was so shocked (as if that never happens). The pamphlet had an image of a woman shooting rainbows out of her eyes on it, and it listed different ways you could be assaulted: when you're unconscious, when you're drunk, when you've said no, when you've been coerced or manipulated, when there's a power dynamic between the two people that confuses consent. I remember reading and rereading this pamphlet. It seemed to speak to some deep place of truth in my body, asking me to pay attention. The butterflies were flapping their little wings as hard as they could. The pamphlet challenged my idea that rape only happened at gunpoint. It suggested that what had happened to me was not, in fact, okay, and that I'd been struggling to swallow something that was as toxic as it tasted.

The second thing that happened was that one of my best friends was raped—yep, by her ex-boyfriend, a friend at the time, whom she trusted. I found myself obsessing about it, feeling much more upset than was appropriate to the situation. Don't get me wrong— it's appropriate to be fucking upset when a friend is raped. It's appropriate to be angry, vengeful, and sorrowful. But I was more like shaking all day and couldn't sleep or exactly breathe. I was breaking out into hives and couldn't stop crying. I was reacting more than my friend was, as if something was happening to me, not to her. I was shaken enough that I called the sexual assault crisis line and found myself explaining that something similar had happened to me. I had to see it happen to someone else before I could acknowledge that it was my story, too. Apparently, it's easier to keep our eyes open with the ones we love than with our own selves.

It certainly didn't feel like it at the time, but I've come to understand that my pneumonias, my anxiety, my startle response, and my nightmares were in a sense my erotic energy trying to bust up against all my doors and duct tape trying to keep them trapped in the basement. It was the butterflies, tired of sleeping, wanting to wake up and speak to me through my vagina. It was the energy of life, insisting on finding a way to live.

Listening to the Nervous System

Your conscious brain may not be willing or able to have certain kinds of conversations with you, but your body may be finding other ways to talk to you. Here are some ways to listen:

+ Write down your dreams as soon as you wake up in the morning. As you retell the story to yourself, think about how the dreams made you feel and if there's anything in your life that makes you feel a similar way. The more you do this, the easier it will be to remember your dreams.

+ Consider the last time you got sick or were injured. Illness and injury can sometimes be understood symbolically as a message from an overtaxed immune system (but not all the time, sometimes we just get sick for no reason!). What did the sickness force you to do or give you an excuse not to do?

+ Where was the illness located in your body? Do you have areas that tend to be more vulnerable to illness and injury? How does that make you feel?

⊕   If you have recurring pain in your body, inquire in a similar way. When does the pain or discomfort arise? What does it need from you? What would happen if you slowed down to rest and take care of your pain?

THE CHANGE PROCESS

Now, years and a lot of healing work later, my butterflies are pretty healthy and hale. They respond very well to being listened to, honored, and allowed to fly freely (but they also make me cry all the time). They have a healthy home where they can rest and regenerate. They survived, too.

I needed to let the butterflies rest for a while. I needed to be in denial and to smoke cigarettes and watch hours and hours of strong female surgeons having their hearts broken on TV. I even needed those wrong relationships I kept getting into: they weren't the right people for me, but they helped me feel secure enough in my life that I could start thinking about getting that mop out and cleaning up what had been defiled. None of it was wasted time. It took exactly as long as it took.

I'm an impatient person, and I always want everything to be better right *now*, but it's taken me a long time to realize that sometimes it takes me a long time to realize things. Everything has its own pace. The stages of change theory (or the transtheoretical model of change[12]) lays out the process that anyone has to go through before they can make any real change in their lives. This theory comes up often in recovery programs where people are addressing an addictive behavior, but it applies to everything from opening up to love to getting your butt to the gym more often. It consists of five steps: precontemplation, contemplation, preparation, action, and maintenance.

In the precontemplation stage, you're living your life with no idea you have a problem. In the contemplation stage, you start to consider that you might maybe possibly have a problem. In the preparation stage, you set yourself up with whatever you'll need to make the change, like buying gym clothes or researching counselors. In the action stage, you're doing it, you're making the change in real time. The maintenance stage is when you keep it going sustainably, when it becomes a new habit you don't have to think about too much. Notice that there are three whole steps before you actually start doing anything differently. That's more than half of the steps! No wonder our New Year's resolutions never work: we don't even start thinking about them until December 31. We need a lot of time to integrate and process the possibility of changing something before anything can actually happen.

Some people include relapse as a stage of change. Inevitably, when we start doing something differently in our lives, we stumble. Our strategies for survival are old and powerful, and we use them because they work. When things are extra stressful, it's natural to fall back on what we know makes us feel better immediately. It's tough if this

12   DiClemente, C. C., & Prochaska, J. O. "Toward a comprehensive, transtheoretical model of change: Stages of change and addictive behaviors." In W. R. Miller & N. Heather (Eds.), *Applied clinical psychology. Treating addictive behaviors* (pp. 3–24). New York, NY, US: Plenum Press.

happens, but relapse can be a valuable stage of change, because once we've laid the groundwork and seen what it feels like to live differently, the relapse can illuminate how far we've come and remind us of why we don't want to go back.

The other night I was talking to my friend who had also been raped about how she felt in the years after her experience. For her, too, there was a long drought of denial and avoidance. I didn't know what was happening for her during that time, but I do remember she was withdrawn and our friendship was very distant for a long time. She knows the trauma fog well. She said, "I think back on that time sometimes, and you know, it was easier. It was less stressful, less confusing, less complicated. But it's better now, even though it's harder. At least now I can feel." I know it's been hard for her, and it still is, but when she started to admit what had happened and what it meant, her desire started to come back. I've seen her joy and her sense of humor returning as she cackles at TV shows or at baseball games. I know she cries and struggles and panics sometimes, but she also laughs now. She laughs all the time. She survived. Her butterflies are alive and well.

So survive we must. However long it takes, we need to create a container of safety before we can start dealing with the devastation of sexual assault. We need to see that whatever we had to do to survive at the time was what we had to do, and we survived, goddammit. It doesn't matter if we smoked ten thousand cigarettes or dated all the wrong people or pushed away everyone we cared about or drank ourselves to the bottom of the ocean. Our desire, our power, our creativity, our ability to love, connect, fuck, and feel don't completely die unless we completely die. Whatever happened, if we're still alive, we can heal.

FEEL

I am lying on my floor with my knees bent, hands on my belly. I am trying to breathe into my belly. This is my homework. A yoga teacher / bodyworker / massage therapist / witch I've been seeing told me that all my feelings were stuck in my pelvis and that if I wanted to feel anything again, I should do this every day.

My mind spins—I think about work, what I'm doing later, the pile of dishes in the sink. I'm supposed to be focusing on my breath. Nothing is happening. I try to focus. I try to let my breath move down lower, into my guts, my genitals, my pelvic floor. I can tell there is tension there, but it is not letting go. I can barely feel that part of my body. It's frustrating. It's all I can do not to jump up and do the dishes before the timer goes off.

Finally, I hear that sweet welcome "ding!" letting me know that my ten minutes is finally up. So I roll over and head to the kitchen to wash those damn dishes. And that's when the tears start.

Every day it's like this. I lie on my back and try to feel my belly, and nothing happens. But then, as soon as I get up to make some coffee or take a shower and get on with my life, I start to cry. I don't even know what I'm crying about, the tears just spring up all of a sudden and spill out. It's a very strange experience, but it's also the small seed of a big change. As I'm incrementally relaxing the tension I am holding in my gut, grief, fear, and anger are unlocking, coming up to the surface and melting all over my face in a mess of unbidden tears.

I do believe we hold emotions and memories in our physical flesh. When something happens, we respond physically—the gut tightens, the jaw clenches, the cold sweats begin. Most of us have physical stress patterns: we tend to respond in the same way every time something stressful happens, and the same old aches and pains tend to come up when we're stressed out. Some of us are in a protective posture all the time without even realizing it, continually sending the nervous system stress signals even when everything is okay. That's why I had to practice breathing into my belly every day for a while and letting myself cry. That's why Step Two in our recovery from sexual assault is to Feel.

TRAUMA AS A SPIRITUAL WOUND

I've come to understand that one of the hallmarks of trauma is that it threatens the survivor's worldview, the core beliefs one holds about the way the world is supposed to work. That's one of the reasons we don't want to talk about it, sometimes for years; it requires facing a challenge to our faith. Trauma is in many ways a spiritual wound.

I didn't grow up super religious, but I was always drawn to various spiritual worldviews. I started getting into yoga and meditation when I was twelve, and, by the time I hit sixteen, I was your classic teenage witch casting spells in her bedroom with scented candles from Walmart. By the time I was assaulted, I didn't exactly believe in a god, but I had a vague idea that bad things happen to bad people and good things happen to good people because the world is fundamentally just. In my recovery process, I had to come to terms with the fact that most events in our lives are generated by random chance. I don't believe anyone "out there" is watching out for me, because if that were the case, I was abandoned on that day. I do believe there are ways we are connected to each other and the world around us that can't always be quantified, but I don't think that's because of any design. I don't believe that I was a target for punishment or that I needed to learn some lesson in order to write this book and share it with you. When something tragic happens and someone pipes up that everything happens for a reason, honestly, I want to clock them. I think we can do good things with what we learn from bad experiences, but there's never some cosmic reason for our tragedies. Things just happen.

When I was sexually assaulted by a close friend, it threatened so many of my beliefs: that I knew how to trust people, that men could be trustworthy, that I was mostly safe in my day-to-day life, that my "no" mattered. If the world was just, I must have done something to deserve what happened to me. When our traumas mess with our core beliefs about the world, they can sometimes bring out the core beliefs we hold about ourselves. Unconsciously, many of us deeply believe we are fundamentally unlovable and worthless. For some of us, this is a childhood wound that still sticks with us late into our lives. For many women, it's part of the message we've picked up from our culture—that women are objects to be used, not human beings worthy of respect and care. For some men, it might be the idea that unless he makes a lot of money and has a lot of women, he's a total failure. For a transgender or nonbinary person, it might be that if they don't fit into one of two strict gender roles, they have no place in this society. Trauma can bring up these core beliefs: If the world is just, then bad things only happen to bad people. A bad thing happened to me, therefore I am a bad person, just as I always suspected!

Core Beliefs

If you find yourself feeling worthless and unlovable from time to time, you are not alone! Most of us feel this way every now and then. The key is bringing these beliefs to our conscious minds so we can have a dialogue with them and practice treating ourselves with kindness anyway. Here are some tips to practice with your core beliefs:

⊕ When you find yourself thinking "I'm so stupid and ugly and horrible and no one will ever love me," don't ignore it. Notice that you're thinking it. Write it down so you can see it in black and white. Acknowledge that you don't believe it (or are working on not believing it) with your rational mind.

⊕ Sometimes negative core beliefs can come out in behaviors. Do you do anything in your life that is harmful to your body, your heart, or your relationships? Behaviors that make you feel bad about yourself tend to perpetuate something you already believe. Notice that this is happening— you may not be able to stop yourself right away, and that's okay, just start to see these behaviors as what they are: self-negating actions.

⊕ Arm yourself with a few affirmations that might help shift these negative core beliefs into more reasonable ones. These should be neutral and true, not fantastic and wild. Don't argue with the mirror and shout "I am beautiful!" while you feel like the ugliest person in the world. Here are a few good ones:

⊕ "I'm normal, with both strengths and weaknesses."

⊕ "I'm human with flaws like everyone else."

⊕ "Everyone makes mistakes sometimes."

⊕ "Feeling bad sometimes is normal and okay."

⊕ Think of one thing you like about yourself. Maybe you're really good at making popcorn. Or you have soft, clean hair. Or you listen really carefully when your friends are going through a tough time. It doesn't have to be a big thing. Just remind yourself that there are good things in you, even if there are also bad things in you. Both can be true at the same time. Try to remember the good when you're being hard on yourself about the bad.

⊕ Prioritize activities that you do just for yourself that make you feel good. Build a skill like cooking, martial arts, bowling, or yoga. Bonus points for movement, because exercise helps us shift the chemicals in our brains toward a more positive outlook. This is one of the best ways to practice self-esteem.

⊕ Start to change your language so that rather than saying, "I'm a failure" or "I can't do this" when something gets hard in life, say instead, "I'm trying," "I'm working on this," "I'm learning," or "I'm practicing."

⌗ Consider others. Negative core beliefs can make us self-absorbed. No one likes it when we talk about how much we hate ourselves, and self-hating behaviors can push people away—not because we're so good at putting walls up, but because we're being assholes and people don't tend to like that. When you find yourself in negative self-talk, think of something you like about someone else (though watch out for comparing yourself to others, which can exacerbate negative core beliefs).

⌗ If you're in a self-negating behavior, see if there's something nice you can do for someone else. It's often much easier to see the good in other people than in ourselves, but sometimes it can help us switch back on our compassion and empathy. We may be able to then boomerang that compassion and empathy back on ourselves.

BODY TALK

In order to ask ourselves the tough questions about how our traumas are affecting our core beliefs, we need to be able to face what we are feeling. I wasn't ready for those challenges to my worldview at first, so I clenched up against them. I held my resistance in my muscles. After years of (medium) success avoiding and denying what happened, I was lying on the floor every day asking my belly to relax and start telling me the truth. My body wanted to let the truth out. My mind wanted my body to shut the hell up and mind its own business.

Thankfully (if unfortunately), my body was always going to win that battle. I can lie to my mind pretty well, but I can't get a damn thing past my body—especially now that I've embraced my sensitivity and made feeling a daily practice. Thinking back, I can see the ways my body was screaming for attention while I was willfully ignoring everything it said. During those denial years, I developed a rare skin condition called dermatographia, a Latin word that means "skin writing." Any scratch on my skin would rise up dramatically into clear red lines. I could draw words or pictures anywhere on my skin with a fingernail. Whatever I'd write or draw would immediately become incredibly itchy, however, and I'd always scratch the images up into a raw red mess shortly after they showed up on my skin.

I remember getting an allergy test around that time. The technician brought in the little vials of allergen essences and poked my skin with them to see which ones would get a reaction. As a control, he also scratched a line above the little dots on my forearm to see how much my skin would react to a stimulus without any allergen present. A little while later, he came back into the room and looked at the inflamed constellation on my arm with the big red welt above them. He proclaimed that I was slightly allergic to apples, pineapples, and tree pollen, but that my biggest allergen was—get this—touch. Yup, after getting sexually assaulted, I developed a literal allergy to human touch. If anyone or anything touched me, my skin would rebel in the form of extreme itching and big red welts. It was as if my nervous system was on a deserted island trying to spell out H-E-L-P in palm leaves.

Allergies and autoimmune disorders seem to have a relationship with trauma, especially if the trauma happened over a long period of time in childhood.[13] An allergy means the immune system is misinterpreting a usually safe stimulus or substance as a threat. For many trauma survivors, one of the things we lose is our sense of safety. We get confused about what people, foods, flowers, and trees are friends and which are trying to murder us in cold blood. We don't trust our instincts, and our immune systems seem to reflect this by reacting with confusion and rejection to normally safe substances in our environment.

Allergies are real. Even if they are created by an imbalance in the nervous system due to a trauma, that doesn't mean we can will them away. No one totally understands where allergies come from and why they sometimes change within our lifetimes, but we know that it probably has something to do with stress, the nervous system, and the microbiome. In my experience, though, when I stopped fighting myself and started listening to the messages my body was sending me that something was wrong, my body started to change. Learning to face everything I felt, including the uncomfortable truths about what had happened to me, helped me create an internal sense of safety. I had to work on my relationship with myself and the not-always-threatening outside world. I strengthened my emotional immune system, and that seems to have bolstered my physical immune system. I still get hives every now and then, especially in pollen-heavy spring, but they don't rise up like they used to in clear red lines. It's no longer dermatographia. I'm no longer allergic to apples or pineapples.

Strengthening the Emotional Immune System

Our physical immune system protects us from invaders like viruses or harmful bacteria. It works best when we take time to relax, to be in the parasympathetic rest-and-digest nervous system state. This can be challenging for trauma survivors, because we don't really believe we can protect ourselves from physical, personal, or psychological invasion. We never really feel safe.

We can't control our environment or other people, but we can cultivate more safety and trust within ourselves. In order to do this, we must develop a loving relationship with our own minds and bodies. This relationship becomes the foundation we can return to no matter what's happening in the world around us. Here are some ways to spend time with yourself with a healing intention:

⊕ Work on your relationship with yourself every day. Prioritize time spent alone. This time should be intentional and enjoyable. I meditate on my couch every morning while the coffee is brewing, and I often still do take

13   Falcone, Tatiana. "Childhood Emotional Trauma Closely Linked to Problems in Adulthood." Consult QD, clevelandclinic.org. Nov 6th, 2014. https://consultqd.clevelandclinic.org/childhood-emotional-trauma-closely-linked-to-problems-in-adulthood/

ten minutes in the afternoon to lie on my back and breathe into my belly. It could also be a quiet walk or drive to work, ten minutes looking out the window sipping a cup of tea, or journaling every morning when you wake up. It can be anything you enjoy doing alone. Limit TV, radio, podcasts, video games, and mind-altering substances during this time—this is time for the real voices in your head and no one else's!

⊕ Meditation is very beneficial, including for trauma survivors, but can also be triggering and very intense depending on where you're at internally. Don't feel like you have to sit; moving meditations like yoga, dancing, or walking might be better, especially at first. If you do sit, you may need an active meditation aid for a while, like a phrase to repeat or a guided audio meditation that you like (without any triggering material in it). Start with short periods—even one minute in meditative reflection can make a difference. In time, it's helpful to connect quietly to what's really happening inside your mind and body, but don't force this. Above all, be kind to yourself, and do whatever works for you.

⊕ Treat these being-alone exercises like you're spending time with your best friend (which you are!). There's no particular thing you need to talk about. You don't need to sit in silence, but you can, if that feels natural. You're not going to force your friend to talk about things she doesn't want to discuss. You're not going to judge her. You can ask questions and respond to what she says, but mostly listen with kindness, even and especially if she's done something you wish she hadn't or is talking about things that upset you.

⊕ Commit to at least ten minutes a day (or whatever you can handle until your tolerance goes up). Forgive yourself if you miss a day. Do your best to be kind and forgive yourself when you're not. Even if this relationship is really bad and full of distrust and hatred right now, keep trying. This is the most important commitment you'll ever make to the most important relationship of your life. It's the only one you'll have until the day you die.

YOGA: HELPING OR HURTING?

For me, yoga has been a major tool for helping me learn how to feel. Unlike most other forms of exercise, yoga is based on the idea of mindfulness: get into a pose and think about how it makes you feel. It was in yoga that I learned that my emotions are absolutely connected to my physical flesh. Yoga taught me that I could observe the emotions that were arising and, rather than reacting to them, embrace them and let them be present and flow in their own way. Yoga taught me how to be okay with being uncomfortable, as well as how movement and breath could help me calm down, slow down, and in many cases ease my physical pain.

Yoga also, however, thoroughly fucked me up. Yoga is a vast practice with many philosophies within it that do not always agree with each other. I had to learn the hard lesson that yoga is not a panacea—especially not for trauma. Some branches of yoga focus on gratitude, contentment, and loving kindness as emotions that we should cultivate, and I think we in the West sometimes misinterpret those practices to mean we should make ourselves *feel* contentment, gratitude, and loving kindness no matter what's going on in our lives. That's a lot of pressure, because we can't make ourselves feel anything we don't feel, and trying *not* to feel is not only impossible but tends to make the emotions we're avoiding even stronger. If you feel angry at your dead mother, envious of your best friend, or still miss that boyfriend who broke your heart five years ago, that's okay. There's nothing wrong with you, and telling yourself you shouldn't feel that way isn't going to change a thing. Sitting there with frustration in our hearts and trying to paste gratitude over our homicidal rage is an exercise in futility. We cannot change our emotions.

What we can do, however, is give ourselves space to feel these emotions and express them in appropriate ways. We can adjust our attention and make choices with our behavior, which is usually what most of these ancient meditation philosophies are actually trying to teach. We do have choices about where to put our energy, attention, and action in our lives. We can feel angry and, at the same time, focus on someone we love or some sweet moment we had that day. We can feel envious and choose to put energy into improving our own lot in life. We're not trying to erase the uncomfortable feeling and override it with gratitude, but when we can shift our focus, sometimes we can shift our internal experience and perspective at the same time. Cultivating mindfulness can help us make choices in our lives that are more supportive to a loving and kind life, but we can't just randomly will ourselves to feel like giving strangers Care Bear Stares and overwhelm everyone with love and gratitude we don't feel. We don't have control over our emotions, but we do have some control over our attention and our behavior.

When I started going to counseling after the assault, a big theme my counselor and I were working on was self-blame. I was having a really hard time understanding that what happened to me was not my fault. My perpetrator had assaulted me after months of asking me for sex, begging me for sex, shaming me for the sex I'd had with other people. It was the sort of nonsense that made me feel that I owed him sex whether I desired it or not—messages that, by the way, are prevalent in the culture I live in. I did say no, I kept saying no, but I didn't fight him very hard when it finally happened, because I had swallowed the Kool-Aid. My counselor was trying to help me believe that I am the only person entitled to my body and that what happened to me was not my fault.

Then there I was in yoga class, lying in *savasana*, the fully relaxed supine pose that ends most classes, after a pretty tough sequence of poses. Everyone was exhausted and so ready for five minutes of rest. During this vulnerable time, lying with my body open to the ceiling, the teacher started playing a recording of a woman saying something like, "You are an incredibly powerful being that manifests everything that happens to you in your life. You may think to yourself, *Why did that person treat me so badly? I didn't deserve that!* Well, you did! You did something in your life that brought that moment into existence! You are just that powerful!"

So.... It *was* my fault. Because of *karma*. I knew it!

I started to cry. Uncontrollably. I left the room to go to the bathroom and choked on sobs, unable to pull myself together for the closing this stupid yoga class. I ran out of the room, pulled my hood over my head, and escaped home. That, my friends, is what we call in the biz a trigger response.

In the West, we think karma means that whatever you do comes back to you, for good or for bad. As it turns out, however, that's a pretty Western interpretation of the concept—one that simply reinforces the idea that we live in a just world where bad things only happen to bad people. It's one of the reasons victim blaming (even when you yourself are the victim) is so common in these situations. If we did something to cause our own assault, that means all we have to do is stop doing that thing and we'll be safe again. We all want to believe we have some modicum of control over our lives. Living in a world where something bad could happen at any time is not a world any of us want to live in. But that's the world every trauma survivor has to wake up to every day.

In India, the word karma means action, and the idea is that every action has a consequence. But we have absolutely no control over what those consequences might be, and they could catch up to us in another life when we are a completely different person. Even good actions can have negative results, and that's never going to be predictable. All we can control is our intentions, never the results of our actions. That's a fundamental principle of Hindu philosophy that we Westerners have deeply misunderstood. It's actually a way of explaining why bad things *do* sometimes happen to good people.

While yoga can be a really effective way to connect with our bodies, some branches of yoga philosophy (and Buddhism, Christianity, and so on) see desire and anger as anti-spiritual and the body as a barrier to communion with the divine. A big piece of my healing included locating my spirituality *in* my body, in my desire, rage, pleasure, and everything else that was going on in there. In order to let the erotic energy come through and give me the courage to change some things, I had to connect to my organs of perception: my feeling, breathing, sweating, bleeding, crying body. I had to practice being with all the emotions and all the pain in my body, the source of the wound and the source of healing.

THE GIFT OF NUMBING

Learning to feel again after an extended period of numbness isn't something that happens out of nowhere. I had to practice feeling my body every day. I had to stop clenching up and shutting down every time I got uncomfortable, which meant I had to learn to be brave about the shame, sadness, and anger that are part and parcel of genuine, holistic feeling. I learned along the way that this practice of feeling is in a sense an act of rebellion.

Our culture would much rather we buy things than feel things. If we could access joy in our connection with each other and the natural world, if we felt that we were enough, and if negative emotions weren't so taboo, we wouldn't need to buy as much stuff. God forbid we let ourselves feel the rage that arises with injustice. Numbness protects us from change.

Connecting to our desire can be risky. Desire is not satisfied with a small, safe, contained life. It wants more. Regardless of whether or not we've experienced a trauma, many of us unconsciously avoid it because it feels easier and safer to do that than to connect to the threat of desire. If we stopped reaching for numbing agents like work, alcohol, and TV and let ourselves be still and feel our feelings, we might discover that we *want* to change. We could destabilize everything. It's in the interest of the status quo that we do not feel our feelings.

We're lucky that we have the capacity to numb ourselves from time to time. Children who have been abused often talk later about the gift of dissociation, the ability to let their consciousness float outside their bodies while a terrible thing was happening to them. Many of us do this on a lesser scale for years in toxic relationships or at a job we hate. Sometimes new parents forget about their bodies because of the intense and immediate work of caring for a helpless being. It isn't always a bad thing to mentally check out. Being fully present to the mundane horribleness of day-to-day life isn't always possible. We need to get through the day. We need to survive. We need to make money. We need to keep it together for the boss, the coworkers, the Joneses, the kids. Our ability to deny how we feel is a gift—that is, until it becomes a poison.

Repression and dissociation dampen our fear and anger, but we can't selectively numb. If one emotion is going to be blanked out, everything must be blanked out: along with anger, there goes joy, pleasure, and certainly desire. All emotions live in our bodies: they are called feelings because we feel them. Besides, we need our negative emotions. They exist for a reason. They warn us that something is not right. My resistance to feeling negative emotions in the years after the assault ironically put me at great risk of getting hurt all over again.

In my trauma fog, I was unconsciously seeking safety and security in a relationship, so I found a guy who wanted a girlfriend and ended up living with him for a couple of years. I had definitely picked up on the message that women are safer inside heterosexual relationships than out there doing it on our own (a myth, in case you weren't sure). This guy wanted to marry me and have a family and the whole thing, which I guessed I wanted, too. But something in me was saying no. Something didn't feel right. I couldn't put my finger on what it was. I had absorbed the message by then that my internal "no" didn't mean anything, and yet, there it was: somewhere in my body, I could feel that something wasn't right. My "no" had survived its burial alive.

When I finally somehow made the decision to leave him, I needed to move out. While he was at work, my mother drove me to our apartment, threw all my shit into garbage bags, and hauled them out while I dithered and second-guessed myself over the curtains and cutlery. Later, I found out not only that my mother had never liked him (which I suspected upon seeing the look of glee in her eyes on moving-out day) but that he had cheated on me and lied about many things throughout our time together. Several times he had tried to sleep with one of my best friends while she continually refused him. When I learned that, I thought back to all the times I'd slept with him when I didn't want to or did things with him sexually that I didn't want to do. I didn't bother saying no because I'd already learned it wouldn't matter. Those experiences were explicitly consensual, but they didn't feel good. And they definitely didn't do anything for reclaiming my sense of safety, let alone my desire.

I'm grateful for the way my body somehow clued me in that this person wasn't good for me and got me out of there. Unfortunately, I was still so unable to listen to my gut or trust my instincts that I went ahead and did the exact same thing all over again: I got together with a new guy barely two months later, lived with him for a couple of years, and left because something that I couldn't put my finger on didn't feel right.

This new guy liked me and wanted to be my boyfriend, which seemed like a pretty high standard at the time. My rational mind was saying, "I'm not ready, I need some time to recover from the last relationship, I don't want to do this," but my safety-seeking, feelings-avoiding mind was stronger at the time. It didn't matter that I didn't want to be in that relationship. It didn't matter that when he got angry, he would throw tantrums and kick at walls. It didn't matter that my body went rigid when we took a weekend away to a beautiful place early in our relationship. I still have a photo of me from that trip, on a beautiful beach, scowling at the camera like it was calling me names. I was like that all weekend. It didn't occur to me that you're not supposed to feel so stiff on a weekend getaway with a new lover. I didn't have a conception yet of what a safe, passionate, loving, connected relationship might feel like in my body. I swallowed my "no"—until right before we got engaged.

My two best friends had both recently set their wedding dates, and my thirtieth birthday was on the horizon, so I figured I should get engaged too, right? My boyfriend never really believed I wanted to be in that relationship (because, apparently, I was better at hiding things from myself than from other people), so I decided to propose to him so he would know that I really did want to be there. I went to my mother to ask her for a ring from our family to propose to him with. As we were driving away from her house, my ring in a box in my pocket, she seemed quiet. I said to her, "I'm getting engaged, mom, aren't you excited?" And she said, "Yeah, well, I'll get excited when it happens." Bless my mother for—again—knowing more than I did about how I felt and keeping her mouth shut anyway.

A few days later, I lost the ring. I couldn't find it anywhere. It eventually popped up in the couch cushions under my best friend's butt. If I wasn't going to pay attention to my feelings, apparently I was going to sabotage my plans unconsciously by losing the engagement ring. It was enough to make me pause and think seriously about whether or not this was what I really wanted. It wasn't. I gave my mom the ring back and ended the relationship. Something in me knew that I'd rather be alone and connected to myself than married to the wrong person just because it fit the narrative of what I was supposed to want. I'll always be grateful to my subconscious (and my mother) for somehow clueing me in that I needed to get out of there. Facing down my thirties as a single woman was a little scary, but that's when I started the real work of healing, and everything has been better (if certainly sometimes bumpy) since then.

I still feel frustrated when I think about how much and for how long I resisted what I really felt during those years. I'm angry at myself for having so much bad sex that buried my desire even deeper. Those years are a loss, and I'll never get them back. I did, though, eventually get out of the safety-seeking spin cycle. My "yes" started coming back for me when I started reclaiming my "no."

How to Feel a Feeling

Emotions come and go all day long. They don't always need us to do anything about them, they just need to be felt. In my experience, when we let them fully come up and feel them as deeply as we can, it's remarkable how quickly they pass. Here's what to do when you feel a feeling:

- Stop. Take a break from whatever you are doing. You might need to get yourself to a private place, and it's okay if this needs to happen at the end of the day if you are at work or otherwise in an unsafe space to feel your feelings. Do your best to make space for it later.

- Put your hand on the place in your body where you feel the emotion, and take a few deep breaths. Close your eyes if you can.

- Relax. The body will tend to tighten up against uncomfortable emotions. My jaw clenches and my belly tightens up, so I try to open my mouth and breathe down into my belly.

- Express. If tears come, let them come (if you're in a safe enough environment). If a sound wants to come up, let it come up. A sigh is a really helpful way to just let the energy move.

- Feel. Notice if your mind revs up trying to explain the emotion, or analyze it, or get to the root of it. There's nothing wrong with that, let your mind do what it's going to do, but try to stay with the sensations in your body in the present moment. Remind yourself that there's nothing to fix.

- Breathe. Our hearts are strong enough to hold the deepest grief for ourselves and each other, and that grief can help us access our compassion. So when we feel it or witness it from someone else, we can breathe it deeply into our hearts, let the heart take it in and do its alchemical magic, and then exhale out of the mouth and let it leave the body. These emotions aren't meant to stay with us for very long, and we need to allow the emotions to flow in but also flow out again. Sometimes I will put my hand on my heart and take three deep breaths into the heart and then exhale out of the mouth, imagining letting the emotion go.

✦ Wait. Some people say that the acute experience of a physical emotion lasts only a couple of minutes. Our experience of emotions can last much longer simply because we're in the narrative of the emotion and we keep bringing it up and repeating the cycle of the emotion. Give yourself a full three minutes (at least) to feel your emotion, and then get on with your day.

SHAME

Why was it so hard for me to face my feelings for those long stupid years? Because of my old friend shame, of course. While guilt is the feeling that arises because you did something bad, shame is the feeling that you *are* bad, right to the core of who you are. Sexual assault is a random act of cruelty and domination that tells us in no uncertain terms that we are not loved or respected by the person assaulting us. If we already believe those things on any level, it can be hard not to take it as proof. Shame loves silence, and I think it takes survivors so long to admit what happened and speak up about it partly because so many of us are positively swimming in an acid bath of shame.

The thing about shame is that it lives in a very primal part of our brains, and when it happens, it can shut down our ability to be rational. I've started to understand that my feelings around my sexual assault are all mixed up with the many bad experiences I've had with men in a patriarchal culture that teaches us all that women are worthless objects. Rationally, we know we're not worthless objects, and many of us actively fight against the way women are portrayed in advertising, the wage gap, or certain laws that imply women should not have control over our own reproductive health. This fight is powerful, and it's working (some of the time, anyway). But we know that women have been treated like shit for generations, and sometimes, when we get tired, we feel pretty sure that's because we are shit, always have been, and always will be.

The key with shame is to recognize when we're in it and take action to bring our rational minds back online. Remember, feelings are called feelings because we feel them: shame, like every other emotion, lives in the body. Shame does not feel good. It is the worst. For me, it feels like a kind of nausea right in my chest and stomach and it makes me want to die in a fire. There is nothing more urgent than shame to make us want to reach for something—anything—to numb the pain. Sometimes the first indication that shame is around is the empty bag of Cheetos sitting right there that we do not remember eating. This kind of knee-jerk numbing reaction can make us feel more shame: staring down the barrel of the empty Cheetos bag doesn't exactly make us feel good about ourselves. So we feel shame about the Cheetos. And then we need to eat more Cheetos. We are merrily on our way down a shame spiral.

I recently stumbled across some information about an ex that I really didn't need. (If you ever want to trigger a cascade of negative emotions, definitely stalk an ex online.) Suddenly that nauseous die-in-a-fire feeling started rising up with a vengeance. Rather than turn away from it and try to tune it out, I greeted it, like, "Oh, hey Shame, what's up." I stopped what I was doing. I resisted the urge to get out the wine bottle.

When the feeling didn't pass after a couple of minutes, I took a breath and asked myself what I was really feeling: what were the core beliefs being triggered by this experience? I was angry at myself for letting my ex treat me with disrespect for such a long time, because on some deep subconscious level, I did not believe I deserve respect. Okay. There it is. The shame-triggering core belief: I am not worthy of respect.

Next, I had a couple of tools I could call on. Firstly, my conscious, rational mind knows I'm as worthy of respect as any other human being. I reminded myself of that mundane truth: all humans deserve respect, even if they are flawed. Then I used a little trick I've found very helpful in the past when I'm judging myself harshly. If this were happening to my best friend, how would I judge her? I've had plenty of best friends treated with disrespect by men before, and I've never thought they deserved it. I texted a few of those friends, too, because talking about shame is one of the best ways to quiet it down.

These things made me feel better, but the shame was still sitting in my stomach. So I used the habits I've cultivated in my daily practice of sitting with myself: I closed my eyes, put a hand on my stomach where I felt the emotion most strongly, relaxed my body, and took a few deep breaths. I acknowledged the feelings, let them be present, and listened to my body with kindness and compassion. I didn't try to push the feelings away. I know it's okay to feel shame sometimes. It doesn't last forever. I let it flow so it could ebb.

Befriending Shame

Making friends with our shame is one of the best ways to stop letting it have power over us. Pushing it away only tends to make it stronger. Here are a few ways to make friends with your shame so it doesn't control your life:

⊕ Learn to identify shame when it's happening in your body. This can happen anywhere down the shame spiral—even if you've been eating nothing but Cheetos for months, or even years. It's *never* too late to get off the Shame-O-Rama roller coaster.

⊕ Take the shame away from feeling shame. So you're feeling worthless. That's okay. It happens to the best of us. So you ate three crates of Cheetos. You did that because you were trying to survive. Your primal brain was reacting to something that happened in the past that was triggered by something in the present, even if it was something relatively small and innocuous. Maybe it was an old trauma. Maybe it was a childhood thing. It doesn't matter. Your system was trying to get you through the day. You got through it. Good for you.

⊕   Call on reasons for your worthiness. Self-love and self-respect are not a given, and they don't come with willpower alone. Practice behaviors that cultivate self-love and try to do them every day. Think of something you love about yourself. If you can't think of anything, do something about it—right now. Sweep the floor. Take a walk. Send someone a nice text. Respect the hell out of yourself for doing that—even if you go right back to the Cheetos afterward. Be as kind to yourself as you can.

THE POWER OF DESIRE

The way my body talked to me (screamed at me, flared up through itchy skin) during these times of repression and suppression meant that my desire had somehow survived within me, and it wanted more than just my flimsy versions of safety. It might be strange to think of our desire manifesting as hives, allergies, pain, chronic fatigue, or other illnesses, but sometimes these symptoms represent the body's rebellion, a refusal to go on as we have been, a desire for something better. Pain is a fantastic teacher because it forces us to change something. It's remarkably common that people resist making a change in their lives until some health crisis forces them to do something differently. The body can be a pain in the ass, but it's always on our side. It's always trying to protect us from something or correct for something, even if that something happened decades ago. That's why the vulnerable experience of feeling is the second, not the first step in our path to recovery. First, we have to survive, and that usually means denial and unhealthy coping mechanisms for a while. We get through that phase in our own sweet time—as long as we don't kill ourselves while we're trying to survive, of course.

The practice of learning how to feel is vital, and it's vulnerable. Avoiding our feelings is fine in the short term, and sometimes we need to buy ourselves a little time to get to a safe place in our lives to begin to deal with our emotions. If we avoid feeling long enough, however, we're almost certainly enmeshed in coping mechanisms that have negative consequences of their own. In its mildest form, avoiding our feelings means repeating our relationship patterns over and over again and never quite accessing joy. In its more serious form, avoiding our feelings can lead to addictions that could literally kill us.

Desire isn't just about sex. Desire is the drive that moves us toward what we want, toward the work we want to do in the world and the things we want to change. Desire isn't satisfied with the way things are and pushes us forward into new territory, even when it's risky. When we're connected to what we want in our bodies and courageous enough to go for it, we not only *feel* more powerful, we *are* more powerful. Several women I've spoken to about this feel that there is a connection between sexual flow, creativity, and financial flow. When the sexual tap is on, energy flows into ideas, energy, intention, and action, all of which are very helpful for doing good work and making good money. Denial also takes up a lot of energetic resources, so when we stop doing that, we free up all kinds of energy that can go to other places.

Regaining sexual flow, I've learned, isn't about forcing yourself to have sex with your partner when you don't really want to. (Don't do that! Stop it!) It's about feeling powerful in your life and connected to yourself. Sexual desire can come when we feel relatively safe and self-determined in who we are. We have to know in our bones that it matters whether we say "yes" or "no" on various levels of our lives, not just in the bedroom. We have to feel this at work, with our families, with our friends. We can't always control that, and having power in our lives is obviously related to the varying degrees of privilege we have in terms of our race, gender, and class, but we have to be able to see, at least in some little corner of our lives, evidence that how we feel matters. We have to be making choices (and sometimes even mistakes) that we can take responsibility for. We can't do any of that if we don't know how we feel in the first place.

Feminist critic Audre Lorde talks about this energy as a force she calls the erotic. She describes it as "firmly rooted in the power of our unexpressed or unrecognized feeling."[14] For me, this means having a direct line to the sensations and emotions that are happening in my body, even if I can't name them or they don't make sense. It means being courageous enough to feel everything I feel, even when it's confusing or painful or steers me away from the life I thought I was supposed to want.

Sometimes, when the erotic drive breaks through our self-suppression, it happens all at once. Several other survivors I've spoken to have shared my experience of living in a quiet fog until suddenly everything changes. The world is dry and gray, and you don't even realize how depressed you are until some tiny spark starts to catch fire. You find yourself crying uncontrollably over the dishes or having a fit of giggles over the most mundane thing. You're up all night writing or painting when you haven't touched your art for months. You might even find yourself making love madly in a late-night alleyway with someone who is definitely not your husband. When the erotic drive has been suppressed, everything has been suppressed. And when those feelings are ready to come back, they can come back with a burn-the-house-down kind of vengeance.

This sudden spark of life can be terrifying. Some of us desperately try to shove our emotions back down into the hole they came from in order to regain some sense of control over the wildfire that is threatening to destroy our life as we know it. Even though, you know, maybe we *should* burn it all down.

The life I had been living at that time wasn't a life I had chosen for myself. I was floating along with other people's decisions, with what my boyfriends or my bosses wanted from me. I wasn't living in my power because it didn't seem possible. When I started to give myself a chance to feel again, I quit my job and broke up with my boyfriend. I started to care about what I wanted and actually take steps to move toward that

---

14   Lorde, Audre. *Sister Outsider: Essays and Speeches.* Berkeley, Crossing Press (2007): 53.

desire. My ability to burn down the life I had accepted for myself and take another path didn't come simply because I was determined or strong or smart enough to connect to my erotic flow and let it wreak havoc on my house of cards. I didn't heal from sexual assault through willpower alone. I feel incredibly lucky to live in a time and place where women's lives are valued at least enough that we do have some choices about things like getting married or having kids. I had a helpline I could call, thanks to a not-for-profit organization in my city (Women Against Violence Against Women) that set me up with a counselor specializing in sexual assault. I had a community filled with yoga teacher / bodyworker / massage therapist / witches telling me to lie down and feel my feelings. My family wanted me to be independent first, married with kids only if it made me happy. I am surrounded by friends and a community that believes in a woman's right to orgasm. If I lived in another time and place where the pressure to be a wife above all other things was stronger, I might not have been able to let that erotic wildfire burn—at least, not in the way that I did.

Getting Support

Trusting ourselves is a tricky business. When that erotic tap finally turns on, it feels so right, but sometimes so totally out of control. We need help—but it has to be the right kind of help. Here are some things to consider:

- ⊕ Connect with the right people. Many of the people who love us in our lives are also attached to the status quo. Sometimes the people who love us the most are also the ones who are most invested in preventing us from changing. You must have people you can talk to in your life when your erotic volcano is erupting, but judgment from others can spark your shame and shut off your tap to vitality all over again. Be careful that the people you talk to listen without judgment.

- ⊕ Avoid enablers. The right people to confide in will encourage you to explore your feelings but not to harm yourself while you're doing it. They will not adhere to some cultural rule or expectation at the cost of your happiness. They will not gasp in shock at the prospect of change. They may not understand what is happening for you, but they will trust you, listen to you, and believe you.

- ⊕ Get a good counselor. I am a huge believer in counseling. Counselors are not your friends or family, so they have no investment in your status quo. It's their whole job to help you live your best life. But counselors are human, and some of them are full of judgment anyway. It's really important that you find someone you trust who shares your values. If you have an organization in your area that focuses on sexual violence, ask them for recommendations.

⌗   Work on your relationship with yourself. Even if you don't have access to
       a crisis line, a counselor, or a supportive community, you still have your
       relationship with yourself, remember? You have that one you're working
       on every day. Talk to yourself about it at the very least. Don't abandon
       your relationship with yourself when you need it most. Keep showing up.

The practice of feeling means paying attention to what your body is saying to you and
resisting the urge to make it stop. Negative emotions are uncomfortable, of course, but
even positive emotions can make us feel vulnerable and trigger a shame response. When
we can befriend our bodies in all their ugly glory, we are cultivating a lifelong relationship
with the flow of sensation inside ourselves. Accessing desire necessarily comes with
accessing everything else. When we practice being in the dirt and shit of our bodies
on a day-to-day level and learn that we are okay and worthy of love as whole beings,
desire can start to flicker back. With time, that little spark of desire can transform into
the life hunger that wants to feel things fully, step away from the places where we feel
oppressed or suppressed in our lives, and change something. Feeling often hurts, but
when we can do it with kindness, compassion, and courage, feeling heals, too.

RAGE

In the dream, he has moved into my house. He has set up in a bedroom between mine and everything else in the house. I can't get to the bathroom, the kitchen, or the front door without walking through the space he's claimed. I scream at him and tell him to get out. He laughs at me. He tells me we're going to be together now, that everyone thinks we've been together all this time, that I have nowhere to run to. My neighbors wander in, asking why I'm so upset, he's such a nice guy, he has a right to live here. I throw plates at him. I push him over. I tell him he assaulted me. Doesn't he know he assaulted me? He can't stay here, this is my house, he has to leave. He laughs. I am shaking with fury. I startle awake to a sore jaw and a shredded mouthguard.

For a long time, my rage only lived in my dreams (and my jaw; I've been through a few mouthguards in my day). In my everyday life I would be calm and measured, and if something difficult happened I'd react with passive sadness or a vague discomfort I wouldn't call anger. But at night, there were beheadings. At night, I would be fighting off monsters and men, saving villages of people from evil despots, a posse of women behind me carrying swords and wooden stakes (the monsters were usually vampires—blame a longtime obsession with *Buffy the Vampire Slayer*). All day I'd teach yoga and meditate and float around and smile at everybody. At night, though, I'd be blood-soaked and vengeful, struggling with my enemy, trying to kill him before he killed me, night after night after night.

ANGER: THE BODYGUARD OF DESIRE

For a long time, my rage didn't talk to me. It was stuck in the same basement corner of my gut where I had shoved my grief, my frustration, and my desire. The erotic drive that was suppressed and repressed after the assault needed my rage to give it the strength to rise up. Anger is the bodyguard of desire. It originates from the fundamental belief that I have a self that's worth protecting, that my desires matter. Connecting with desire requires connecting with anger.

Desire is a force of attraction. It arises when we are drawn toward something or someone. The force of attraction requires an equal and opposite force—it's a law of emotional physics. Knowing what we want means also knowing what we don't want. Our desire points the way while our anger protects us from stumbling off the path.

It's appropriate to be angry after assault or violation. When we feel threatened and our anger arises naturally, the power of our erotic energy is awake and ready to do its best to protect us. When we are in contact with our anger, that means we are in contact with our deepest feelings. Some of us do get angry when we are assaulted or violated. I didn't.

Anger is an emotional language with a very limited vocabulary: the word "no." After what happened to me, I learned in a very deep way that my "no" didn't matter. So why would my anger matter? If my boundaries were never going to be respected no matter what I did, why would I bother sticking up for them? My rage, defeated, curled up into the fetal position and went to sleep somewhere far, far away. My desire had lost her number one defender, supporter, and best bud. She went to sleep, too. Everyone went to sleep.

Our culture is kind of weird about anger. Men who express it are seen as violent, and women who express it are dismissed as shrill. If you practice yoga or meditation, as I do, you might have heard somewhere along the line that anger is somehow antispiritual, that it's an emotion you're not supposed to feel. Any expression other than beatific gratitude, essentially, is "not very yogic" of you. Bookstore shelves are lined with titles on how to tame or calm anger, not how to work with it generatively. In some spiritual circles, anger is about as dangerous as desire.

That's really too bad, because anger is a key to healing. Anger can help us define and express our sense of self and the boundaries around that self, which can actually help us cultivate trust and intimacy. Trauma and violation can cause us to lose our voices, and anger is a hero that that can pluck them from our strangled throats and set them free. Welcome to Step Three for recovering desire after sexual assault: Rage.

One of the best things about rage is that it reduces the amount of fucks we give about what other people think of us. The scariest thing about it, though, is that characteristic lack of fucks: it puts the self ahead of relationships and is perfectly willing to destroy any emotional bonds that get in its way. When it is expressed reactively, it can push the people we need the most away from us. When we can work with it compassionately and with mindfulness, however, it can actually draw those people closer.

Anger is often described as an inhibitory emotion. It shows up to help protect us from some other emotion—usually grief, hurt, or fear. Anger definitely sometimes shows up when there are other difficult emotions present, but I think the idea that the anger is somehow less real than the other emotions or should be discounted because grief or fear are present is unfair to this formidable emotion. It's not an either-or sort of thing. When there's grief or fear, sometimes there *should* be anger. It's valid to be angry about a loss that also hurts and that you feel sad about. It's valid to be angry that your safety is being threatened. If anger shoves aside the fear of what other people might think of you, that's a great favor. That's when we can really get some shit done.

Listening to Anger

Take an inventory of your relationship to anger. It can show up as mild irritation, frustration, or full-on rage in response to pretty much anything. Journal on the following questions:

⊕   Where does your anger show up? In dreams, in traffic, with your partner, at work?

⊕   When was the last time you felt anger? What happened?

⊕   Is your anger usually fleeting and situational or about one big thing?

⊕   What do you do when it shows up? Do you talk about it? Keep it inside?

⊕   How would you like to respond when anger arises? Is that different from how you tend to actually respond?

TWO FORMS OF ANGER

There are (at least) two distinct forms of anger that come up in our lives. Righteous anger is clean, clear, and calm, capable of shoving aside anything that stands in its way. Anxious anger is more confusing and is commonly mixed up with other emotions that can cloud the way forward. Both are useful in their own way.

Righteous anger usually comes up in the face of injustice. When we see a wrong being perpetrated against us or against someone else, we can get an incredible surge of energy to fight that injustice. Our "no" comes out clear as a bell. This is the anger that drives community organizers, human rights lawyers, and artists who focus on social issues. Change is hard and scary, and our righteous anger can help us refuse to accept things as they are. It helps us believe in the possibility of a better world.

My favorite description of righteous anger is from the comedian Tina Fey in her book *Bossypants*. She explains what happened when her colleague, Amy Poehler, felt a hint of oppression in the *Saturday Night Live* (SNL) TV show's writing room. Fey writes:

> *Amy Poehler was new to SNL, and we were all crowded into the seventeenth floor writer's room. […] There were always a lot of noisy "comedy bits" going on in that room. Amy was in the middle of some such nonsense with Seth Meyers across the table, and she did something vulgar as a joke. I can't remember what it was exactly, except it was dirty and loud and "unladylike."*

> *Jimmy Fallon, who was arguably the star of the show at the time, turned to her and in a faux-squeamish voice said, "Stop that! It's not cute! I don't like it."*

Amy dropped what she was doing, went black in the eyes for a second, and wheeled around on him. "I don't fucking care if you like it." Jimmy was visibly startled. Amy went right back to enjoying her ridiculous bit. [...]

Amy made it clear that she wasn't there to be cute. She wasn't there to play wives and girlfriends in the boys' scenes. She was there to do what she wanted to do and she did not fucking care if you like it.[15]

Righteous anger is about injustice. There's no confusion or anxiety, it's clear as day what must be done. Amy Poehler was able to speak up against someone trying to silence her with terrifying black-eyed clarity. She got her point across and moved on.

This type of anger feels awesome. It's a high, but it's also incredibly calm. You know exactly what you need to do, and you will do it no matter what anyone says. I've only felt it a couple of times in my life, but it was remarkable, a fantastic sense of confidence and inevitability. I cheerfully quit a yoga teaching job at a big studio under the influence of righteous anger when one of my managers offered to "make me a star" by changing everything I liked about my teaching. This came after weeks of manipulative behavior from the corporate level. I knew I wasn't the only teacher who was being pushed around and that most of us were underpaid women. The male teachers were getting raises and prime-time slots, and the women were getting confusing feedback and shifting schedules that made them wonder if they were any good at their jobs at all. I needed the money, and I was trying to build my career, but I knew if I'd stayed I would have compromised my values. As soon as my manager said the phrase about making me a star, I felt my eyes go Amy Poehler black. I said with a smile, "No I don't want this job, thanks. What I want is for you to understand that what you're doing is not okay." My manager went speechless as the power dynamic flew out from under his feet. It felt great.

Unfortunately, this black-eyed, clear-tongued, ass-kicking rage is the rarer of these two types of anger. Righteous anger shows up in situations of injustice, while anxious anger usually arises in our intimate relationships. Anxious anger asks us to stand up for ourselves and push back against the people we want and need in our lives. This type of anger almost always indicates that a need is not being met or that a boundary has been crossed. It's a little internal fire alarm that tells us there's smoke somewhere in the vicinity of our sense of self. In this way, our anger protects our autonomy, our boundaries, our needs, and our choices. When we suppress and avoid this type of anger, we risk losing ourselves in our relationships, becoming enmeshed or codependent, and letting our relationships rule our lives and even our sense of identity. Psychologist Harriet Lerner explains in her brilliant book *The Dance of Anger*:

Anger is a signal, and one worth listening to. Our anger may be a message that we are being hurt, that our rights are being violated, that our needs or wants are not being adequately met, or simply that something is not right. Our anger may tell us that we are not addressing an important emotional issue in our lives, or that too

15   Fey, Tina. *Bossypants*. New York: Little, Brown and Company (2011): 143–144.

much of our self—our beliefs, values, desires, or ambitions—is being compromised in a relationship. Our anger may be a signal that we are doing more and giving more than we can comfortably do or give. Or our anger may warn us that others are doing too much for us, at the expense of our own competence and growth. Just as physical pain tells us to take our hand off the hot stove, the pain of our anger preserves the very integrity of our self. Our anger can motivate us to say "no" to the ways in which we are defined by others and "yes" to the dictates of our inner self.[16]

When anger arises, then, it is not simply an annoying emotion tricking us into thinking we feel something we don't feel. It's not something to be contained, tamed, and then swallowed. Expressing it doesn't make us mean or violent (or non-yogic) people. Anger is a powerful indication that we are in contact with our feelings, our boundaries, our sense of self, and our desires.

WHAT HAPPENED TO ANGER?

In the best kind of rape situation (yes, I know how ridiculous that sounds), a violation takes place, everyone sees it and understands it as a violation, friends, lovers, and community members believe the survivor, they express their anger and solidarity, and they make the perpetrator take responsibility. The violation is understood clearly as a violation not only of the survivor's boundaries but also of the social code. It's understood as an experience that was outside the realm of anyone's reasonable expectations and should never have happened. Ah. What a fantasy.

Unfortunately, it more often goes like this: a violation takes place, some people believe the survivor, some people think she was lying or asking for it, and some people try to silence her (and it is usually, but not always, a "her"). The perpetrator goes free of any consequences at all, and our brave survivor is left wondering why her experience feels so incredibly at odds with the reaction she got from the people who are supposed to love, protect, and support her. All her feelings freeze in her guts, and she sleepwalks around for the next few years. If the survivor is male, his assault may be minimized and he may be ridiculed for having a negative reaction to the experience. If the survivor is transgendered or nonbinary, they may feel even more thoroughly silenced and lack resources where they can safely get help.

We don't really understand rape in our society. In her book *Trauma and Recovery*, psychologist Judith Herman points out that sexual domination by men against women is permitted and even encouraged in some areas of our society. She writes, "Women quickly learn that rape is a crime only in theory; in practice the standard for what constitutes rape is set not at the level of women's experience of violation but just above

---

16   Lerner, Harriet. *The Dance of Anger: A Woman's Guide to Changing the Patterns of Intimate Relationships.* New York: HarperCollins (2005): 1.

the level of coercion acceptable to men."[17] Experiencing a trauma that no one around you seems to understand as a trauma is a strong message that the integrity of your self doesn't matter. When anger has nothing to protect, it can have no part to play. It might as well hang its hat for a decade or so.

When I was assaulted, I was a little confused at first, but not *that* confused. I knew something was wrong. But when I started talking about it, I lost my conviction. My counselor at the time did some vague gesturing and implied that it had happened because of my boundary issues, and that if I could just stand up for myself better this sort of thing wouldn't happen to me. So, then, what happened was my fault. My stomach fell to my shoes and stayed there for the rest of the hour. I left the appointment and barfed into some bushes a few blocks away.

My counselor wasn't the only one who implied it was my fault. The person who violated me was a close friend with relationships to other people in my life. Those people listened to what I was saying but didn't seem to absorb the information. They went back to hanging out with him like nothing had happened. Maybe they thought I'd lied or misunderstood. Maybe they blocked it out. Or maybe they just didn't care. He was such a nice guy, a nerd, not very good with women. Maybe it just didn't compute for them.

Herman argues that trauma is always, on some level, relational. It is about a betrayal, whether it happens on the intimate level or that of community or social systems. For a traumatized person, the reaction of the community really matters and can go a long way toward helping the person heal or deepening the wound. Herman writes, "In the aftermath of traumatic life events, survivors are highly vulnerable. Their sense of self has been shattered. That sense can be rebuilt only as it was built initially, in connection with others."[18]

Many survivors are not believed after the attack and/or are refused help or protection. This is a phenomenon psychologist Jennifer Freyd has called institutional betrayal.[19] When the schools, hospitals, police officers, shelters, or community systems we rely on don't believe us or take the perpetrator's side, that can create a secondary trauma in addition to the first and slows our healing way down. It matters a lot what happens after an assault. If we are believed and get help right away, our concept of the world as a reasonably safe and just place can remain relatively intact. But when we are betrayed by our perpetrator and then the systems that are supposed to help betray us, too, we feel even more abandoned, alone, and hopeless. Going through my experience was bad enough, but when my counselor, my family, and my group of friends dismissed me or didn't believe me, that *really* hurt. It made it much harder to trust myself that what happened really had happened. It made it much harder for me to get the help I needed.

---

17   Herman, Judith. Trauma and Recovery: *The Aftermath of Violence*—from Domestic Abuse to Political Terror. New York: Basic Books (1997): 72.

18   Herman, Judith. Trauma and Recovery: *The Aftermath of Violence*—from Domestic Abuse to Political Terror. New York: Basic Books (1997): 61

19   Freyd, Jennifer J, Melissa Platt and Jocelyn Barton. "A Betrayal Trauma Perspective on Domestic Violence." E. Stark & E. S. Buzawa (Eds.) *Violence against Women in Families and Relationships* (Vol. 1, pp. 185–207). Connecticut, Greenwood Press (2009): 201.

Many women who have been raped or assaulted are told they must have been asking for it. Many of us already agree with that assessment anyway. It's easier to believe we had a hand in our own abuse, because that means all we have to do is change something about ourselves and it will never happen again. Victim blaming is easier than acknowledging the world as a chaotic and cruel place where we can't control a damn thing. Fixing my boundary issues sounded a lot more doable than admitting to myself that I actually have no control over when and how people violate my boundaries.

I have no doubt that my counselor had my best interests at heart. We tend to think of counselors as authority figures who can see us better than we see ourselves, but they're just humans, raised in the same culture we were raised in, confused and upset by the same things we are. My counselor's reaction was damaging, but my first reaction wasn't anger. It was just to barf in those bushes and never go back to that office again.

If you've ever gotten awkward and said the wrong thing around someone going through something hard, let me tell you: you are not alone. I've done it, too. When a good friend told me about an experience she'd had with an ex, I blurted out, "I mean... that's rape!" She wasn't ready at the time to name her experience that way, and it wasn't my place to name it for her. She needed to go through her survival phase before she could define for herself what had happened. Later (like, years later), she told me she was glad I had said that word because it eventually validated a truth she hadn't always felt supported to express. But in the interim, we barely talked. I didn't know what to do. None of us do. Even our counselors don't always know how to help someone who's been raped. We never talk about this stuff!

Supporting Someone after Trauma

When someone has gone through something terrible, it can be really hard to know what to say or do. Here are some tips to keep in mind:

⸶ Listen to them. Don't rush to change the subject, try to cheer them up, or find solutions. If you don't know what to say, keep eye contact and a relaxed posture and stay silent. You might feel uncomfortable, but stay in the room. If you try to change the subject or leave, that may compound their sense of shame.

⸶ One of the best things you can say when someone tells you they went through something awful is, "I'm sorry that happened to you." You can also reflect back the words they are using to describe what happened: "That sounds so scary," or "That sounds horrible," depending on what they said. Sometimes people describe what happened without using any emotional words. You can ask them, "How did that make you feel?" Be careful not to put words in their mouth.

⸶ Believe them. Hearing about someone else's trauma can be upsetting, to put it mildly. If you jump to assuming they are at fault, lying, or that they misunderstood what happened, especially if you feel they are accusing someone you know, that's normal, but keep those thoughts to yourself and work them out on your own later. It is exceedingly rare that people lie about these things. It's possible that the perpetrator will have a different story, but your friend is telling you a truth from their perspective. Believe that truth.

⊕ Some people have the urge to comfort with touch. This is exactly what some people need, but depending on the trauma, they may not want to be touched. If you feel the urge to touch your friend in a comforting way, ask them: "Can I put my hand on your back?" You'll be modeling consensual touch, and this could go a long way toward helping your friend heal.

⊕ Don't name what happened to them until they name it themselves, even if, for example, it was very obviously a rape. It's not for you to define their experience, that's their journey. Don't take their story away from them.

⊕ In the days and weeks following the experience, your friend may be acting differently. Check in with them in a way that lets them know you're thinking about them but doesn't require anything from them, even a response. Rather than "How are you doing?" You can say "I'm thinking of you."

⊕ Offer help in concrete ways, and keep consent in mind. Rather than "Let me know if I can do anything to help," try, "I'd like to come make you dinner tonight, would that be okay with you?" Don't offer anything you don't have to give, and don't insist on doing things for them that they don't want. Stick with things you really do want to do to help, and offer first rather than doing without asking. This helps take the pressure off them from knowing what they need, which they may not. It also continues to model consent and that you respect their needs, desires, and boundaries.

⊕ There are some amazing resources for people going through traumatic times. You and your friend may have no idea what to do, but support groups, crisis lines, and counselors more likely will. It might be helpful to do some research for your friend, like finding the number of a local crisis line, asking them if they'd like help looking up counselors, or offering a ride to an appointment. Don't push them. Let them go through the experience however they are going to go through it and be careful not to micromanage. Remember that everything has its own pace. Sometimes the pace is slow!

Women aren't the only ones who suffer from our misunderstandings about sex, violation, and consent. One in three women will have experienced some kind of sexual assault or violation in her lifetime, and for men the number is a not-super-encouraging one in six. These numbers are even higher for the transgender and queer community, probably because sexual violence is often motivated by hate and stigma. Around half of transgender people will experience some form of assault in their lifetimes, and rates of assault tend to be higher for gay men, lesbians, and bisexual people than for the heterosexual population. We have, at least, a cultural narrative for assault of a woman by a man. It's not always an accurate or useful narrative, but at least we know what that is. There are visible resources available for women who have experienced this stuff. Queer, transgender, and gender non-conforming individuals may avoid accessing resources like going to the hospital or the police because they may be shamed or turned away—institutional betrayal is much more common than it should be, especially for certain minorities. There are resources, however, from groups like the federally funded organization FORGE (forge-forward.org) which has published a survivor guide for trans, nonbinary, and gender non-conforming individuals online (at https://forge-forward.org/wp-content/docs/Lets-Talk-Therapist-Guide.pdf). These resources are always going to be limited and may not always help the way we want them to, but at least they are out there.

When men experience sexual violence, it can be confusing in a whole different way. It messes with our cultural myth that men are insatiable beasts who always want sex and women are passive beings who can choose to submit or not but never really want sex. When a man is sexually violated by a woman, people may not see it as a violation, because a man would never say no to sex, right? Men also tend to get the message that expressing hurt or vulnerability is unmanly or weak. In fact, men who express tenderness might be at a higher risk of sexual violence because sometimes man-on-man assault is about keeping men in their "proper" place.

In his study *Love and War,* Tom Digby argues that rape is a tool of what he calls "misogynistic terrorism."[20] The idea is that we must agree, as a society, that women are inferior to men in order to maintain a strict gender binary. When a man is raped, it is a violent form of feminization that aims to teach the victim what it "means" to be a man. Digby writes:

> **The misogyny of rape does not depend on the victim being female. When rape of a male is a way to make him symbolically female, and thus reviled, that dynamic works only if females are inherently reviled. The stigma inherent in femaleness becomes attached to the raped boy or man.[21]**

Most women who experience violence at the hands of men never report it, but at least we have a social understanding of heterosexual violence against women. We're aware that it's a thing. It confuses us that women can sometimes be perpetrators. Men who are violated by a woman might never tell anyone at all for fear of how people might react. They might not admit even to themselves that they've had nonconsensual sex which was unwanted and hurtful (which—guys—it always is, that's the meaning of nonconsensual).

The famous 1990s TV show *Friends* came up in its entirety on Netflix not too long ago, so I rewatched the whole series as an adult, curious about what my young mind was

20   Digby, *Love and War: How Militarism Shapes Sexuality and Romance.* New York, Columbia University Press (2014): 133.
21   Ibid, 145.

absorbing at the time. In one season, Monica and Chandler are a couple trying to have a baby. Monica became a classic shrew pretty much the minute she got a ring on her finger, which is a trope that I guess was supposed to be funny. Many of the jokes in this particular arc of the show involve her trying to essentially steal Chandler's sperm against his will. Several times, Monica wheedles Chandler by negotiating a quick fuck with no talking, no cuddling, and no foreplay (foreplay was apparently really uncool in the 90s). In one episode, the two are in a nasty fight. Monica is furious with Chandler but wants to have sex anyway because she's ovulating. He resists, telling her he doesn't want to conceive a child in the middle of a horrible fight. She softens and apologizes, so they make love. The minute it's over she starts yelling at him again and tells him she didn't mean the apology and she's still angry. Chandler is understandably extremely upset. His body was used under false pretenses and he felt violated. "I feel so used!" He exclaims against the laugh track. Chandler tries to express some of these feelings to his best friend Joey, who can't understand what's so upsetting. He says to Chandler, "So? You got to have sex, right?" Chandler shakes his head and immediately responds, "What's the matter with me, why am I such a *girl*?" The episode basically ends with a high-five.[22]

This episode is disturbing for a few reasons, not the least of which is the total dismissal of Chandler's valid feelings about being sexually manipulated. Men have just as much of a right to consent and bodily autonomy as women do. The use of the word "girl" in the pejorative here is a clear message that any man who feels this way is displaying a shamefully feminine vulnerability. The heartless portrayal of Monica as a baby-crazy shrew who hates sex and only wants it for procreation is hurtful too, and represents, I think, a certain misogynist fear our society sometimes has about women. Toxic masculinity is dangerous for all of us on so many levels. It's no wonder it's such a challenge to see each other as humans when this is the prime-time TV we watched as kids and young teens.

For Male Survivors

Consent matters, whatever your gender. We all have the same right to want the sex we're having, and we all have the right to have our "no" respected. If you are a man who has experienced a violation of any kind that made you feel hurt or confused or upset, there are resources out there for you.

- ⊕ In the US and Canada, you can contact the 1in6 online or phone helpline for men who have experienced assault at https://1in6.org/. There may be local resources as well.

- ⊕ If there isn't a specific crisis line in your region for men, there is usually a general mental health crisis line you can call. The person on the other end

22   *Friends.* "The One With Phoebe's Birthday Dinner." Season 9, Episode 5. Directed by David Schwimmer. Written by David Crane, Marta Kauffmann, and Scott Silveri. Bright/Kauffmann/Crane Productions, Warner Bros. Oct 2002.

of the line has (hopefully) been trained in listening sensitively. They should believe you and validate your feelings about what happened.

⊕ It may be helpful to remember this first response when and if you choose to tell the people in your life what happened. You can't control how others will respond, and our cultural mythologies are powerful and pervasive. The crisis line should be able to refer you to further resources like support groups or counseling.

For Queer, Trans, and Gender Non-Conforming Survivors

Sexual assault and domestic violence are common for LGBTQ+ individuals, and it may be harder to access mainstream resources where you may encounter discrimination and institutional betrayal. Here are a few organizations that can help and may be able to help you access local resources:

⊕ forge-forward.org is a federally funded resource for transgendered individuals.

⊕ The Gay, Lesbian, Bisexual, and Transgender National Hotline is free and confidential. 1-888-THE-GLNH (1-888-843-4564)

⊕ The Human Rights Campaign at www.hrc.org has lots of articles and online resources for LGBTQ+ people.

ANGER AND ADDICTION

In general, men are twice as likely to be alcoholics as women[23] and four times as likely to take their own lives.[24] Women are almost twice as likely to be depressed as men,[25] however, and anywhere between two and eleven times as likely to suffer eating disorders, depending on what you're measuring.[26] There isn't as much reliable data on these factors for trans or gender non-conforming individuals, but there's evidence that hazardous substance use may be twice as high in the gay and trans communities (20–30 percent vs. 9 percent of the general population[27]) and that eating disorders

23   "Fact Sheets—Excessive Alcohol Use and Risks to Men's Health." The Centers for Disease Control and Prevention. March 7 2016. https://www.cdc.gov/alcohol/fact-sheets/mens-health.htm

24   O'Regan, Ellish. "Men four times more likely to die by suicide than women." The Independent, March 16, 2018. https://www.independent.ie/irish-news/health/men-four-times-more-likely-to-die-by-suicide-than-women-36710994.html

25   Albert, Paul R. "Why is depression more prevalent in women?" *Journal of Psychiatry and Neuroscience 2015* Jul; 40(4): 219–221. https://www.ncbi.nlm.nih.gov/pmc/articles/PMC4478054/

26   Tetyana, "Eating Disorders: Do Men and Women Differ?" *Science of Eating Disorders*, July 3, 2012. https://www.scienceofeds.org/2012/07/03/eating-disorders-men-women-differ/

27   Hunt, Jerome. "Why the Gay and Transgender Population Experiences Higher Rates of Substance Use." Center for American Progress. March 9, 2012. https://www.americanprogress.org/issues/lgbt/reports/2012/03/09/11228/why-the-gay-and-transgender-population-experiences-higher-rates-of-substance-use/

may be four times as common in transgendered college students than their fellow cisgendered female students.[28]

Some of the gender divide between alcohol use and disordered eating could be due to differences in the way men and women describe their experiences and tend to be diagnosed, but something is obviously up here. Psychologist Terrence Real points out that, while all humans have the same capacities for love and hurt, it matters that we are socialized differently according to our sex and gender. "The stable ratio of women in therapy and men in prison has something to teach us about the ways in which each sex is taught by our culture to handle pain," Real quips.[29]

It has been well documented that women tend to internalize their pain, keeping it contained to their own bodies, while men will act out, sometimes with violence against others. Men may not be diagnosed with depression as often as women not because they are happier, but because the depression looks different from the outside. Real writes:

> *Overt depression, prevalent in women, can be viewed as internalized oppression, as the psychological experience of victimization. Covert depression, prevalent in men, can be viewed as internalized disconnection—the experience of victimization warded off through grandiosity, perhaps through victimizing [others].*[30]

Men often get the message that the most important thing is their status, expressed through money and power. Many men understand that anger is the only appropriate emotion to express, because being a feared boss or father (or god) gives you power over people. This doesn't make it okay to victimize people, of course, but perhaps looking at the limited ways men have been taught to express their pain might illuminate some more generative ways to work with men's anger. In her book *The Will to Change: Men, Masculinity, and Love*, feminist cultural critic bell hooks points out that:

> *The first act of violence that patriarchy demands of males is not violence toward women. Instead patriarchy demands of all males that they engage in acts of psychic self-mutilation, that they kill off the emotional parts of themselves.*[31]

Considering the prevalence of risky alcohol use and suicide, male disconnection and self-isolation may very well be killing them.

Women, on the other hand, tend to get the message that the most important thing in their lives is their relationships with other people, their identities as wife, girlfriend, mother, daughter, sister, and so on. Anger is dangerous: not only will we get called shrill if we speak above a normal tone, anger can threaten emotional and relational connection. Anger can push people away. Harriet Lerner's book *The Dance of Anger* was written in 1985 but continues to be popular because so much of what she says still rings

---

28   Gordon, Allegra R. "Shining a Light on Gender Identity and Eating Disorders." *National Eating Disorders Association.* 2017. Accessed Dec 2018. https://www.nationaleatingdisorders.org/blog/shining-a-light-on-gender-identity-and-eating-disorders

29   Real, Terrence. *I Don't Want to Talk About It: Overcoming the Secret Legacy of Male Depression.* New York: Scribner Paperback, Simon and Schuster (1997): 83.

30   Ibid, 83–84

31   hooks, bell. *The Will to Change: Men, Masculinity, and Love.* New York, Washington Square Press (2004): 66.

true. Times have unquestionably changed, but the following passage still resonates, at least for me:

> *Why are angry women so threatening to others? If we are guilty, depressed, or self-doubting, we stay in place. We do not take action except against our own selves and we are unlikely to be agents of personal and social change. In contrast, angry women may change and challenge the lives of us all, as witnessed by the past decade of feminism. And change is an anxiety-arousing and difficult business for everyone, including those of us who are actively pushing for it.*[32]

When we define ourselves by our relationships, we know we'd better swallow our anger rather than risk the relationships that define who we are. Tend and befriend, the stress response that exists primarily for female animals, is literally based on the instinctive assumption that we cannot protect ourselves so we must befriend allies to protect us instead. We can't piss off our allies when we've got helpless babies to feed.

For men, on the other hand, no allies are invited to help with the pain of a trauma or the existential awfulness of being a human in the world. Women can't express anger because we rely on our allies, and men aren't allowed to have allies at all to help them carry their pain. We are, then, stuck at opposite ends of an unhealthy anger spectrum.

I've often wondered if women are likelier to use food to manage stress in part because it's a way of containing emotional damage to the space of one's own body. It's a way of protecting the kids and the husband and everyone else's feelings while we punish our guts with too much or not enough food. Drinking too much, on the other hand, might be a way to express emotions without having to take responsibility for one's own vulnerability. Alcohol can have a numbing effect, which is helpful when you know you're not supposed to share your emotions, but it can also loosen inhibitions, which might give men a chance to express all those difficult feels in the ironically more socially acceptable realm of being falling-over drunk than, I don't know, talking about it with a friend. Bonus if you don't remember what you said the next day. Maybe eating disorders help women swallow socially unacceptable emotions while alcohol helps men barf them out on anyone who will listen.

I do think these gendered lines of suffering are changing. Women are stepping into many more positions of power and finding more ways to speak up and be seen and heard. Many men in my life and in the public eye are paying attention to what's happening out there in the world, considering their own behavior, and finding ways to express how they feel without acting out. There is certainly more space for people to reject their gendered conditioning and express themselves in whatever way feels most true, though it might still be a bit of a cramped space. I've had the privilege in the last couple of years of meeting several men who have gone through various forms of recovery programs, mostly from substance use. These men are some of the most emotionally present people I have ever met. Many of them have rich emotional

---

32   Lerner, Harriet. *The Dance of Anger: A Woman's Guide to Changing the Patterns of Intimate Relationships.* New York: HarperCollins (2005): 3.

vocabularies and are often able to clearly express what they want and when something makes them feel uncomfortable. Their recovery programs help them get incredibly close to each other and many of them obviously deeply value their friendships, mentors, and allies. Meeting these men made me wonder if it wasn't just the substance use but also the toxicity of modern masculinity that had pushed them into their predicament and treatment. It was almost as if they'd gone through recovery from patriarchy.

From what I understand, many recovery programs for men include a lot of skill building in the realms of emotional expression, vulnerability, and asking for help—asking for allies. Men in recovery programs have a chance to talk honestly about their feelings with other men, completely and expressly protected from judgment. They meet male role models who show emotion and affection in a way that they may not have experienced from their father figures (or prime-time TV). These were some of the kindest, most compassionate, and most interesting men I've met.

Of course, as one of these men explained to me, they also struggle to maintain this level of emotional vulnerability because it's not supported by the culture. They learn that in order to be healthy people, to maintain their recovery, to be better lovers and good men, they must be honest about their feelings, ask for help, and surround themselves with as much love and tenderness as they can. At the same time, the culture tells them they are being weak and "soft," that they should suppress those feelings and go back to being angry jerks. From the outside, it looks to me like these men have it all figured out, but as my friend told me, this tension between being the man the culture wants them to be and being free is something many of these men struggle with on and off all their lives.

We all suffer from this ambient cultural toxicity. As the psychologist Terrence Real has written, "If traditional socialization takes aim at girls' voices, it takes aim at boys' hearts."[33] Maybe we need some Patriarchy Anonymous groups that could help women sustain their boundaries, encourage men to express their feelings, and help us all make space for those who don't want to identify in either gender group. We could all use some deprogramming, here. No wonder so many of us drink our feelings and eat our anger.

ANGER AS THE KEY TO VOICE

When we are violated, our boundaries are, by definition, disrespected. When that violation isn't understood by our community as a violation, our feelings are invalidated. When we feel we have no right to our feelings about something that happened, our sense of self becomes fragmented. When anger arises, even if only in dreams or in traffic when people don't signal their goddamn lane changes, it means some part of us knows that we have a self worth protecting. Even children who have never known anything other than abuse and violation express anger. Even without a previous context for an integrated, valued, appropriately boundaried self, we are born with the desire to

33   Real, Terrence. *I Don't Want to Talk About It: Overcoming the Secret Legacy of Male Depression*. New York: Scribner Paperback, Simon and Schuster (1997): 123.

protect our own bodies and hearts. If there's anger, even if it's deeply buried, there's a spark. There's the potential to heal.

My anger feels hard-won to me. It isn't always my first reaction, even when it should be. When someone does something hurtful, my first response is often shame and sadness, like I deserved the mistreatment. But I root around for my anger, I invite it, try to get it to talk to me. Sometimes, on the other hand, I'll misinterpret a text, and my rage will bloom up suddenly and violently and I cannot focus on anything else. It's not always easy for me to know when I'm reacting to something in the present or a trigger from the past. I'm still learning my boundaries, so sometimes I have to draw them out thickly until I know my loved ones will honor them. Once that trust is in place, I can soften the lines a bit. Then again, if a lover is too cool and distant, I start to feel fearful and abandoned. Boundaries are so fun!

My anger isn't always easy to deal with, but it is my key to intimacy. It helps me clarify what I feel and pushes me to communicate. It will not allow me to fall into a relationship and lose myself. It reminds me that I can do this alone if I need to. My rage is a powerful aspect of my healing from what happened in the past, and it is a good friend that keeps me connected in the present. It is a living animal cuddled at my feet, ready to jump up and guard me when things get out of hand. My anger has my back—as long as I continue to allow myself to feel it.

Feeling our rage is only the first part of the equation, of course. Whether it's a tiny spark or an inferno that keeps exploding all over the place, we need good tools to channel it, so we don't accidentally explode our lives. Expressing our anger by yelling or punching things, which is usually the urge, might actually have the opposite of the intended effect. In a 1999 study published in the *Journal of Personality and Social Psychology*,[34] researchers did an experiment with two groups of people. They instigated anger in both groups by getting them to write an essay and then telling them their work was crap. The first group was sent to hit a punching bag while the second group was told to sit down and be quiet for a while. Afterward, the groups were tested for aggression using a little game that allowed them to give their opponent annoying little horn blasts. The idea was that the bag-punchers would be less aggressive with their horn-blasting because they'd had a chance to express their anger, while the group made to sit quietly should be more aggressive because their anger was still sitting there waiting to be expressed. The researchers found the opposite to be true—bag punching exacerbated feelings of anger and expressions of aggression, while sitting quietly seemed to provide a kind of meditative cooling-off period that afforded the participants more calm.

Violent or aggressive expressions of anger aren't super helpful, but neither is swallowing or suppressing our anger. So what should we do, just hang back and shred our mouthguards to pieces while we dream about assholes who don't know how to signal their lane changes? I hate it when people don't signal their lane changes.

---

34   Diamond, Stephen A. "You Can't Punch Your Way Out of Anger." Psychology Today, Sept 24, 1999. https://www.psychologytoday.com/ca/blog/ulterior-motives/200909/you-cant-punch-your-way-out-anger

Anger needs action. It craves expression. But the key to getting it out it isn't in our fists. It's in our voices.

One winter solstice, I went to a three-hour grief ceremony (I really do know how to have a good time). Participants were invited into the circle to express their grief in whatever way they liked. The circle had four corners: one for emptiness, represented by an empty bowl, one for sadness, represented by a pile of dead leaves, one for fear, represented by a large rock, and one for anger, represented by two sticks that could be banged together. People banged the sticks about all kinds of things—the state of the world, the way children are raised, lost opportunities or lost time, the betrayals that happen in our relationships. Invariably, the anger had a distinct choking sound. People trying to let their anger out would grip the sticks, freeze and vibrate, try to open their throats and the sounds would barely strangle out of them. One person stepped up, stood in silence for a moment, and then simply repeated, "NO NO NO NO NO NO NO!" in a voice that sounded like she had a hand wrapped around her neck. The roar of rage came out like a whimper.

Anger needs voice. It needs us to speak up and express whatever is wrong. When we have been swallowing our anger for fear of social judgment or pushing people away, our rage voices atrophy and our throats get tired. We open our mouths to speak, we choke, and then depression swallows us instead. When it's time, we must speak up. We just have to figure out how.

CHANNELING ANGER INTO INTIMACY

I can't change anything about what happened in the past. But working with my anger in the present in my intimate relationships helps me feel more powerful in my self and more intimate with my others. It feels good to keep getting better at clarifying and nurturing my boundaries, to keep finding ways to teach myself that my internal "yes" and "no" signals matter. This is a practice, for me, of protecting my self within the context of connection.

When two people come together in a relationship, there's a bit of math I think everyone should do. Count the entities: there's you, there's me, and there's the relationship between us. One plus one equals three. A lot of people in our culture count everything up and find that one plus one equals one: one being, one relationship, one enmeshed thing with no individual self belonging to anyone. This is the monstrous We, a two-headed beast stomping all over everyone's yards and gardens. It doesn't have to be this way.

In intimate relationships, each person has a responsibility to his or her own self as well as to the relationship, the being they create together. The We coexists with two separate Is. No doubt this gets a whole lot more complicated in family dynamics with more than two players, but there should always be a self separate from any number of relationships.

Anger helps us find the lines between the entities, ensuring a healthy constellation of separate selves.

When anxious anger arises in intimate relationships, we must be careful about lashing out against the other person, which can cause things to escalate and then solidify whatever relationship dynamic needs to change. Instead, we can pause to reflect on what the anger alarm is pointing to. The fact that we are angry does not necessarily mean that our loved one intended harm. It just means we're feeling something. We must ask ourselves what need is not being met or what boundary is being crossed. We must take responsibility for how we feel and what we want and need without expecting anyone else to meet our needs for us. We have a right to our own needs and boundaries—and so does everyone else. When we're ready, we can communicate how we feel to our loved ones, not with violence or reactivity, but simply by explaining our feelings and asking for their help. Certainly this kind of conversation could turn into a fight, but, more often than not (in my experience, anyway), it helps us get to know each other better and clarify how we feel and what is happening in the relationship. Most of us absolutely want to meet our lovers' needs and respect their boundaries. We just don't know what they are.

Using anger to express our needs is a useful strategy for women who tend to sacrifice their own feelings at the altar of their relationships, but as our gender roles shift under our feet, men need to find ways to express their needs and boundaries, too. Many of the heterosexual men I know and love in my life are very aware that an expression of anger might be interpreted as a form of violence by the woman in their lives. These men have no interest in having power over a woman or victimizing anyone, but without any good role models from their father's generation (or on TV) for how to be in an equal partnership, many of them are feeling a little lost.

A popular strategy for these men seems to consist of agreeing with everything his girlfriend thinks, going along with whatever she wants, and apologizing when she's upset even when he doesn't know what he's apologizing for. The intention is to be kind and loving and keep the relationship going, but these well-meaning men keep getting dumped. I'm not blaming the girlfriends: it's not much fun being in a relationship with someone who doesn't stand up for himself and doesn't bother bringing any energy or intention to the relationship. There's no challenge, no friction, no distance for cultivating desire (which often means sparse, lackluster sex). This doesn't mean a couple needs to fight all the time to keep the passion alive, of course, but rather that each individual in a relationship must work to maintain their own sense of selfhood rather than a vague blobby "coupleness." As my brother pointed out when he was reflecting on the demise of his last relationship, agreeing with everything his girlfriend wanted wasn't only ineffective, it was lazy. "I never took the time to really think about what I wanted for us," my brother told me; "I was letting her do all that work."

For therapist Esther Perel, this is the source of missing passion for many couples who get along well and agree on everything. When intimacy stops being about sharing one's self with another and instead absorbs that self into the "we," the couple loses their erotic tension. Perel writes:

> *My belief, reinforced by twenty years of practice, is that in the course of establishing security, many couples confuse love with merging. This mix-up is a bad omen for sex. To sustain an élan toward the other, there must be a synapse to cross. Eroticism requires separateness. In other words, eroticism thrives in the space between the self and the other. In order to commune with the one we love, we must be able to tolerate this void and its pall of uncertainties.*[35]

As scary as it might sometimes seem to stand up for what you want and communicate about the ways you and your partner see things differently, it does a service to the love, intimacy, and eroticism in the relationship. It might seem selfish, but we have a responsibility to know ourselves and take care of ourselves. Otherwise we'll have nothing to bring to our lovers.

A lot of women in this generation are getting tired of the heavy load of emotional labor we inherited from our foremothers, who did absolutely fucking everything for their men and families. Most of today's men never learned from their forefathers how to interpret and predict other people's needs or how to make everyone's plans while cooking a healthy meal in a clean kitchen. Going along with whatever she wants isn't as generous as it sounds. It also requires a degree of disconnection, since being super cool and laid back all the time also probably means never standing up for your needs or boundaries or maybe never even questioning what they might be. Just as women have to learn to stand up for themselves, so do the men trying to love us. As silly as it sounds, the concept of an equal heterosexual relationship is kind of a new thing. It takes a little getting used to, but I believe in us!

Steps to Using Anger in Intimate Relationships

Anxious anger usually means intimate anger. When we can channel it toward improving intimacy and trust rather than simply reacting and exploding, it can really help us learn more about ourselves and our loved ones. Here are the steps:

- ⊕ Feel and validate your anger. Name it. It might very well come along with other emotions you can also name.

- ⊕ Take a time-out for yourself away from your loved one. This can be as long as you need. I often need a few days.

- ⊕ During this time-out, ask yourself, *What need is not being met or what boundary has been crossed?* Find an effective way to process the question. I like journaling and talking to my trusted friends, but whatever method you use to clarify your feelings is great.

---

35   Perel, Esther. *Mating in Captivity: Unlocking Erotic Intelligence.* New York: Harper (2007): xv.

⊞   See if you can pull apart boundaries, needs, and desires. Needs are needs—they are requirements. If a need is not being met, something must change. By definition the relationship is not sustainable if there are unmet needs floating around. (Keep in mind, though, that we can usually meet our own needs; sometimes our partners should simply get out of our way.) What you discover here may be a preference or a desire instead of a need. Ask yourself how important the preference or desire is. Remind yourself that you are allowed to have preferences and desires in a relationship.

⊞   Take responsibility for your own needs, preferences, desires, and boundaries. These things are your problem. No one is obligated to meet your needs for you, and you can't control other people's behavior. You can't force anyone to meet your needs. It's completely reasonable for your partner's refusal to help to be a deal breaker for you.

⊞   Decide whether or not you want to communicate with your loved one about this problem. Sometimes it's enough to clarify what you are feeling for yourself, and you may find it's not such a big deal. Communicating needs and boundaries is always a little bit threatening to the relationship because you are standing up for your separate self. Ask yourself if you can solve your problem alone or if you need your loved one to assist you. Let your anger remind you that you don't need people in your life who don't respect your boundaries or who have no interest in meeting your needs.

⊞   Communicate with your loved one if you decide to. Tell them what your problem is, what your desires are, what your need is that's not being met, or what boundary has been crossed that must be respected in the future. Be careful to use "I" statements. Don't tell your loved one how they feel or why it's their fault or how they have to change their behavior.

⊞   Ask for help. You can literally say, "I would like your help with this problem I have."

⊞   Listen to your partner. They may have their own needs and boundaries and desires that you had no idea about. Generally using "I" statements and taking responsibility for your feelings is pretty good at preventing a fight, but you never know—your loved one might get angry. Often, we get angry when our intimate ones threaten to change on us. It might feel very threatening to your loved one to discuss needs that are not being met. Try your best to give your loved one space to express what they need to express. If you end up in a fight, it happens! Fighting is sometimes useful, especially if you can come back later and try the conversation again.

⊞   If your loved one is willing and able to help you meet your needs, discuss what that might look like. You might have specific ways you'd like things to change between you and so might your loved one. Remember that your loved one may have limitations on what they are willing and able to do.

⊞   If your loved one is unable or unwilling to help you with your problem
     directly, consider if there is a way they can facilitate you meeting your
     own needs. If, for example, you need more time on your own away from
     the kids and your partner can't or won't take on more time for childcare,
     perhaps your partner can help pay for a childcare worker to come once a
     week so you can get your alone time. If you like to get your work done at
     home in the morning and your partner keeps interrupting you even after
     you explain the boundary, leave your partner with the kids' meal prep,
     leave the house, and work in a cafe. Needs are needs and boundaries are
     boundaries! Find a way. If the only way is to leave the relationship, do it.
     You will be okay.[36]

I know that most people in my life don't see me as a very angry person. Some of my
best friends have told me that I need to express my anger more often, more loudly,
more clearly. They could be right, but I think I do express my anger, all the time actually
(at least now I do). It comes out in my writing, in conversation with my loved ones,
and in the way I move my body (and jam down on my mouthguard). Most often my
anger looks like a really calm and loving conversation where I tell my partner what I'm
feeling and carefully avoid telling him how he should feel or what he needs to change.
I do my best to take full responsibility for what I feel and need and want, and I ask him
for his help. My anger reminds me that if I need to separate from the relationship, I
have the power to do that and I'll be okay. That's my style, and it works for me. Other
people have different styles of communication and might find more value in fighting
more explicitly or having different kinds of conversations than I do. That's totally fine.
Communication and relationship are a lifelong journey, and these things can shift and
change. Finding any sustainable way to express our anger without hurting others is vital.
The method we use matters a lot less.

Anger can start a conversation—first with the self, and then with others. It's not always
peaceful or easy to communicate, and it can make a mess—but that's just relationships.
Relationships are hard, and we're not born knowing how to do them well. When we
can connect to our anger, however, and find some way to express it in our intimate
relationships, we can create a different kind of world for ourselves and our loved ones.
In a way, this work is a rebellion against the oppression we've all grown up with in
our society. I have to admit I laughed out loud when I read this passage from Judith
Herman's book on recovering from trauma:

> *Because of entrenched norms of male entitlement, many women are accustomed
> to accommodating their partners' desires and subordinating their own, even in
> consensual sex. In the aftermath of rape, however, many survivors find they can
> no longer tolerate this arrangement. In order to reclaim her own sexuality, a rape
> survivor needs to establish a sense of autonomy and control. If she is ever to trust*

---

36   These tips are condensed from Harriet Lerner's fantastic book *The Dance of Anger*. If you want more on
this, do read that book.

again, she needs a cooperative and sensitive partner who does not expect sex on demand.[37]

I mean really! We ask for so much.

Herman is dead on, though. One of the best things about being raped (stick with me) is that when you can get to the other side of the pain and fear and grief, your old buddy anger shows up to remind you you have a self to protect and care for and that self matters. There is no longer any reason to put up with bad sex or partners who aren't deeply invested in your safety and your pleasure. After having been through the shitstorm of traumatic recovery, a few social norms don't hold you back from asking for what you want and saying no to what you don't want. The sex gets way better.

Channeling Anger

Sometimes we need to channel anger within intimate relationships, but sometimes our anger is about more than that. We might feel angry about the state of the world or about something that happened in the past that we can't do a damn thing about. Anger wants action, voice, movement, and expression, but it's not always appropriate or possible to directly communicate with the person or people who instigated our rage. Here are other possible ways to channel your anger:

- Exercise—run, jump, dance, take up martial arts. Move your body.
- Journal.
- Create art, whether through dance, music, poetry, painting, whatever you like to do. Anger is excellent fuel for creativity.
- Communicate your feelings to a friend or a counselor.
- Volunteer for or donate to an organization that fights the injustice you are angry about.
- Adjust some of your work toward fighting injustice, whether that means setting up a funding drive, creating a volunteer program within your workplace, or offering your services to certain underserved populations— whatever is doable.

ANGER AS THE POWER OF CHANGE

My first real job after I moved away from my childhood home was in the summer between my first and second year of university in Montreal. I was young and plucky and trying to make it on my own. I worked at a coffee shop with a boss who would ask to have meetings with me and, when I agreed, would take me shopping instead and make

---

37   Herman, Judith. Trauma and Recovery: The Aftermath of Violence—from Domestic Abuse to Political Terror. New York: Basic Books (1997): 65.

me try on outfits while he watched. He bought me clothes and jewelry I didn't want. It made me feel deeply uncomfortable, but I did not yet have a strong enough sense of what was okay and not okay coming from a boss figure (*Lean In* did not yet exist, guys).

One day I sat down with him in the empty coffee shop and told him I thought it was time for me to have a raise. He said, "You know what, give me a kiss and I'll give you a raise." I sat there stunned. It was the most explicit thing he had said to me. It hadn't been totally clear to me before that moment what boundary was being crossed in all those other vaguely creepy situations (thanks for looking out for me, anger!). He repeated his request, with a few admonitions of "Come on, just one little kiss!" A little part of my brain that understood something was wrong piped up. While I laughed nervously (hi, tend and befriend!) and said, "No, no, I'm not doing that!" my internal dialogue went something like this: *Did he just ask me to kiss him for a raise? Is he serious? Is this a joke? It doesn't seem like a joke. Should I do it? I don't have to do this, right? Isn't this sexual harassment in the workplace? I think it is. I don't have to. I'm not going to do this. Should I?* Finally, he took my no for an answer and said, "I'm just joking. Sure, you can have a raise." I think I ended up with another twenty-five cents an hour, after all that.

I left work shaking with no one but a summer dorm roommate at home and my parents a province away. I called my roommate and told him what had happened. He was very sweet and supportive, and I'm sure had no idea what to say. That was it. I didn't say anything to anyone else. I didn't quit. I didn't go to any other higher-ups at this huge coffee chain, which I won't name. It took me years to consider that he probably did that to a ton of other girls before anyone stopped him. That felt like my fault for not speaking up when I should have. Why didn't I get his ass fired?

Well, among other reasons, because women are taught from a very young age that our voices don't matter. People don't listen to us when we talk. I didn't know for sure that anyone else in the organization would have believed or supported me, and if experience is any indicator it probably would have just gotten awkward for me and I would have ended up being fired. Which, by the way, did happen to me a few years later after refusing to sleep with a different boss (yoga studios, am I right?), but that's another story. When you know in your bones you don't have any power, you act like you don't have any power. I didn't feel safe speaking up at the time, but maybe if I had I would have helped someone else avoid that situation in the future. It feels like my fault that it probably happened to a bunch of other girls before and after me. Once again, shame and silence showed up to shut my mouth and take down my story.

One of the things that can happen when you have experienced trauma or violation, especially if your community blames you or doesn't believe you, is that you can lose your sense of the right to your own story. A lot of trauma survivors struggle with guilt—for having survived when others didn't, for having participated in some way in their trauma, for not speaking up early enough, or on some other level. Getting past self-blame is a real challenge, and it can prevent us from feeling that we have a right to what we feel, let alone to share our stories.

Sometimes we need to get through the self-blame phase by going through a period of total and utter other-blame. Taking responsibility for our lives, our boundaries, and our choices is a huge piece of healing, but we can't get there before we stop blaming ourselves for what happened. Sometimes we need to own the identity of victim before we can own the identity of survivor. It's a relief when we can stop self-flagellating and instead discharge our anger against some group of people that had a hand in the violation—like guys with beards, CEOs, poets, skateboarders, or, I don't know, all men. When you can put bad people into a category, it makes it feel a hell of a lot easier to avoid being hurt again.

That's fair enough. It happens a lot. People feel a lot more fathomable when they are safely in a category. It's a way of putting up boundaries around other people instead of around the self (which is, by the way, where they belong). Directing our anger at a group of people might feel really good, especially when it helps us redirect the blame away from ourselves, but it's dangerous, too—not to mention fundamentally wrong (hello, racism!). Eventually we will need to find that strange line between blaming ourselves and taking responsibility for our lives. This takes as long as it takes.

There are a lot of big conversations happening right now around consent, sexual violence, and what it all means, which is wonderful. But this is also the first time many of us have put words to our experiences of trauma and violation. There is a huge rush of expression and a whole lot of rage, too. The rage is what is creating the space for the conversations to happen. It's a huge and exciting energy, but it's also incredibly volatile. A lot of our anger about our own assaults is compounded by the anger we feel that it's been happening to everyone else, too. We don't always get angry when we're the ones being violated, but when we see it happen to other people, the rage comes in bright and thick.

Trauma is not the only thing that steals our voices. Living in a society that silences girls' anger and boys' vulnerability sets us all up to be unable to speak out and express how we feel. It makes sense to me that a certain systemic silence is being broken through social media, where all people have to do is type out "#metoo" and they have joined a conversation; they've gotten a story out without having to get into the details and be judged and go through the shame of everything all over again. These kinds of social movements free us from the details, but they also pop the rage genie out of the bottle. Collective rage genies are even more unpredictable than personal rage genies. They want a target. Directing that rage against a category of people feels as good as scratching an itch, and it's an important part of healing, but it can't be the final act.

Lots of men have violated women, yes. There is a systemic problem at play when white, straight, rich, cisgendered, Christian (etc.) men categorically have more power than pretty much anyone else. I am a big believer that if we're going to heal as a society, everyone has to be involved, straight white men included. We have to figure out how to communicate with each other in generative ways without losing ourselves in reactionary anger. We have to avoid shame while being honest about what really happened, what really happens to us all the time. We all need Patriarchy Anonymous.

I struggled a lot with starting to write this story. My voice got caught in my throat when I thought about all the other women who have been violated in much more violent and repeated ways than I have been. What right do I have to tell my story when there are so many other stories that aren't being told? As I've spoken to other survivors, however, I've noticed that this is a bit of a theme: so many of us honor and acknowledge the magnitude of the issue even while minimizing our own stories. It's hugely healing to see our violations as an aspect of a systemic problem and not as an isolated incident that happened to us alone, but then we swing back to our training as women and overfocus on the fact that it happened to other people, pushing our own stories to the side in the process. Our shame and silence prevent us from speaking out under the pretense of making space for other people's stories. We don't feel we have the right to our own private pain when there is so much injustice in the world. We don't think it's okay to feel pleasure or enjoy sex when women who have less power than we do are being violated every day. We feel we are letting down our people if we let go of our anger, grief, or rage. We don't tell our stories because other people aren't able to tell theirs. Besides, telling the truth is fucking painful.

Doing our healing and telling our stories ain't easy, but it matters that we do these things. We're not doing anyone any favors by voluntarily keeping ourselves stuck in the weeds of trauma with our fallen comrades. The more of us can get up and get through it, the more of us there will be to offer a hand into those weeds and help everyone else out. Healing isn't selfish. It's an act of resistance.

We need to understand and acknowledge what happened as a community. We need public agreement that what happened was not okay. Survivors of combat situations often have war memorials to visit that help them to understand the context of their pain and remember that they are not alone. Survivors of sexual violation, on the other hand, are often isolated with their truth. Judith Herman writes:

> *Only 1 percent of rapes are ultimately resolved in arrest and conviction of the offender. Thus the most common trauma of women remains confined to the sphere of private life, without formal recognition or restitution from the community. There is no public monument for rape survivors.*[38]

That's not to say that combat violations aren't as severe as sexual violations. We don't need to get into a trauma competition and try to prove who has it worse. Any gender can have combat trauma or sexual trauma, but there is a historically different treatment of these two traumas in our society that runs along a gendered line. It's only recently that sexual trauma has begun to be recognized as the devastating violation it really is, and that impacts the way we heal and if we heal at all. Herman goes on to say:

> *In the task of healing, therefore, each survivor must find her own way to restore her sense of connection with the wider community. We do not know how many succeed in this task. But we do know that the women who recover most successfully*

---

38   Herman, Judith. *Trauma and Recovery: The Aftermath of Violence—from Domestic Abuse to Political Terror.* New York: Basic Books (1997): 73.

are those who discover some meaning in their experience that transcends the limits of personal tragedy. Most commonly, women find this meaning by joining with others in social action. [The most successful survivors] became volunteer counselors at rape crisis centers, victim advocates in court, lobbyists for legislative reform. [...] In refusing to hide or be silenced, in insisting that rape is a public matter, and in demanding social change, survivors create their own living monument.[39]

My intention in telling this story isn't to take up space that should go to someone else. I'm very aware of the many layers of privilege that supported my ability to heal and write this book. I know I'm one of the lucky ones. I'm not trying to tell anyone else's story here but my own, but it is my deep hope that if you have a story to tell, reading this one helps you consider that your voice matters, your expression matters, and your experience matters. This book is my attempt to create a living monument for myself and anyone else who has gone through something similar (and I know there are a lot of you). My anger is helping me tell my story. I hope your anger can help you find a way to tell yours.

---

39   Ibid.

FORGIVE

I have forgiven my perpetrator.

Well, sort of. We don't hang out and gab about the old days. If I saw him in the street, I'd probably run away or throw my coffee at him or something. I don't exactly wish him well.

For me, forgiveness doesn't necessarily mean forgetting or letting someone back into your life. It doesn't have to mean trying to have a relationship with the person again. Forgiveness isn't about the other person at all, really. It doesn't require an apology, punishment, compensation, or even justice (though those things definitely help!). All it means is that the weight of the other person's betrayal no longer sits on your heart day after day. The fear and constriction of the experience exist in the past and no longer hold your body hostage. You can see the other as a human being with pain, just like you. The perpetrator is not a source of fear. They do not loom large in your mind. They do not have power over you.

Forgiveness is a form of freedom. Forgiveness can release our powerful sexual and existential desire from the tangle of pain from the past. It can help us remember the possibility of real, full-hearted intimacy with another human being. We can't rush this kind of forgiveness. Before we can get there, we have to be able to fit what happened into a narrative that makes sense to us. We have to find our way back to safety. We have to mourn what we've lost. We have to find a little bit of compassion for ourselves, however we handled our own survival, as well as for the person who tried to destroy our lives.

It took me a long time, but I do feel some compassion for my perpetrator now. I think I understand why he did what he did. I don't believe he intended to hurt me, which doesn't change the fact that he did. I'm quite sure he hates women in his deep dark insides, but I doubt that hatred is conscious or chosen. What I needed to understand in order to get to that compassion is that what happened to me wasn't a random event that took place because there's something wrong with me. What happened to me fit into a much larger social narrative that both he and I participated in, in different ways and to different degrees. I pity him, actually. Doesn't mean I want to see him. Still wouldn't be that mad if he died in a fire. His existence just doesn't really matter that much to my healing, my desire, or my ability to fully participate in my life.

ME, TOO

One Sunday night, vaguely bored and too tired to do anything in particular, I opened up my Facebook feed. The phrase #metoo was splashed across my newsfeed, over and over and over and over, scrolling as far as a thumb could scroll.

The campaign was created by Tarana Burke, a black civil rights activist who first used the phrase to raise awareness around 2006, but I and many others (of course) found it through a white actress, Alyssa Milano. She popularized the phrase in the midst of allegations of sexual misconduct against Hollywood producer Harvey Weinstein. On Twitter, Milano invited her followers to reply to her tweet with the words "me too," quoting an unnamed friend: "If all the women who have been sexually harassed or assaulted wrote 'Me too.' as a status, we might give people a sense of the magnitude of the problem."[40]

Magnitude, indeed: within a day, more than fifty thousand people had responded to that one tweet,[41] and the conversation went on for weeks and weeks across various social media platforms. When I first saw Milano's tweet, I snorted a little at the invite to every woman who has been "sexually harassed or assaulted," because honey, that's every woman. We haven't all been violently attacked, but have we been catcalled? Put down at work? Lost a job or a promotion because of our baby-making vulnerability or because we wouldn't sleep with our boss? Called a slut? Been *almost* raped? Had our nudes leaked? Been hit on at work? We don't always make a big deal out of these things because they seem so normal. They are normal. They are a normal part of the human female experience. They happen all the goddamn time.

Just before I started to roll my eyes, though, at another futile attempt to make anyone care, I scrolled a little further and hit that sneaky ol' magnitude. I already knew that all my close friends have experienced some form of assault or harassment, but here was every woman on my Facebook feed, a few men, and several trans and nonbinary people. Acquaintances, work colleagues, friends' moms, and my second cousins once and twice removed. Literally everyone and their mother had joined the online survivor party. Some people simply wrote, "Me too." Others added pieces of their story: "It started when I was nine." "It was my stepfather." "My mom and aunt said I deserved it." "I never talk about this because most people blame me." I remember sagging into my old red couch. I felt like my heart had deflated and landed in a pile somewhere in the vicinity of my shoes. I settled into the couch cushions and stared into space for a while. I pretty much stayed there for the next couple of days.

---

40   Milano, Alyssa. "Status." twitter.com. Oct 15, 2017. https://twitter.com/alyssa_milano/status/919659438700670976?lang=en

41   Sayej, Nadja. "Alyssa Milano on the #MeToo movement: 'We're not going to stand for it any more.' " The Guardian. Dec 1, 2017. https://www.theguardian.com/culture/2017/dec/01/alyssa-milano-mee-too-sexual-harassment-abuse

SHAME, SILENCE, AND ISOLATION

One of the things that struck me about the many responses to the Me Too movement is how much shame and silence surrounds these experiences. We all have so many stories we never tell. We're afraid of what other people will say—and we're right to fear that; people sometimes say really shitty stuff when we tell our stories. For some of us, including me, it feels too heavy to try to acknowledge *all* the things that have happened. I found myself tallying up all the times I'd been harassed, violated, manipulated, and sexually intimidated, and it was *so many times* I had to stop before my tallying fingers cramped up. Not all of these experiences were violent or traumatic; plenty of them are par for the course of being a human female out here on these streets. But it's high time we give our heads a shake and acknowledge that it's messed up that being dominated, humiliated, and fearing for our lives on the daily is something we think of as normal.

Every now and again I encounter a well-meaning man who has no idea how common sexual violation is for women. He might know one or two people who've been through it or seen it on the news, but he doesn't realize that four out of five women in his life (and around two in five of the men)[42] have had these experiences. Women tend to talk to each other about this stuff, but we don't always talk to our brothers, our fathers, or our boyfriends about it. Maybe we should. Maybe we should stop protecting our men from the realities of the world we live in and let them suffer with us under the burden of our "normal." Women are tired—not only from trudging through our own experiences, but also from holding each others' stories and secrets, supporting each other through the pain, and protecting our families and bosses and partners from our anxiety and exhaustion. Maybe it's high time to let a dude hold our stories once in a while.

Breaking the silence might be scary, but it's deeply important for our personal and collective healing. The Me Too campaign is one of several that have come up over the years which attempt to reveal a very important truth: what happened to you wasn't a one-time act of violence that occurred because there's something wrong with you. What happened was a part of a much larger social structure in our society that we must all participate in changing. It happened because there's something wrong with all of us.

Breaking the Silence

Telling your story is a vital stage in your healing. A good place to start this process is with a professional who has experience helping people heal from sexual trauma. Once the narrative takes a shape you can understand, you have some choices about what to do with your story. Tread carefully—you may want some control over your audience so that you don't have to face judgment or not being believed. A supportive audience may help remove some shame, but judgment might be very upsetting, and you can't control

42   Chatterjee, Rhitu."A New Survey Finds 81 Percent Of Women Have Experienced Sexual Harassment." National Public Radio. Feb 21, 2018. https://www.npr.org/sections/thetwo-way/2018/02/21/587671849/a-new-survey-finds-eighty-percent-of-women-have-experienced-sexual-harassment

others' reactions. Be gentle with your audience—they may resist your story because they don't want to believe it, and you may trigger others' stories if you choose to share your own. You don't need to go into details to get the essence of the story across. If you do share, then you'll likely notice that what happened fits into a social narrative that's shared by many others and much larger than your individual experience. Here are some options:

⊕ Keep it to yourself. It's your story, and your choice.

⊕ Write it down as a short story, a journal entry, or a poem. Get clear on what happened, but also focus on how you got through it, where you found support, and the many possibilities of your life as a survivor.

⊕ Don't worry about details. It doesn't matter exactly when or specifically what happened. It's notoriously hard for survivors to remember this stuff, and unless you are taking legal action, it's unnecessary and might be retraumatizing. Focus on how you felt and still feel.

⊕ Write a book about it (oh, wait, that's me, I'm doing that! Hi!).

⊕ Make it into a piece of art using metaphor, so the details of the story are obscured by shape, color, imagination.

⊕ Tell a friend.

⊕ Tell a lover.

⊕ Tell your family.

⊕ Tell someone who thinks sexual assault isn't a problem in our culture.

⊕ Join a group of others who have been through something similar, and tell them. Listen to their stories with compassion.

THE PATRIARCHAL LIE

In order to forgive my perpetrator and stop seeing him as some kind of evil monster with power over me, I had to dig deep into the musty depths of my heart to find a little compassion. I had to consider what we had in common, how we share a culture and a set of social narratives. I had to be able to think of him as a flawed human being, just like me. I had to be able to see his suffering.

I think my perpetrator is like many men in this culture: angry that patriarchy did not deliver on its promises. We may not realize it or think about it all the time, but patriarchal societies operate under the fundamental myth that men are people and women are objects. A lot of people think the word "patriarchy" means that we live in a world where men have power over women. That's sort of true, but it's also based on a lie: that if men hide their vulnerability effectively, make enough money at their jobs, and jump through whatever other hoops they think will prove their manliness, then they will have earned sexual access to any woman they want. In her book *The Will to Change: Men, Masculinity and Love,* feminist cultural critic bell hooks writes:

> **Lying about sexuality is an accepted part of patriarchal masculinity. Sex is where many men act out because it is the only social arena where the patriarchal promise of dominion can be easily realized. Without these perks, masses of men might have rebelled against patriarchy long ago.**[43]

It's a painful lie for all of us. Many men believe (consciously or not) they have to shut down their natural emotions and struggle to make money at a job they hate in order to have access to women's bodies. Women are taught (consciously or not) that their desires don't matter. It's no wonder we're so confused about sexual assault, consent, and its consequences.

The lie is problematic not only because men think they are owed something, but also because women are taught over and over again in many different ways that we are not powerful and don't have any sexual agency. Men's sexual desire is seen as potentially dangerous, and women's sexual desire is seen as funny, embarrassing, or inconsequential, if it's seen at all. Writer Naomi Wolf points out that many feminist campaigns have had to lean on "constructing a narrative of helpless female sexual victimization by predatory, brutal men" in order to make any progress.[44] This narrative was useful for a time and is certainly true in some cases, but it "almost entirely failed to develop a companion discourse that included female sexual desire and sexual agency."[45] Wolf continues:

> **The trouble is that most date rapes today happen after a nuanced encounter— in which a woman wants *this,* but emphatically does not want *that.* If we are unable ever to talk about sexual agency without fearing that this makes us "fair game" for anything that follows, we will never be able to prosecute real rapes successfully.**[46]

We need more of an understanding of what and how complex sexual violation is and that it occurs on a wide spectrum. We have to believe and support survivors while understanding that yes, sometimes women want to have sex, but when they do, that doesn't mean they were asking to be hurt or violated.

I thought about this trouble with nuance when I heard on the news that Asia Argento, one of the first women to accuse Harvey Weinstein of sexual misconduct, has herself been accused of sexually assaulting a seventeen-year-old man. Weinstein's lawyer jumped to the conclusion that Argento is a hypocrite and therefore all allegations against him should be seen as suspect. When we think women are innocent victims and men are evil perpetrators, we can't hold the possibility that what Weinstein did to Argento was wrong and what Argento did to the young man was wrong. We forget

---

43 hooks, bell. *The Will to Change: Men, Masculinity, and Love.* New York, Washington Square Press (2004): 73.

44 Wolf, Naomi. *Vagina: A New Biography.* New York, Ecco (2013): 153.

45 Ibid.

46 Ibid, 153–154.

that hurt people sometimes hurt people. We get so lost in the narrative we don't put responsibility in the right places. We can't tolerate nuance.

When only evil monsters can assault innocent women, some men are picking up on the possibility that calling themselves feminists might protect them from persecution. Learning something about feminism has become one of the patriarchal hoops that men believe they can jump through in order to entitle them to women's bodies. There's a whole brand of guys out there who have learned a bit of vocabulary about feminism and then use it to try to get women into bed. My friends and I call them Ians; their namesake is an Ian who started a sexual relationship with a friend of mine while in a polyamorous relationship with his wife and a few others. His version of polyamory seemed to be less about expanding his capacity for love and more about using as many people as he possibly could for his own gains without facing any consequences. This particular Ian would come over to my friend's house late at night, mansplain feminism to her, fuck her, then quickly shower and get the hell out of there before she could get a word in edgewise. He knew something about the theory of feminism but hadn't really integrated the fundamental idea of the movement: the radical notion that women are people. (PS: sorry to all the good Ians out there, I'm sure you're not all like that! #NotAllIans)

The man who assaulted me was not the big, strong jerk you might imagine when you think about a rapist. He was a skinny, awkward nerd who had picked up his version of the patriarchal lie: that "nice guys" should get a chance to finish first. He had listened to me complain about all the jerks I'd slept with, including the guy who had locked me into a dark room and intimidated me into having sex with him (it was a yes that time, but a yes born of 100 percent pure fear). After a while, he seemed to think all this listening and being a good friend-ing meant I owed him sex (and he once "playfully" pushed me into a dark room and locked the door in some sort of menacing echo of the story I'd told him only days before). Here he was, a nice guy, totally different from all those jerks. I'd given it away to so many assholes, he pointed out, why couldn't I just give it to him? (Note to any guys reading: slut shaming is not a great way to get a woman to sleep with you.) He understood that it was unfair that big, strong, popular men got to have sex with whoever they wanted and that skinnier guys didn't always get that prize, but, he felt, women still owed him sex, one way or another. What he did not understand was the radical notion that women are people.

These aspects of the patriarchal lie turned murderous in the mind of Elliot Rodger, an infamous twenty-two-year-old who killed six people and injured fourteen in a spree that he described in a long, disturbing YouTube video in 2014 as his War on Women. He was speaking for a group of people called "incels," or involuntary celibates, who mostly complain about how women owe them sex in that delightful corner of the Internet called the manosphere. Rodger stated, "I will punish all females for the crime of depriving me of sex [...] They have starved me of sex for my entire youth and gave that pleasure to other men."[47] Those other men, the good-looking guys who get all the sex, Rodger termed Chads, and the withholding women who fuck them were called Stacys. This angry young man clearly did not see the Stacys (let alone the Chads) as people.

In 2018, Alek Minassian drove a van into a group of people in Toronto, killing ten of them. When I heard about this on the CBC News: World at Six radio show, the host asked the reporter whether or not this was a terrorist attack. It was definitely *not* a terrorist attack, the reporter explained; the motive seemed to be related to Elliot Rodger. Minassian had written in a Facebook post just before the attack, "The Incel Rebellion has already begun! We will overthrow all Chads and Stacys! All hail the Supreme Gentleman Elliot Rodger!"[48] So, definitely not a terrorist attack. Terrorists have to have brown skin, apparently, and speak a non-English language. Violently attacking a group of people based on an oppressive ideology with the explicit purpose of terrifying that group of people: no? Not a terrorist attack? Okay.

Some people argued that Minassian's attack couldn't be terrorism against women because he targeted both men and women, the Stacys, but also the Chads with the right to fuck them. Again: the implication that anyone is entitled to a woman's body outside of individual, personal consent is an oppressive ideology that targets women. It is terrifying. It is terrorism.

In his book *Love and War*, Tom Digby lays out the ways in which acts like this are indeed forms of terrorism. It's not just about bombs or machine gun fire, either: for Digby, even the everyday threat of misogynist violence is a way to keep women in their place—which is, of course, inferior to men. This inferiority is, in turn, what keeps *men* in place, defining themselves as the superior gender who, de facto, should have rights over the inferior sex's body. Digby writes,

> *The threat of rape, which is perhaps the ultimate expression of misogyny, terrorizes virtually every woman in the United States. Few men, and not all women, are aware of the pervasive effective of the threat of rape in women's lives.*[49]

This misogynistic terrorism is another one of those normal things about life in a woman's body that are so common we often forget that they are not okay. Regardless of the realistic likelihood that a specific person of any gender is about to be raped on the street (and how many times more likely it is that our date will be the one to rape us?), every woman I know thinks about it every single time she's alone outside in the dark. Most of us have a plan for what we'll do if and when we are eventually attacked. We have strategies for what happens if we get separated at a club or a party or if someone gets roofied. Some of us carry pepper spray or rape whistles in our purses, and many of us

47   Winton, Richard, Rong-Gong Lin II and Rosanna Lia. "Isla Vista shooting: Read Elliot Rodger's graphic, elaborate attack plan." *LA Times*. May 25, 2014. https://www.latimes.com/local/lanow/la-me-ln-isla-vista-document-20140524-story.html

48   Yang, Jennifer. "Facebook post linked to Alek Minassian cites 'incel rebellion,' mass murderer." The Star. April 24, 2018. https://www.thestar.com/news/gta/2018/04/24/facebook-deletes-post-linked-to-alek-minassian-amid-questions-about-its-authenticity.html

49   Digby, Tom. *Love and War: How Militarism Shapes Sexuality and Romance*. New York, Columbia University Press (2014): 133.

slide our keys between our fingers when walking alone. We talk about these strategies, plan with each other, and generally move through the world with an awareness of the possibility of violation, or even death, at any moment. Not so long ago I was watching a friend's baby and we went for a walk, my dog's leash in my hand and the baby strapped to my chest. Adjusting for the weight of the squiggling baby with his tiny hand wrapped around my thumb, I felt this sudden, intense vulnerability, this knowledge that I wouldn't be able to run very fast or fight if a man suddenly decided to try to take me down. What's the word for what I felt in that moment? Oh, right. It's *terror*.

As a culture, we're quick enough to notice that there is a pattern that some people who set off bombs identify as Muslim. That's easy (not to mention lazy): they are "other," so we can quickly place the enemy. A long history of white supremacy has caused us to unconsciously fear non-white people to the point that president Donald Trump justified his plans to create a border wall by calling Mexicans "rapists"[50]—despite the clear lack of evidence that immigrants are any more violent or criminal than anyone else in the US.[51] In fact, 56 percent of the mass shootings committed since 1982 in the US were committed by white people, while only 16 percent were committed by black people and 8 percent by Latino people.[52] Of 106 shootings, 102 were committed by men.[53] The problem isn't with immigrants, here. Maybe the problem is with men. Specifically, young white men.

Tom Digby suggests that these young white male terrorists are acting out against the patriarchal lie. They have been taught that in order to be "real men," they must be warriors, capable of protecting women, providing for their families, and procreating (or, at least, performing the acts related to procreation). When this burden becomes heavy enough on a man who is not making much money or getting laid very often, these men don't know what their place is supposed to be in society, and this masculine insecurity can become toxic. However, Digby writes:

> *attacking people is something every boy or young man can do. And if he attacks for the sake of a larger cause, that enhances the sense that he is acting as a warrior. Thus the barriers to entry into a career as a terrorist are really quite low.[54]*

Elliot Rodger and Alek Minassian are a part of a movement. It is a movement of misogynist terror that keeps women afraid and inferior and that ensures men are stuck for the rest of their lives striving to define themselves as warriors, superior to the women they control. The "incel" movement isn't about sex. It's about power.

50   Wolf, Z. Byron. "Trump basically called Mexicans rapists again." CNN Politics. April 6, 2018. https://www.cnn.com/2018/04/06/politics/trump-mexico-rapists/index.html

51   Flagg, Anna. "The Myth of the Criminal Immigrant." The New York Times, March 30, 2018. https://www.nytimes.com/interactive/2018/03/30/upshot/crime-immigration-myth.html

52   "Number of mass shootings in the United States between 1982 and November 2018, by shooter's race and ethnicity." Statista, Nov 2018. https://www.statista.com/statistics/476456/mass-shootings-in-the-us-by-shooter-s-race/

53   "Number of mass shootings in the United States between 1982 and November 2018, by shooter's gender." Statista, Nov 2018. https://www.statista.com/statistics/476445/mass-shootings-in-the-us-by-shooter-s-gender/

54   Digby, Tom. Love and War: *How Militarism Shapes Sexuality and Romance.* New York, Columbia University Press (2014): 166

Don't get me wrong. I don't think my perpetrator was about to take a machine gun out on a sorority or anything (pretty sure). But I felt his frustration and righteous indignation, the sense that I didn't have the right to say no. So he showed me that I did not have that right. He took away my power and proved that nice guys could finish first. And he did. He got what he wanted and never had any consequences. His friends didn't really believe me. He never responded to my strongly worded letter (and it was very strongly worded. Lots of big words. Highly intimidating.). He never apologized in any way. He just went on to live his life, and probably makes 26 percent more income than me, too.

I doubt, though, that he feels particularly powerful. Honestly, if he felt powerful, he probably wouldn't have needed to show me how he was powerful. We live in an era where people keep telling men—especially white, straight, rich men—that they are powerful. They might not be healthy or happy or have genuine, intimate love with another they see as an equal, but they should at least have a couple of people in their lives they can boss around. This narrative shifts, however, when class and race come into the picture. bell hooks points out that feminist authors with class privilege "express surprise that most men do not see themselves as powerful," since in their white, rich families, their fathers were, pretty much, all-powerful.[55] That's not everyone's experience: "women who have been raised in poor and working-class homes have always been acutely aware of the emotional pain of the men in their lives and of their work satisfactions," hooks writes.[56] Power can exist in a lot of different ways, and race, class, and gender are interconnecting factors.

hooks argues for the fundamental truth that what human beings crave is love and connection, being seen and heard in intimacy with other human beings. In a twist of patriarchal sleight-of-hand, we are offered domination instead. She writes:

> *That love and domination can coexist is one of the most powerful lies patriarchy tells us all. Most men and women continue to believe it, but in truth, love transforms domination. When men do the work of creating selves outside the patriarchal box, they create the emotional awareness needed for them to learn to love.*[57]

Domination is no substitute for love, and everyone wants love, no matter how straight, white, and rich they may be. Learning love is hard work. It requires seeing the ways in which we've participated in the lie and acknowledging how much time we lost chasing power when what we really wanted was connection. Some men take out these frustrations on women. Some are starting to see how they've been cheated by the patriarchal lie, how their desire for love has been traded in for the false promise of domination. Some men are fighting back against this lie by figuring out how to choose love.

---

55   hooks, bell. *The Will to Change: Men, Masculinity, and Love.* New York, Washington Square Press (2004): 99.

56   Ibid.

57   Ibid, 123.

Privilege is a funny thing. Its hallmark is its invisibility. It means not having to think about something other people have to expend a lot of energy worrying about. It means not noticing your race, gender, or class because it doesn't obstruct you in any way. It's really hard to see your own privilege. Men certainly have some power in our society, but that wavers with other factors like whether they are straight, rich, white, cisgendered, attractive, able bodied, or mentally well. Women have power in some contexts, too, specifically in the emotional realm. Women are encouraged to focus on their interpersonal relationships, which makes it easier for us to create supportive networks, talk about our feelings, and ask for help. Considering that social isolation and its attending loneliness may be worse for us than smoking fifteen cigarettes a day,[58] women's emotional privilege may contribute to our tendency to live almost seven years longer than men.[59] We all have some power in some contexts, and it is our responsibility to figure out where and when so that we can use our voices to help each other out.

Forgiveness is, in a sense, about taking our power back. When someone has made us feel powerless, we have to consider the zones in our lives where we do have a voice, even if it's not anywhere near the perpetrator's orbit. We may not have been trained to think of social connection and compassion as particularly powerful, but they are. Being able to see ourselves and each other as whole but flawed humans with the capacity to change isn't always easy, but it sure is hopeful.

In order for me to forgive, I needed to believe in the possibility of change. Change requires that I see myself clearly alongside all these assholes hurting other people—as someone who is also, sometimes, an asshole. I needed to be able to be angry while also taking responsibility for the ways I participate in the lies of the patriarchy and contribute to a culture that creates people like Elliot Rodger. As uncomfortable as it is to admit, Elliot Rodger is one of my people. We live in the same culture, watched the same movies, grew up with the same prime-time TV. Elliot and I (and you, as well) have been indoctrinated into patriarchal ideology—along with capitalism and white supremacy and probably a whole bunch of other stuff too—from our first moments of consciousness. We are breathing the air of this stuff. All of us. No one gets to say they aren't affected. No one gets to say they don't participate.

FIRST AND SECOND THOUGHTS

A lot of people think of patriarchy as something men do to women. It's actually something we all do together in a sort of unconscious collusion. Certainly some men use their power and privilege to use, put down, or violate women, but it's a myth that the fact of our chromosomal makeup excuses us from taking part. Women are taught to collude with our own abusers. We protect our men when they commit violence and willfully forget what they've done. We fail to keep our children away from the men

---

58   Sunnucks, Jack. "Being Lonely Is Worse Than Smoking 15 Cigarettes a Day." Vice, May 2, 2018. https://www.vice.com/en_asia/article/ywxypm/being-lonely-is-worse-than-smoking-15-cigarettes-a-day
59   Ginter, E. And V. Simko. "Women live longer than men." Bratisl Lek Listy 2013; 114 (2): 45–49.

who hurt them. We dismiss other women's claims of wrongdoing and make fun of men who say they've been sexually assaulted. We blame other people for their misfortunes. Sometimes we use men sexually without considering that men's consent matters just as much as anyone else's. Sometimes we do this stuff because we are trying to grasp for our own little piece of power. Sometimes we do it out of fear. Mostly we do it because it's all we've ever learned. It's natural to react first with what our culture taught us. It's pretty near impossible to stop the reflexes of our first thoughts.

What matters much more than our first thoughts, however, is our second thoughts. The problem of violence against women isn't something individual women can solve by taking a bunch of self-defense classes and somehow making themselves less rape-able. It's not something individual men can solve by, I don't know, quitting being rapists (though that would probably help). Most of us aren't explicitly sexist or racist, but we've all grown up swimming in sexist, racist waters. We don't even realize how much knee-jerk assholery is floating around the edges of our subconscious minds. We have to unlearn these things actively. We have to take responsibility for our own assholery and try harder to see each other as people. That's all it is: the whole thing. It's seeing people—all people—as human beings with strengths and weaknesses, and, if you can stand it, the potential for change. None of this is easy. It's something we have to practice. We've got to try to be kind to ourselves and each other while we figure out new ways of being in the world.

Art for a Better Second Thought

It's natural for human beings to see each other in social categories rather than as individuals. This may have been an adaptive strategy at some point in our species' survival, but it's not useful when we're trying to connect with other human beings, learn from each other, and co-create a more egalitarian society. It's important to acknowledge our own blind spots when we can, including the fact that, by definition, we usually don't even know they are there. That's okay, but we can also do the work of trying to root out those blind spots and see each other as individuals rather than as stereotyped representatives of some social group. Art is the most fun way to work on our own blind spots. Here are some suggestions:

⊕ Go to events where a diverse roster of people have the opportunity to express themselves. If you're at an open mic, for example, keep track of how similar the performers look, and pay attention to your own reactions when you see someone speak who looks different from you. Notice if you tend to have judgments and assumptions about them. Listen to them.

⊕ Hunt down photo campaigns that show different bodies as beautiful. For example, Substantia Jones's Adipositivity Project (https://theadipositivityproject.zenfolio.com/about.html) and Mariana Godoy's empoderarte-me series (http://empoderarteme.tumblr.com/) showcase fat bodies as beautiful, sensual, and diverse in their own right.

- Make a resolution to see more films, read more books, and/or listen to more podcasts by an underrepresented group, such as women, indigenous writers, or trans and nonbinary people. Make a point to see popular movies showcasing non-white romantic leads. Notice whether or not the films and books you're consuming pass the Bechdel test (two women talk to each other about something other than a man—more on this below).

- Be willing to observe your own first thoughts when you experience these forms of art. Be kind to yourself. Give yourself a chance to let your mind open and keep working on your second thoughts.

- Be kind to other people when they say something that might reveal some biased first thoughts. You can talk to them about what they said, for sure, but remember that we're all ignorant and our biases are powerful. It takes work to do better, and getting mad at people for their views only tends to make them hold on harder. Wherever you can, open a conversation with kindness and compassion and stay aware of your own blind spots.

FORGIVING OURSELVES

For many of us, forgiving our perpetrators isn't so hard—it's forgiving ourselves that's the real issue. Getting beyond the identity of helpless victim without turning to self-blame is incredibly challenging. Trauma isn't always traumatizing because of explicit violence. Sometimes it's traumatizing because it shows us in a light that makes us hate ourselves: weak, stupid, vulnerable, miserable, powerless, and so on. Finding compassion for someone else is okay, but when we need it for ourselves, it might as well be buried at the bottom of the ocean.

As we talked about in the last chapter, anger and rage are vital pieces of the healing puzzle because they help us figure out how to protect and care for ourselves. Being honest with ourselves about our anger, hurt, and betrayal is a non-negotiable first phase of the forgiveness process. We need to learn what our needs and boundaries are and find a way to stand up for them. When we first start dealing with and acknowledging our pain, however, that anger can rage like a wildfire and threaten to burn all the houses down. Rage doesn't always land in the right place. Blame can land on the people who didn't get hurt, the people who didn't help us enough after the violence happened, or people the perpetrator looks like. Sometimes we forgive our perpetrators far too quickly and our rage and pain get redirected onto the wrong people—or straight back onto our own selves.

Having compassion for someone doesn't mean blindly forgiving them or suppressing all your feelings about how they let you down. It just means seeing them as a flawed human being doing the best they can with the resources they have available. We have to work at turning this compassion toward ourselves. Whatever we did, however we survived, we have to remember that there are reasons why things went down the way they did. If we could have made better choices in the moment or in the aftermath we would have. It wasn't our fault we were hurt. It wasn't our fault if we didn't know how to deal with it after the fact. Maybe we've made some mistakes, but that's a natural function of having choices. There are no right or wrong choices, just actions that have consequences, not all of which are predictable. It sucks that we live in a world where our stumbles can make our lives explode, but there are always more choices coming down the line in some form or another as long as we're still alive to fuck things up. As Gil Scott-Heron sings in his song "I'm New Here," recorded at age sixty-one after a period of struggle with drug use: "No matter how far wrong you've gone, you can always turn around."[60]

When we use our anger mindfully, it can help us set up appropriate boundaries and figure out how to meet most of our own needs. Then we can figure out where the anger actually needs to be directed. When someone is mean to me, my first reaction is often to apologize for being a horrible person who caused their cruelty through some far-reaching tendril of my own stupidity. It can take me a day or two to clue in that someone crossed *my* boundaries and that I actually need to stand up for myself. That anger is still useful, even when it comes after a delay. It still helps me find my boundaries even if I dropped them for a minute there.

Compassion and forgiveness are only advisable once we've created some sense of safety within ourselves and our relationships. This is important, because compassion requires softening the walls around the self, an easing of our hard-won boundaries. It can only happen after the anger has had its time, and that's not to be rushed. We can't think ourselves past anger—we have to let ourselves feel it in our bodies for a while before compassion and forgiveness become possible. Compassion requires a willingness to see a perpetrator as someone you have something in common with, as one of your people. This is incredibly confronting, and it doesn't have to happen at any specific time (or ever). But again, forgiveness isn't about the other person. It doesn't matter if the other person has apologized, paid you a million dollars, self-flagellated in pain and remorse, or if he spends his days not thinking about you in cream-colored cafes reading stories written by straight white men all day. Justice isn't the same as forgiveness. Forgiveness is about finding your own power and trusting it enough that you can let go of your attachment to the other person and what they did to you.

Inviting Empathy

A few years ago, I learned an empathy cycle from New York yoga teacher Eric Stoneberg that has served me many times over (and that I wrote about in my first book, *Secrets of the Eternal Moon Phase Goddesses: Meditations on Desire, Relationships and the Art of Being Broken*). It is adapted from the Shakta Tantric worldview, a goddess-worshiping philosophy originating in India. It goes like this:

---

60   Scott-Heron, Gil. "I'm New Here," 2010, *I'm New Here,* XL Recordings.

⊕   "I'm not you": When someone makes us angry or does something we don't understand, the first place we go is to separation. This is where the anger arises. This is an important stage where we need our boundaries to protect us.

⊕   "I'm something like you": If we can consider one thing we have in common with the person who hurt us, that can help us soften the wall between self and other. We start to put ourselves in the other person's shoes and consider how the other person might feel.

⊕   "I'm nothing but you": The small opening in the second step allows us to remember that we are all connected in some way or another. From this Tantric perspective, this is an expression of oneness, that we are all a manifestation of the divine Goddess energy. From a more secular perspective, we can remember that we're all human beings doing the best we can with the resources we have available. When we can get to this step, we can go beyond compassion and consider how we are literally as well as metaphysically a part of the world that created the pain that led to the person's wrongdoing. We might even consider how we could help lessen the other person's pain for the sake of the whole.

⊕   It's important to note that these three steps exist within a cycle, and each stage lasts as long as it lasts. We're not trying to rush to oneness, and oneness is no more valuable than any other stage, including anger or contemplation. We can't stay in oneness forever, either, it's not safe or useful to do so. We have to go back to "I'm not you" and remember ourselves as individuals with choices and responsibilities. The cycle can repeat itself over and over in our lives, over the course of a moment or a decade. Each stage is useful in its own right.

It's easy to want to head straight to the soothing tones of forgiveness where what's past is past. But if we jump to this part too quickly, we might miss the part where we find and stand up for our boundaries. Opening our boundaries to compassion is incredibly dangerous until we know how to keep ourselves safe.

Skipping over anger also does a disservice to love. Jumping straight from hurt to the all-encompassing wholeness of the universe is false forgiveness, a form of blind compassion. In his book *Spiritual Bypassing*, Robert Augustus Masters warns of the dangers of avoiding the difficult work of connecting with our unhealed wounds and trying to fix everything with a too-eager compassion. He writes:

> **When we are driven by blind compassion, we cut everyone far too much slack, making excuses for others' behavior and making nice in situations that require a forceful "no," an unmistakable voicing of displeasure, or a firm setting and**

maintaining of boundaries. These things can, and often should, be done out of love, but blind compassion keeps love too meek, sentenced to wearing a kind face.[61]

Love means a lot of things, but it definitely doesn't mean never saying no. Love doesn't forgive all, but it can sometimes help us heal—as long as we let it be fierce from time to time. Love must not be sentenced to wearing a kind face.

For me, forgiveness can mean holding someone responsible for their actions while also acknowledging their humanness. People rarely intend to do us wrong. People often act out because they themselves are hurting. That helps us feel for them, but it doesn't make bad behavior okay. Sometimes we need to figure out how to hold our empathy, compassion, and even love for someone who has hurt us alongside the truth that they did us wrong and might very well hurt us again. This is hard work.

Let's be honest—we don't like hard work. We like things to be simple. Our subconscious minds are sweet little children who like to think that people are either good or evil, monsters or rescuers, safe or dangerous. Sadly for the naive babies of our minds, life isn't like that. People can be good and do something bad. People can promise us that we'll always be safe and not have the slightest idea of what they are promising. People can be so sorry for what they've done and do it again anyway. People can be really well-intentioned parents and make an absolute psychological mess of their unsuspecting children. When we let that freaky little "and" into the room, we can come to a much more mature and complex understanding about what's happening.

I believe my perpetrator was hurting *and* that what he did was wrong. I believe he hated me *and* had no idea that he hated me. He wanted me to be his girlfriend *and* he treated me like a vending machine after he had put a dollar in and then kicked it when the bag of Twizzlers was not immediately forthcoming. All those things are true at once, which means that if he wanted to do the difficult work of looking at his own subconscious belief systems, he could probably change them. He could probably find a way to see women as people, to love them as flawed human beings just like him. I have to believe that's possible. The belief that people can change and do better is the only way to survive the merry-go-round of assholery that is life.

MONSTERIZING

When sexual violence happens, especially male-on-female violence, our knee-jerk reaction is to side with the perpetrator. We've been conditioned by decades of popular movies to see men as heroes and women as objects that push the men's plot along. Only 49 percent of Oscar-winning films for Best Picture pass the Bechdel test—a simple measure that started out as a joke in a 1985 comic strip by Alison Bechdel. The test requires that a film have 1) two (named) female characters on screen at the same time 2) talking to each other 3) about something other than a man. The Bechdel

---

61   Masters, Robert Augustus. *Spiritual Bypassing: When Spirituality Disconnects Us from What Really Matters.* Berkeley, North Atlantic Books (2010): 21–22.

test's official database houses 7,760 films to date, and the percentage of films that pass this simple test sits at an underwhelming 57.8 percent.[62] We tend to take the male perpetrator's side partly because we are so used to looking at things from a man's perspective. We only consider women's inner lives and perspectives as an afterthought— even if we're women ourselves.

This plays out in real life. After a group of students raped and humiliated a young woman in Steubenville, Ohio, two sixteen-year-old football players were convicted of raping a minor in juvenile court. CNN's Poppy Harlow stated that it was "incredibly difficult, even for an outsider like me, to watch what happened as these two young men that had such promising futures, star football players, very good students, literally watched as they believed their lives fell apart."[63] Many other reporters, male and female alike, jumped to sympathize with the boys, apparently somehow forgetting that a young woman had been raped, filmed, and *peed on while unconscious on the front lawn.* These reporters aren't bad people. They just went with their first reaction. It takes a little work to see things from the survivor's perspective. As silly as it may seem, we need more popular, accessible Hollywood movies that tell different kinds of stories from a woman's perspective (not to mention all the other perspectives we're missing, including those of people of color, people with different sexual orientations and gender expressions, differently abled people, non-neurotypical people, and so on). We need more practice seeing a range of different kinds of people as *people.*

Of course, when we can get past our tendency to side with the perpetrator, we tend to then go to the absolute opposite extreme. Now, we all agree the perpetrator is an evil monster. We pile all of our social anxieties about rape and violence onto this one person. We fire him, jail him, socially isolate him, sometimes even kill him, if we can get him on death row. This is monsterizing: making a human being who did something bad into an evil monster who must be destroyed. Remember how good it felt to see the man-hunting shark in *Jaws* get blown to bits by a couple of well-meaning Americans? As Slavoj Zizek points out in his film *The Pervert's Guide to Ideology, Jaws* was a *great* place to put our nebulous anxieties about immigrants, natural disasters, and the Soviet Union at the time.[64] When there's evil in the world, we need a monster we can blow to bits so we can feel like we have some control over an unpredictable world. This is completely reasonable and natural, but it's also not helpful. Not for us, and not for the sharks: sharks are actually pretty cool about not killing people, but partly thanks to *Jaws,* people are not that cool about not killing sharks, and now the animals are largely endangered.

Monsterizing in sexual assault cases gives us the illusion that taking revenge on this one person and getting rid of him will somehow solve the problem of violence against women in our society. When we do this, we miss the point that violence against women

---

62   "Bechdel Test Movie List." Dec 2018. https://bechdeltest.com/statistics/

63   Wemple, Erik. "CNN is getting hammered for Steubenville coverage." The Washington Post. March 18, 2013. https://www.washingtonpost.com/blogs/erik-wemple/wp/2013/03/18/cnn-is-getting-hammered-for-steubenville-coverage/?noredirect=on&utm_term=.3452633bee1e

64   *The Pervert's Guide to Ideology.* Directed by Sophie Fiennes. Ireland: Blinder Films and the British Film Institute, 2013. Film.

is a social and cultural problem, that it's embedded in our everyday lives. As Tom Digby points out:

> *To focus revenge or punishment on individuals can distract from a broader, crucial, specifically philosophical project: identifying, describing, explaining, and critiquing the cultural programming that systematically produces the perpetrators of misogynistic terrorism.*[65]

These assaults and attacks aren't rare. They happen all the time. It feels so good to find, accuse, and punish someone for them that we feel our work is done. It allows us to stop feeling uncomfortable and skip the part where we have to consider how big and far-reaching the problem actually is. We can skirt that sneaky ol' magnitude.

That doesn't mean perpetrators shouldn't have to face consequences for their crimes. They should. The problem is that when we focus on pointing out and punishing these people, we think that absolves us from looking for the pattern and actually changing things.

Paul Gilmartin is a survivor of childhood covert incest who was interviewed on the podcast *I, Survivor*. He acknowledges the damage his mother caused him and the damage he caused to the women he mistreated in his own life. He shows a fantastic ability to hold empathy and responsibility at the same time, and he insists that while we must have consequences for our actions we must also try to see each other as human beings and have empathy for the reasons we sometimes hurt other people. "If these were forest fires breaking out," he points out, "we wouldn't just say, 'Oh, fire is such a piece of shit!' We would look, we'd go into the woods and go, 'Okay, what is causing this?'" That doesn't mean people wouldn't have consequences—Gilmartin adds, "We wouldn't say, 'Welcome into our home for Christmas, Arsonist!'"—but we'd take the time to consider why the fires were starting and how to prevent them in general, rather than simply punishing a single person who caused one. We must remember that, as Gilmartin phrases it, "Compassion and consequences are not mutually exclusive."[66]

Perpetrators should face consequences, and sometimes they should be big ones. No doubt some people intend harm and should be stopped and possibly imprisoned. But so many assaults are much smaller than that. They are mini power plays that might not even leave a visible mark but can devastate the survivor's life anyway. They are strange, confusing experiences where one person thinks everything is going great while the other is thinking about escaping out the bathroom window. The consequences of these actions are devastating, but excommunicating a perpetrator from his community, imprisoning him (or killing him) may not feel like appropriate punishment for the crime—even to the victim.

Our tendency to turn people into monsters is part of the reason these experiences are so cloaked in shame and silence. It perpetuates the myth that rape is always a violent

---

65   Digby, Tom. *Love and War: How Militarism Shapes Sexuality and Romance*. New York, Columbia University Press (2014): 136
66   *I, Survivor*. "Covert Affairs." Wondery, Oct 9, 2018. https://wondery.com/shows/i-survivor/

bloody affair committed by an unhinged asshole. We have different legal definitions for the various ways you can kill someone: causing death by accident is called manslaughter, and when it is intended and premeditated it's called first-degree murder. These are different crimes that have different legal consequences, but at the end of the day, someone is still dead. We've thought so carefully within our legal system about what it means to cause death and how much intention matters, but we haven't put nearly as much serious attention into understanding sexual assault. Whether there was intent, malice, premeditation, brutal force, and so on matters, but at the end of it, someone was still sexually assaulted. However the punishment is meted out, the survivor is still stuck with it for life.

Sometimes we talk about how rape isn't sex because sex is about love and connection and rape is about power. This is a useful narrative in some ways, but, for some of us, an experience of nonconsensual sex was both nonconsensual as well as sex. It looked a lot like something we might want to consent to from time to time. We may have even had a sexual response during a sexual experience that we were coerced or manipulated into, and it's confusing to try to think of that as not-sex. It's a lot harder to explain to the authorities that someone raped you when it took you awhile to realize that it was rape. You might not even think of it as rape because even though you said no, you went along with it because that seemed like the safest option. Many of us end up with sexual difficulties after a rape, which means we were wounded in a sexual place. We need a better vocabulary to understand the difference between painful, physically forced rape and the less physically obvious mentally or emotionally coerced rape. They are different experiences and have different healing journeys, but as Naomi Wolf points out in her book *Vagina: A New Biography*:

> **Rape tends to be understood and even prosecuted—if there is no weapon involved, and no additional physical assault, no visible bruising and no blood—as if it is "just" forced sex, rather than a highly violent act resulting in potentially lasting damage. But this new science shows that "mere" fear and "mere" violation, when imposed on a victim through a "nonviolent" sex assault, even a date rape, can imprint and harm the female brain and body in measurable, long-lasting ways.[67]**

Most women don't report their rapes because, around 85–90 percent of the time, the perpetrator is a friend, a former partner, or a schoolmate. Half the time it happens on a date.[68] We might be angry and want revenge, but we don't want to be responsible for destroying someone's life. Maybe that's because we can see their humanity even when they can't see ours. Maybe it's because we know we'll be more likely to be blamed and shamed for putting someone away rather than actually getting any sense of justice or support from the community. Maybe it's because we blame ourselves. Or maybe it's because we need a different set of consequences than what's currently on offer.

67   Wolf, Naomi. *Vagina: A New Biography*. New York, Ecco (2013): 105–106.
68   "Most Victims Know Their Attacker." National Institute of Justice, Oct 1, 2008. https://www.nij.gov/topics/crime/rape-sexual-violence/campus/pages/know-attacker.aspx

I think a lot about what happened with comedian Aziz Ansari in 2018. In the midst of the flurry of allegations in Hollywood against sexual predators, a woman spoke out about her bad date with the then-newly famous comedian and TV star. To make a long and super uncomfortable story short, she consented to go out with Ansari and went back to his place, and he then pressured her aggressively into some really awkward sexual activity that she did not consent to—including, at one point, a couple of fingers going into her mouth in what I guess you might think was sexy, you know, if you'd never had sex before.[69] When the story went live, Ansari put out a bewildered statement saying that he had thought everything had been consensual and half-apologized for something he was pretty sure he hadn't done.[70] Up until then, Ansari was a champion of women and often dealt with issues of race, class, and gender in his work. His award-winning TV show, *Master of None,* was cancelled. If he had any deals for upcoming comedy specials on Netflix, they were cancelled, too. I'm sure no one ever picked up his part-comedy, part-sociology book, *Modern Romance,* for a light read in public ever again. At least, not until his comeback—which he has begun not a year after the whole thing went down.

This story is, in many ways, the crux of our problem. We totally get that women are sometimes raped and violated. Totally. We get it, it's really bad, rapists are bad, we'd never be rapists, let's kill all the rapists and then all our problems will be solved; all righteous citizens get yer pitchforks out. Right? Sadly, it is not that simple. What happened to the young woman Aziz Ansari went on that date with has happened to so many of us (I've had that date, like, four times, and I'm pretty sure you have, too). We may or may not have experienced it as traumatic, but it might have made us want to hide in our basements forever and never date again. Bad dates should be funny stories we can tell our friends later. They should never be situations where things are happening to our bodies that we didn't consent to. A bad date shouldn't mean fearing for our lives or bodily integrity. The difficult thing to swallow here is that Aziz's date was telling the truth about her experience of violence while Aziz was probably also genuinely confused about what happened and never intended to force his date into anything. A man might see Aziz's downfall and think to himself, "Have I ever done something like that?" The truth is, yes, you possibly have, bro.

Aziz's sudden rise to fame probably brought a lot more dates into his life all of a sudden. Short, non-white men don't often get a swipe right on dating apps (for a whole other set of problematic social and cultural reasons), so his popularity in the dating world might have been somewhat new and overwhelming. I don't mean to imply that people who get fewer swipes for artificial reasons like race are necessarily going to be any worse at consent than someone with a ton of experience; if anything, non-white men may have had more opportunities to think critically about sex and dating because they don't tend to fit the white-oriented standards of beauty in our culture. But fame comes with a lot of attention and a degree of power that may have skewed Aziz's sense of entitlement

69   Way, Katie. "I went on a date with Aziz Ansari. It turned into the worst night of my life." Babe. Jan 13, 2018. https://babe.net/2018/01/13/aziz-ansari-28355
70   Thomas, Megan. "Aziz Ansari responds to sexual assault allegation: 'I was surprised and concerned.' " CNN. Jan 16, 2018. https://www.cnn.com/2018/01/15/entertainment/aziz-ansari-responds/index.html

and awareness of his own behavior. Maybe, like so many men of his generation, Aziz saw someone in a porn stick their fingers down someone's throat once and thought that's what women wanted. The heady mix of sudden fame and power plus a bit of awkwardness created a situation that was received as violence by his date, who, by the way, knew his fame meant he had more power than she did. He had probably swallowed the patriarchal lie with the rest of us and figured that now he was famous, every woman would obviously reward him with total access to their bodies. Probably quite a few were doing so at the time. He may have been coming from a place of ignorance and innocence, but, for his date, it was violence. Both can be true at the same time.

So what do you do when the limits of your knowledge and abilities cause you to commit violence against someone you never intended to harm? Take a year off and then book a comeback tour? This is an important question. I don't think Aziz Ansari should be imprisoned, but I also think we need to believe his date and collectively acknowledge the hurt and pain she experienced as a result of his actions. I want a better solution for these everyday violations. I want a way for men to concretely unlearn the entitlement they have picked up from generations of films about men where women barely talk to each other in the background. I want kids of all genders to learn what consent is in school and how to spot it before things go off the rails. I want us all to feel that our "no" matters. I want us to stop assuming that if we excommunicate every person who has ever been violent toward a woman that we will solve the problem of violence against women. I want us all to look honestly at the ways we participate in the toxicity of patriarchy and stop doing it, goddammit.

Dr. Adi Jaffe is a mental health professional who wrote a book called *The Abstinence Myth.* Jaffe argues that abstinence as the only treatment for addiction may actually be preventing a lot of people from getting help. When success is measured solely by the intimidating goal of consecutive days of sobriety, there is a huge amount of shame in relapse. Jaffe acknowledges that an addictive behavior might be someone's only coping mechanism and that asking them to quit before they can get any other kind of help could end up being counterproductive. For many people, he says in an interview, "using, in whatever way they are doing it, is the only thing that's making their day survivable," and telling them they can't get any help until they quit is like telling someone with two broken legs, "Okay, I have physical therapy for you, it's right at the other end of the building—you just can't take your crutches or your wheelchair."[71] Helping people improve their stress management and relationship skills rather than focusing on abstinence might support them enough for them to be able to let go of an addictive behavior. If we could take the shame away a little bit, Jaffe believes, and let people bumble through a recovery process in a less intimidating way, more people might get help and actually get better. I think this principle applies to our collective problem with consent. It is unreasonable to expect us to know what consent is and treat each other with respect when we've never seen it in our own lives, let alone in porn or

---

71   *Getting Curious with Jonathan Van Ness.* "Why is Abstinence Still Being Used to Treat Addiction? w/ Dr Adi Jaffe." August 14, 2018. https://www.earwolf.com/episode/why-is-abstinence-still-being-used-to-treat-addiction-w-dr-adi-jaffe/

in Hollywood movies. We're not born with that kind of skill. We're terrified to even consider the possibility that we perpetrated a nonconsensual act or said something racist or perpetuated some stereotype, and denial and defensiveness aren't super helpful for positive change. If we could acknowledge that we've had bad training without spiraling into shame, we could learn new things about each other and how our bodies and minds work. We could avoid the shame spiral when we mess up along the learning journey. We could listen to each other and communicate about what we want and don't want. We could get better at seeing each other as people. We'd definitely be having better sex.

So let's admit, collectively, that we have a problem here. We were born mainlining toxic masculinity and we need to figure out together how to break the pattern. Feeling shame about our mistakes or the ways we've participated in the whole situation prevents us from actually looking at ourselves and being willing to try it a different way. Let's set aside the shame and start doing the uncomfortable work of figuring out what it might mean to have loving, connected sexual experiences that aren't about power. We can't try new things if we're too terrified of fucking it up. No one taught us how to do this!

So yes, Aziz Ansari must take responsibility for his actions. He is someone who, before this story came out, was a self-described feminist who worked out some of his own questions and confusions on his show, in his book, and in his comedy routines. He has an opportunity now to let people watch him learn what it might look like to do better, to take responsibility without the debilitating effects of shame. Unfortunately, as I write this, the news from his comeback tour is dismal: his comedy seems to have turned away from his focus on social justice and is now centered more on making fun of people who are too politically correct. Even Orbey notes in the *New Yorker* that

> *The amused but progressive spirit that once informed Ansari's commentary on current events seems to have crusted into suspicion about wokeness and its excesses. Without ever mentioning the #MeToo movement—or his own experience as one of its most disputed casualties—Ansari decries the destructive performativity of Internet activism and the fickle, ever-changing standards of political correctness.*[72]

I wanted Aziz to spend his time off in counseling (with a feminist therapist), looking honestly at himself and his actions and learning something he could share in his comedy acts and TV shows. I wanted him to take the opportunity to teach a generation of men who are terrified and confused about what sex is how to go through the process of learning this stuff. I wanted him to use his fame as a power for good. It would have taken some courage, to be sure, and undoubtedly he would have made himself more vulnerable to the fire of wokeness and its excesses, but we could have learned something from seeing the process of atoning for his mistakes and blind spots and committing to do better. Now *that* is a Netflix special I would watch. Be better, Aziz Ansari. Help the rest of us.

---

72   Orbey, Eren. "Aziz Ansari's New Standup Tour Is a Cry Against Extreme Wokeness." The New Yorker, Oct 4, 2018. https://www.newyorker.com/culture/culture-desk/aziz-ansaris-new-standup-tour-is-a-cry-against-extreme-wokeness

THE COMPLICATIONS OF CONSENT

Consent is kind of a new idea in our culture. We are slowly unlearning the idea of owning or being entitled to each other's bodies in romantic relationships, and we're starting to figure out what it means to ask whether or not someone wants a certain kind of touch and how they might feel about what we are doing. All our romance narratives are focused on this wild, untamed passion that grabs/pins down/takes rather than asks/checks in/respects. Sexual desire is something we often think of as nonverbal, animalistic, and out of our control, but when we just take what we want without concern for the consequences, before we know it, we've assaulted someone. It's not okay.

One solution we've found to this problem is using our words. Yes, asking permission is helpful, but it's complicated, too. More than one of my male-identified friends who date women have told me the same story—they practice what they learned in their consent workshops and ask their date permission before they do anything. And does she tear up with gratitude that someone is finally asking her how she feels? Nope, she gets frustrated and says, "stop talking, and just kiss me!" Now that, my friends, is confusing.

This is partly a problem of our cultural narratives that tell us that men always want sex and that it's a woman's job to either say yes or no. For a lot of women, having a choice at all is kind of a new thing, and it's incredibly, painfully difficult to say no. We've been conditioned to say yes to men even when we mean no. When consent workshops focus only on men and teach those men that their job is to ask and a woman's job is to agree or dissent, we're perpetuating the myth that sex is a man's choice and a woman has to deal with it; it simply adds a clause where a woman is allowed to say no sometimes—which is something she may not feel completely equipped to do. There isn't any space for her desire in this narrative. Consent that boils down to him asking, her responding, is still gendered, power-based, and not very playful. It implies that all initiative belongs to men, just as it always has, and that women are not in a position to participate in choosing what happens next. Besides, men aren't the only ones who need to learn about consent. Women and other genders not only need to learn how to feel their desire and own their "no" but also how to respect other people's sexual boundaries and desires. Being sexually assaulted a lot doesn't automatically teach us how to treat others with sexual respect.

Taught in the right way, consent workshops can be incredibly effective, especially when they are given to mixed genders. Consent classes for mixed genders that have been going on in Nairobi, Kenya, for the last decade have reduced the incidence of rape in that region by 51 percent.[73] Boys do probably need some extra help unlearning the cultural pressure to chase girls and get as many conquests under their belts as they can, but as we figure out what's most effective in these workshops, we have to be teaching all genders to participate in consent together and to communicate effectively about it,

73   Singh, Anisha. "How 'Consent Classes' In Kenya Reduced Cases Of Sexual Harassment." NDTV, Oct 27, 2017. https://www.ndtv.com/education/how-consent-classes-in-kenya-reduced-cases-of-sexual-harassment-1767943

not simply reducing it down to a formula where he asks and she either says yes or no. It's much more than that.

It doesn't help, either, that a lot of us have a nonconsensual romance narrative very deeply embedded in our skins and feel that sexual passion is a non-verbal, dominance-oriented "taking." Some women expect that and are confused when it doesn't happen (especially if they've never been to a workshop about it). You can't just tell someone to unlearn everything they thought they knew about desire and romance in one conversation. Besides, there should still be room for passionate abandon when we're not analytically thinking through every step of our sexual experience.

Verbal consent is probably the gold standard for what we have currently come up with in terms of consent, but this model has its limitations. In the thick of things, someone may not be sure how they feel. They might want to do some things but not other things. They might be into it in the moment and then realize the next day they were only trying to get back at their ex and be full of regret. They might really want to have sex with you, but for some other reason (like, say, a monogamous relationship with someone else or a recent breakup) they resist, which can lead to mixed signals. There may be cultural differences between two people that affect how we read body language, tone of voice, silence, or verbal cues. Someone might, for any reason in the world (like having you stick your fingers down their throat), change their mind in the middle of everything. Not to mention that women often unconsciously fear the consequences of saying no to a man. As the old adage goes, men are afraid women will laugh at them, and women are afraid men will kill them. There are a lot of hidden power dynamics in our world, many of which aren't even available to our conscious minds. Men have historically had power over women, so even if everything else is equal between a heterosexual couple—same age, same income, same status at work, same physical strength—there's still a power dynamic there. Asking and saying yes or no out loud is a lot more complicated than it might seem.

A further complication with verbal consent is what happens in our brains when we are sexually aroused. If things are going well in a sexual encounter, our rational, analytical brains quiet down, allowing us to be fully present with sensation in our bodies so we can surrender to pleasure and orgasm. It's well documented that women (at least) have a harder time orgasming when they are in an analytical state of mind; surrender is a prerequisite for letting go into pleasure. Notoriously, being turned on can make us want to do things we wouldn't do in a more sober, rational state. It's a fun place to get to, but it's also vulnerable: behavioral economists Dan Ariely and George Loewenstein studied a group of male college students to find out what effect sexual arousal had on their decision-making skills, and, predictably, it significantly changed them.[74] Under a state of sexual arousal, the subjects were much more willing to make reckless decisions, including agreeing to unsafe sex practices. That means we might be much more willing to say yes to something when we're aroused than when we're not, so even if you get

---

74   Ariely, Dan, and George Loewenstein. "The Heat of the Moment: The Effect of Sexual Arousal on Sexual Decision Making." *Journal of Behavioral Decision Making* 19 (2006): 87–98.

verbal confirmation in the heat of the moment, there's no guarantee someone might not regret it in the morning. Desire has its dangers, so we must take seriously each other's physical and emotional fragility as best as we can. At the same time, we must take that surrender seriously, too, and not interrupt it every three seconds to bring our verbal, analytical minds back online.

For me, that kind of surrender can only happen when I know that my consent matters and I can trust the partner I'm with. When it does, it's like my words are at the bottom of a well, and it's a bit of a struggle to pull them up to the surface. I can nod or make sounds, but it's kind of a challenge to string a sentence together. For me, consent conversations need to happen *before* sexual contact begins, and then we can get into a nonverbal groove together. Even then, however, it's still useful to use our words from time to time: something might come up that requires a verbal check-in, and it's always okay to pause, come up for air, talk it out, and then dive back into nonverbal playland.

I'm still sorting out my own understanding of consent, but I know that I need to feel safe enough with someone to know that they will be responsive to my reactions, which include tensing up, holding my breath, or verbally saying, "wait," "stop," "slow down," or "no." I'm listening for the same sort of reactions from my partner and want to make sure they are staying present with me throughout the experience. Consent happens in the nonsexual realm, too: does my partner respect my space and my decisions? Do we decide together when we want to hang out and what we want to do? Is there respect in this relationship in general? I don't think asking permission before every single touch within a sexual experience is the most effective (or most fun) strategy, but I do want some degree of verbal confirmation before anything gets started. I find it quite romantic when someone asks for a first kiss because it indicates respect and it means the other person cares how I feel. I think respect is romantic. But the deeper I go with someone in a sexual encounter, the less able I feel to verbally gauge my consent levels. I need to know I can stop and go back into my analytical mind if I need to, but I want to trust enough not to have to.

I've started to think of consent not as a blanket "permission granted" status, but as a space that two people co-create together. We learn about each other's body language, preferences, and verbal and nonverbal cues over time. There is work involved in learning someone's sexual language. That's one of the reasons sex tends to get better when you get to know someone—the first time with a new partner is almost never the best time. Simply relying on a verbal "yes" and then plowing ahead no matter what else happens isn't a complete form of consent.

Sex is fundamentally unstructured adult play, and there needs to be space to explore, to try things, and for some things to not work perfectly. There need to be some rules in place but not too many. I need to be able to laugh with a partner when there is awkwardness and know that they will stop if I indicate that I need them to. I don't expect my partner to read my mind, and I certainly wouldn't want someone to think I can read theirs. I do, however, want them to be paying attention, both to their own pleasure but also to how I am responding to what they do. We are exploring each other together, playfully, and by the same rules—like, for example: anyone can call for a time-out at any time for any reason, and there's no pressure for any particular thing to happen in any specific way. The problem with Aziz Ansari and his date may have been very simple: Aziz was so focused on his own experience and his own goals for the evening that he wasn't paying any attention to what the human being in front of him was feeling, experiencing, and expressing with her words and body language. Staying present and caring about the person in front of you goes a long way toward keepin' it consensual.

Reading Consent Cues

Obviously a verbal yes and no are helpful to maintain consent, but there are many other signals you can be listening, watching, and feeling for to make sure your partner is enjoying what you are doing and feeling safe. Here are a few things to look out for:

- Flirting: Flirting can be hard to read. Sometimes people seem to be flirting when they don't mean to. Others may be awkward but really do intend to flirt. Before you physically touch them in a sexual way, ask them if it's okay or tell them you want to and let them make the next move. If they don't, let it go.

- Protection: Someone may want to have sex with you, but not unprotected sex with you. This requires a conversation, even a short one in the moment, like, "Let's get a condom!" Contraception and protection from STIs are consent boundaries that must be respected.

- Power: We all know the obvious power dynamics that can mess with consent, like those with bosses, sports coaches, teachers, counselors, and movie villains who are blackmailing you. But it's pretty hard to avoid all power dynamics in all relationships. Before you get involved with anyone, ask yourself if you have power over them in any realm. Are you physically stronger? Do they need you for work? Money? Even emotionally? If they do, they might think they owe you or be afraid of what you'll do if they say no. They might be using *you* for your power. Tread carefully here. Again, we can't avoid all power dynamics, but it's helpful to be aware of them. Consider using your own "no."

- Breath: Is the person breathing deeply, sighing, or moaning when you do something in particular? That's usually a yes. Did their breath suddenly go completely quiet? That's probably a no. You can stop and see if they ask you to keep going. You can ask them if they are okay.

- Touch: Initiate contact slowly. Give your partner a chance to swat your hand away, pull back, groan, press back into you, or respond with a verbal "yes" or "no." Even if you're sure they like a particular kind of touch, teasing is fun and can create a little consent buffer, giving your partner time to respond to what you're doing.

⊕   Tension: Are they relaxing with your touch, pressing back into you, moving with your rhythm? Those are generally yeses. Are they tensing up suddenly, pulling away, physically pushing you away, wincing, or going rigid? That's probably a no. You can slow down or stop and check in.

⊕   Context: Did they say just a minute ago that they didn't want anything to happen, but now something is happening? Even if they initiated it? This is a really important moment to use your words. Don't just go with it. They might be trying to please or placate you, or instinct might be overriding their wiser minds. Remind them that they said they didn't want to just moments before and ask if they are sure they want to keep going.

⊕   Words: Listen for words like "wait," "hold on," "slow down," or "ouch!" Check in verbally from time to time if you're getting any "no" body language. Simply saying something like, "Are you okay?" or "Is this okay?" is really helpful—it doesn't need to be a long conversation.

⊕   Let it go: keep in mind that if someone doesn't want to have sex with you, flirt with you, do a certain act with you, or date you, it's okay. If you check in and a "yes" has for whatever reason morphed into a "no," be respectful. Give your partner space. Don't guilt them or pressure them—they will want to have sex with you far less if you do! Sex can be vulnerable, and people may need to be reassured in various ways that they are safe and their boundaries are protected, especially if they've been sexually violated before.

THE POSSIBILITY OF RESTORATIVE LOVE

We are living in a time when our anger is moving us forward. It's helping us notice victimization, create a vocabulary for what that means, and empower survivors. We may not be ready yet as a culture to think about what it might mean for a perpetrator to heal. Forgiving a single act of violence is one thing, but as I'm trying to point out here, sexual violence against women isn't a collection of unrelated unfortunate acts. It is a systemic issue. There is a time, of course, when the focus must be on the healing of survivors. That takes priority. But we won't be able to truly move on as a society and genuinely stop the cycle of violence until the perpetrators heal, too.

Seeing a perpetrator apologize, pay a fine, lose custody of his children, get fired, or be escorted out of the courtroom to jail can be useful for a survivor. Appropriate consequences can bolster healing. Unfortunately, of course, that's not usually what happens. In her book *Trauma and Recovery*, Judith Herman points out,

> **Genuine contrition in a perpetrator is a rare miracle. Fortunately, the survivor does not need to wait for it. Her healing depends on the discovery of restorative**

love in her own life; it does not require that this love is extended
to the perpetrator.[75]

My perpetrator has never apologized, and it doesn't matter. I can forgive him, feel compassion for him, hope he finds a way to do better, and still never want to see him again. As survivor Paul Gilmartin has pointed out, "You don't have to have somebody in your life to have love or compassion for them. Sometimes that's the only way you can have love and compassion for them."[76] Destroying my perpetrator's life might help him clue in that he has some work to do on himself, but it wouldn't necessarily protect other women from him. It wouldn't necessarily help me move on. I'd rather he do the work of thinking about what went wrong and try to do better.

In 2018, Eliana Dockterman wrote an article in *Time Magazine* on sex offender therapy. She points out that "Most people find it difficult to reconcile the hope that rehabilitation is possible with the impulse to push these men to the periphery of society forever. Punitive measures alone, however, have not been found to meaningfully increase community safety."[77] Punishment, isolation, and excommunication are meant, at least in part, to protect others from getting hurt. Unfortunately, punishment doesn't really do that; 70 percent of incarcerated individuals go on to reoffend within five years of their release, and there's some evidence to suggest punishment and imprisonment may contribute to a cycle of illegal activity.[78] Therapy, on the other hand, might help.

The social workers in Dockterman's story work hard to listen to the sex offenders that come to them and to see them as people, but also to help them take responsibility for their actions at the same time. The offenders often rationalize their behavior. They don't relate to the famous men who abuse their power, thinking that their situation is different, that perhaps their victims actually wanted their attentions, or that their desires were more important than anyone else's. With time and effort in therapy, they start to see why they did what they did and understand that it was wrong. One man, who was caught repeatedly masturbating beside women in movie theaters, "believes that he exposed himself in the hopes of making a human connection, however irrational that may sound. [...] 'It took me a long time to figure out that women don't want to see that. They find it disgusting,' he said."[79]

It's difficult to try to see these men as human beings instead of as monsters, especially if we've been hurt by people like them. Some certainly may be sociopaths devoid of empathy, but a lot of them are flawed human beings choosing the absolute worst ways to try to make sense of the loneliness and powerlessness of life. Learning life skills in

75   Herman, Judith. *Trauma and Recovery: The Aftermath of Violence—from Domestic Abuse to Political Terror.* New York: Basic Books (1997): 190.

76   *I Survivor.* "Covert Affairs." Wondery, Oct 9, 2018. https://wondery.com/shows/i-survivor/

77   Dockterman, Eliana. "Can Bad Men Change? What It's Like Inside Sex Offender Therapy." Time. May 14, 2018. http://time.com/5272337/sex-offenders-therapy-treatment/

78   Kelly, William R. "Why Punishment Doesn't Reduce Crime." Psychology Today, April 25, 2018. https://www.psychologytoday.com/ca/blog/crime-and-punishment/201804/why-punishment-doesnt-reduce-crime

79   Dockterman, Eliana. "Can Bad Men Change? What It's Like Inside Sex Offender Therapy." Time. May 14, 2018. http://time.com/5272337/sex-offenders-therapy-treatment/

therapy might help these human beings live their pain without hurting other people along the way.

We need to focus on our own healing, of course. Survivors need support, too, all kinds of it, more than we are getting. We need to focus on the power of restorative love in our own lives. But finding a little piece of compassion for our perpetrators (and certainly for ourselves) is key to finding forgiveness. Forgiveness can release us from the past so we can remember the possibilities of love and intimacy.

We don't need to love our perpetrators to forgive them. We don't need to talk to them or see them trying to be better. We don't need to stop holding them accountable for what they did. We forgive them when they stop being evil monsters with control over us, when they shrink back into regular old human beings who are hurting in their own ways. We can forgive them when we can forgive ourselves, when we can start seeing ourselves as worthy of love, no matter what we've done or what's happened to us in the past.

My friends are tough. They've been abused, sometimes by their own family members. They've been stalked, chased, raped, humiliated, oppressed, and manipulated. They've gotten depressed living with boyfriends who subtly put them down for years until they finally got out and found their joy again. We congratulate ourselves and each other on our hardness, our resilience, our ability to survive the terrors of love, sex, and living in a world that hates women. As much as I admire us all for being the badass bitches we've had to become, it shouldn't have to be this way. We shouldn't have to prepare ourselves like soldiers to survive the field of love. We should be able to be soft sometimes, tender, and vulnerable. We should be able to hang out with the wrong guy for a minute without our lives exploding. We should be able to see the rose-colored glasses that come with a new crush as a fun accessory, not a life-threatening liability. Every time I fall in love (or even lust), I have to do it alongside the terror of abuse, manipulation, or outright rape. I do it in spite of the parts of me that fear certain annihilation. I do it because I'm full of courage (or stupidity). And I wish I didn't have to be so brave. This is not the world I want to live in. I want the right to love without fear.

Each one of us that heals enough to reclaim some tiny sliver of compassion in our own lives contributes to the possibility of a better world. When the time comes to set aside thoughts of revenge long enough to focus on restorative love, we begin to take control of our own healing. My badass bitches are not only impressive because of what they've survived, but because of how they've chosen love, even when their own pain wanted them to choose something else. One created a monthly women's group for connecting with a spiritual intention. Another runs dance classes for little kids and teaches them how to ask for consent when they want a hug. Another flew across the country to be a witness for a woman in the process of pressing charges against her abusive ex. Some of the men I know are gathering in groups to do their own learning and think critically about what it means to be a man in this world. Some of us create these mini-cultures of love simply by having open and honest conversations with each other. We do it by joking around, by having fun with each other, by making mistakes, and by being confused and seeing different perspectives. We do it when we nakedly engage in the excruciating task of intimacy with another human being. This type of healing doesn't have to be big and dramatic. It is a daily practice of self-love and compassion for other human beings. The work of restorative love helps us forgive. Forgiving sets us free.

PLEASURE

One late summer afternoon, I found myself high up on the bleachers at a Superdogs show at Vancouver's Pacific National Exhibition. The PNE is basically a large-scale county fair, complete with rides, a petting zoo, and as much bright pink cotton candy as you could hope to want (which is, inevitably, a lot). As I watched the dachshund Tater Tot and the fluffy white mixed breed Kleenex run through an obstacle course with pure joy in their little dog feet, I felt so happy I could die—literally. I almost had a panic attack. I stopped breathing, and tears started streaming down my face. I felt my heart racing, and I thought the pink cotton candy might be about to make a repeat appearance (which, to be fair, might have been because I'd eaten a lot of cotton candy). By the time the dogs finished their antics and got up onto short podiums so groups of adorable little kids could pet them reverently, I felt so exhausted I had to go home.

On that sunny day at the county fair in the terrifying joy of watching hilarious dogs jump around, I realized something must really be wrong with me. I called my doctor as soon as I got home. I can't remember if I tried to explain about the Superdogs, but I did end up with a diagnosis of Generalized Anxiety Disorder and a prescription for some benzodiazepines so I'd stop freaking the F out anytime I came across a cute animal.

The Superdogs, in all their glory, completely destabilized me. They gave me a moment of brightness in the wash of gray that was my life at the time. It had been a year or so since the assault, and I was with a boyfriend who was constantly pressuring me to have sex and subtly manipulating me on the daily. I hadn't faced my grief, my fear, or the loss of the color in my life, so the sudden blast of joy from these delighted dogs sent a shiver through the straining floodgates. If I could feel pleasure, the subconscious terror cried out, maybe I'd have to feel everything else, too. I did not want to feel everything else. I clutched my little blue pills like a lifeline.

THE PAIN OF PLEASURE

Everyone wants pleasure—it feels good, gives us energy, helps us manage stress, and keeps us hopeful. Pleasure is the food of desire, which is why it is Step Five in our road to recovery. But pleasure has a dirty little secret: sometimes it is unavoidably linked with pain. Opening to pleasure means opening to the truth of our bodies, and suddenly all the crap we've been repressing rises up to the surface. I wonder if that's part of the reason why anhedonia—literally meaning "no pleasure"—is such a common feature of depression. Depression is a complex experience, but for some of us it involves subconsciously suppressing anger or grief. Depression isn't always about sadness; it's often about numbness, about not really feeling anything at all. Every emotion is flattened, and the color goes out of the world. If we could feel pleasure in this state, all the anger and grief we'd swallowed might make a repeat appearance (along with the cotton candy).

For years, I've noticed a phenomenon with my girlfriends when they are in unhappy relationships. I call it going gray. They stop wanting to come out, instead staying home all the time watching TV with their stupid boyfriends. Their style shifts from whatever unique playful thing they like to wear to sweats and T-shirts. Their skin seems to take on an actual tinge of gray, and their eyes go kind of flat. Then, inevitably, they break up with the guy, they mourn, and a few months later their color starts returning. They start to look you in the eyes again. They wash their hair. They start showing up again at parties, bright and shiny as new pennies.

I thought of this when reading Naomi Wolf's fascinating book *Vagina: A New Biography*, which argues that the dopamine response related to female sexual pleasure can make us more creative, more focused, more connected, more powerful, and yeah, more colorful. New scientific studies are exploring how the pelvic nerves work differently around a vagina than around a penis: the nerves bundle up in different areas within a female pelvis, like around the clitoris, cervix, or anus, but not in the same exact way for any two female pelvises. This suggests that female sexual pleasure is more varied than that of males, which involves pelvic nerves that tend to be more straightforward and uniform across the board. This might explain why some women seem able to have clitoral, vaginal, and even cervical orgasms, while others don't. Wolf argues that there is a clear link between the brain and the vagina that affects women differently than it does men. For that same reason, when there is physical or psychological damage to the vagina or the pelvic nerves (as in any form of sexual assault), it messes with our dopamine flow. She notices again and again that women who have experienced sexual violation have a "flat affect" and that "the light [has] gone out of their eyes."[80] These women had gone gray.

I don't know if every woman I've ever known who has gone gray in this way was assaulted (I mean, it's not unlikely), but it does seem to happen when we don't feel safe enough to feel our bodies in a pleasurable way. I've probably been biased by looking for it only in women who are in relationships with dudes I don't like, but it probably also happens when we're in jobs that don't fulfill us or when something else is happening in our lives that makes us feel powerless and oppressed. It probably also happens to men stuck in the narrow scripts of modern masculinity, to closeted gay or lesbian people, and to trans people unable to express themselves in their truly felt gender. I bet I'd see a few more gray faces out there if I was looking more carefully. When we're trying to protect ourselves, on whatever subconscious level, we're not free to feel pleasure, let the dopamine flow, and live our lives in full color.

---

80   Wolf, Naomi. *Vagina: A New Biography*. New York, Ecco: (2013): 113.

Feeling pleasure requires being present. It is a physical experience that happens in the body. It's a rush of warmth up the center of the chest, a tingling in the feet, a flush of the cheeks. It's the full-body shake of laughter, the total release of orgasm. If we let ourselves feel it, we have to be in our bodies. If we're busy surviving after a sexual assault, that might be the *last* place we want to be.

The body is the location of our pain and trauma, which is stored in our nervous systems. When pleasure pokes us to feel, it threatens our ability to keep everything safely contained under the surface. Pleasure, then, is a practice, and it's not always easy. Eventually, I started trying to find ways to safely engage with it without panicking and barfing cotton candy. I'd go to movies by myself and eat double-buttered popcorn. I'd go to a cafe and curl up in an old armchair with a good book and a shot of Baileys in my Earl Grey tea. I'd literally smell the flowers—full on, with my eyes closed, nose nestled into the petals. These pleasurable moments were mixed—they felt good, but sometimes the grief they triggered would make my legs want to give out. I tried to keep breathing, to let the moment be bittersweet. I knew that if I was going to find my way back to pleasure, it would be on the back of my pain. I had to trust that everything I'd swallowed did not, after all, have power over me. I had to work to get my color back.

ADDICTION TO STRESS

Our culture is weird about pleasure. North Americans have a bit of a collective Protestant hangover (even with variations in individual religious upbringing) that tells us that pleasure is sinful and that we're not really good people unless we feel bad most of the time. When something good happens to us, we worry about whether or not we deserve our success. We wait for the other shoe to drop. We fear failure so much we don't even try. Vulnerability researcher Brené Brown calls this "foreboding joy," pointing out that feeling happiness is a very real sort of vulnerability because when we have something we want, that means we have something to lose.[81] Feeling happiness and satisfaction is kind of the worst, because when we inevitably go back down the garbage chute that is life, the pain of that loss will be much worse than when we were hanging out in our boring but familiar crappy lives with nothing to lose but time.

I remember having drinks with a couple of girlfriends recently, talking with them about being in a new relationship. I was struggling with some guilt about moving on from my last relationship and obsessing about how to manage my ex's feelings. One of my friends pointed out that maybe the familiar thing was the stressful thing, and was I possibly maybe avoiding giving myself a chance to enjoy being in a new relationship? She asked me, "What would you say to either of us if we were in your situation?" I paused, then piped up with the sudden brightness of the lightbulb going off in my head, "Girl, enjoy a nice relationship for once in your *goddamn life*!" Everyone at the bar briefly turned to look in my direction as my girlfriends solemnly nodded. It was true: I was a little addicted

81   Brown, Brené. *Daring Greatly: How the Courage to Be Vulnerable Transforms the Way We Live, Love, and Lead.* New York, Gotham Books (2012): 124.

to what I know best—stressful, high-drama romantic relationships—and was missing out on an opportunity to feel safe and connected to someone who treats me with kindness. I had to give myself permission to focus on the source of pleasure instead of the source of stress.

The familiar thing is often the stressful thing. We're more comfortable with stress and pain than with joy because it's what we've always known; it's a pattern we keep laying down, over and over. We tend to focus on stress rather than ease, because at an instinctual level we are more concerned with survival than comfort. Our brains are already primed to overfocus on negative information. The stress pattern is even stronger if we grew up in families where tension was the order of the day. If we learned as little kids that love meant fighting, yelling, or stony silence, we'll tend to seek those things in our adult relationships. Tenderness and affection can feel overwhelming and alien, so we unconsciously resist that form of love. Feeling good can feel uncomfortable because it goes against some very old conditioning about what we think relationships are supposed to feel like.

Pleasure, then, can threaten the negative emotions that we don't even realize we're attached to. Letting ourselves feel pleasure can seem like a betrayal when grief and pain feel necessary. Maybe, for example, we're not ready to let go of the story of our victimhood. Perhaps we feel we deserve the pain—another gift from our old friend shame. Trauma and sexual violation always come with grief. We may not acknowledge the loss right away or be able to identify exactly what it is, but there's always loss. The self that existed before the trauma is gone, and it can be hard to conceptualize who we're supposed to be now. The story we held about what we thought the world was has been irrevocably broken. The old story and the old self must be mourned.

Grief is also appropriate when we've lost someone. It is an aspect of love: we don't grieve if there wasn't love. Mourning means we care. Grief is a form of holding on, it helps us honor what we've lost. What grief does not require, however, is that we never feel pleasure. We can be deeply mourning a loss and have a moment of joy, sweetness, and sensual pleasure. The pleasure won't erase the grief or sedate our anger for long (even if sometimes we wish it would).

A moment of joy is not a betrayal of our loss or resistance. As human beings, we contain multitudes: when we let there be pain and pleasure, joy and grief, deep connection and heartrending loneliness all at the same time, we are expressing the fullness of our humanity. Having a moment of happiness inside a period of deep grief won't interrupt the mourning process, which is always uneven anyway. We don't need to be loyal to any of our emotions; they're not going to run out on us until they are ready, even (and especially) if we try to force them out. You can trust me on that one.

PLEASURE IS RADICAL

Pleasure has always been policed in some way or another in cultures across the world. That's because pleasure is, in a way, a source of resistance. Naomi Wolf's theory is that women have a special relationship with pleasure in that, when we have the right kind of it, we are feisty, powerful, and strong, and when we don't, we can lose our will to stand up for ourselves. She argues that dopamine, which generally arises when we seek and receive a reward, especially with certain kinds of sexual pleasure, is "the ultimate feminist chemical. If a woman has optimal levels of dopamine, she is difficult to direct against herself. She is hard to drive to self-destruction, to manipulate and control."[82] On the other hand, when dopamine is too low, women tend to stop fighting back and become easier to subjugate—they go gray. Wolf interviews neurologist Dr. Burke Richmond at the University of Wisconsin, who found that his female patients with balance difficulties or proprioception issues such as vertigo have almost always been sexually violated at some point in their past. Dr. Richmond explains:

> **If you lightly push most people, they will resist. They won't sidestep or fall over, or be grossly off balance. But these women will. If you push them, they will keep falling over; you have to catch them. [...] They have normal strength, normal reflexes, normal physical functioning, [...] but their bodies are reacting as if they _do_ have a neurological problem.[83]**

These women had quite literally lost their ability to stand their ground. The physical damage to their sexual bodies seemed to create damage to their brains. According to Dr. Richmond, it is evident that sexual violation makes women easy to push over, literally and figuratively. In part because of this effect, Wolf makes the argument that rape is not an unfortunate effect of individual men's perversion, but rather "a technique to suppress revolution and tamper with the very chemical makeup of potential revolution."[84] If raping turns women into pushovers, then rape is a highly effective weapon of war.

This theory that sexual violence makes women easier to subjugate was something of a revelation to me. It gave me a reason why I became so colorless after the assault, why I felt so unable to _try_ at anything. It also addressed a certain dark thought I've rarely admitted out loud: Why have women been so thoroughly subjugated for so long? Did we agree to our own inferiority in some way? Do we somehow deserve our own oppression?

This thought first rose up for me in middle school, while I was watching a slideshow about ancient religions. Slight, sweet-faced Mr. Deacon had dimmed the lights and was showing a range of goddess statues, many with prominent breasts or pregnant bellies, sometimes even with vulvas on full display. He explained how most early cultures thought god was a woman because obviously women can create life from their bodies,

82   Wolf, Naomi. Vagina: A New Biography. New York, Ecco: An Imprint of Harper Collins Publishers (2013): 59.
83   Ibid, 96.
84   Ibid, 203.

seemingly from nothing. I had only ever grown up in a world where god was a man, where women had been oppressed, repressed, and mistreated as far back as anyone could remember. It made so much sense to me, in the dark in that plastic high school chair, that everyone would assume god was a woman, that people would see women as powerful and magical. For just a moment, I thought of myself as powerful and magical. Then Mr. Deacon flipped on the lights and pointed us toward the Judeo-Christian era in our textbooks, and reality sank back in. What the hell happened?

Respect and honor for the feminine seems to have been the standard for a lot of earlier religions and cultures, at least based on the proliferation of feminine-oriented art and iconography from earlier times. Then we lost it to a host of worldviews that insisted on the primacy of man. This came along with cultural and religious colonization (often by Christians) that sometimes literally whipped the feminine worship out of the body of the people. And it's mostly been like that for what, five thousand years?

Hearing about the long-lived suppression of women in most cultures across the world over thousands of years (alongside other forms of racial, religious, and class discrimination, of course) sparked a dark thought: why didn't we fight back more? Women are obviously generally smaller than men, so we have a bit of a physical disadvantage, but that never quite felt like enough of an explanation for me. It made me feel small and stupid, like maybe I deserved to be in the dustbin of history with the rest of my gender.

Wolf's argument is that there is a physiological reason why women have been suppressed for so long: the powers that be knew, probably from experience, that if you damage the vagina, essentially, you damage the brain. Mess with our dopamine flow and we'll stop fighting back. Rape has always gone along with pillaging not (only) because colonizers are assholes, but because when you can quickly and easily shut down half the population, you cut your colonizing hours in half. They didn't need a scientific study to prove what they could see with their own eyes: rape a woman and she'll turn gray. This shone a little light on my dark thought: If women have been subjugated for so long, it's not because we were weak-willed or didn't mind being dominated. It's certainly not because we didn't fight back (we're still fighting back). It might simply be because men have a weapon against us that we, apparently, do not have against them. I admit it's kind of weird that this made me feel better, but having a concrete reason for five thousand years of patriarchy made me feel a little less like, you know, it was our own fault.

There's good news here, too, from Wolf's perspective. The unique vagina-brain connection might also make people with vaginas *more* powerful. Wolf writes:

> *I don't like any kind of feminism that sets one gender above another, so I do not mean this in any way as a value judgment. Neither gender is "better." But one gender is theoretically able to get more of a certain kind of dopamine and opioid/endorphin activation during sex, which has a very specific effect on the brain and even the personality. We cannot escape what this math implies for female sexuality, in its unmediated, un-messed-up state: nature constructed a profound*

> *difference between the sexes, which places women in, potentially, a position of*
> *greater biochemical empowerment.*[85]

Great sex, Wolf explains, boosts women's dopamine, endorphins, opioids, and testosterone. It makes us more willing to take creative risks, to give fewer fucks about what other people think of us. It makes us want to take over the world. And have more sex. Wolf goes on, "So the fear that patriarchy always had—that if you let women have sex and know how to like it, it will make them both increasingly libidinous and increasingly ungovernable—is actually biologically true!"[86] From this perspective, it makes sense that suppressing and policing female sexuality has always been an aspect of patriarchal society. Knowing our sexual bodies and being unafraid to use them might have made us so full of spunk and fire that our subjugation wouldn't have been possible.

Maybe, then, we had to be oppressed so thoroughly, cut off from the power that is fed by pleasure, not because we are powerless but precisely because we are powerful. This also makes sense alongside Audre Lorde's theory that the erotic drive that lives within us is a source of power that women have been cut off from due to systematic oppressions. Lorde describes this internal power as a "resource within each of us that lies in a deeply female and spiritual plane,"[87] and I've often wondered why this erotic power had to be specifically female, or what female meant in this context. It feels intuitive that there's a revolutionary energy inside that needs to be supported, but I don't necessarily feel that its source is my vagina, my pelvic nerves, or my gender identity.

So of course, I had to ask the guys. Wolf doesn't comment specifically on how sexual violence might affect men, but I can't imagine that having pelvic nerves in a different place would make someone any less despondent after being raped. Women's bodies are more physically vulnerable, we're certainly more frequently targeted for rape, and we have different experiences in the culture, so there are material differences here. Still, it makes sense to me that the felt experience of erotic energy must be possible for anyone. Wolf argues that the boost in creativity that comes with orgasm is uniquely related to having a vagina—and specifically to having what she calls "high orgasm," or

> *that kind of orgasm that most intensely induces the most complete possible trance*
> *state and that most involves all the body systems, so that afterward the woman*
> *feels the most replete and also experiences the highest level possible for her of the*
> *positive brain chemicals' activities.*[88]

I asked a few self-identified men in person and on social media if they felt there was a connection between their sexuality and their creativity. A few men said no, but more of them said yes. One described exactly the type of orgasm Wolf says only women can have, in his case usually involving the prostate. He described it to me as "that deep, mind-numbing, world-shaking kind of orgasm, where after, you feel like your

85   Ibid, 60.
86   Ibid.
87   Lorde, Audre. *Sister Outsider: Essays and Speeches.* Berkeley: Crossing Press (2007): 53
88   Wolf, Naomi. *Vagina: A New Biography.* New York, Ecco: An Imprint of Harper Collins Publishers (2013): 25.

perspective has shifted and shaken loose the creative blocks."[89] Another man told me how erotic energy is present when he's writing music or cooking, and that for him, sexuality and creativity feel deeply linked. Another, the poet Jeremy Radin, told me about his complicated relationship with his body and his erotic self. He wrote to me:

> *I write to try to reconnect with the body, to rebuild those broken pathways and reclaim my body and its desire as something worthy and potentially beautiful, to unweaponize myself and divest from patriarchal modes of thinking about sex and longing which seem always to be rooted in violence. I am trying to write myself always into care and tenderness, which I think of as an act against my straight white maleness and my imposing physical size. I guess much of my work, even when not explicitly about this, is about renavigating sex and desire—the way my body interacts w[ith] the world.*[90]

For Radin, the oppression that comes with patriarchy has damaged his erotic flow. He wants to feel connected, vulnerable, and alive in a world that wants him to be shut down or even violent. Through his writing, he not only rejects the suppression of his own erotic energy, but also the legacy of violence that comes with patriarchy. Erotic energy, at least as I understand it, clearly lives through these men and their experience of sexuality and creativity. Whatever our physical organs or gender expression may be, I believe we all have access to this potentially powerful erotic energy. It makes sense that sexual violence would make anyone feel cut off from it, at least for a time.

Wolf's argument is based on new science about female pleasure, and this realm has always been racked with controversy. All new science needs time to go through the wash of the scientific method and see what stands the test of time. As Cordelia Fine persuasively argues in her book *Delusions of Gender*, the very concept of a "female brain" may just be a comforting way to keep women in their place. All our brains are, actually, different from each other and different every day. Claiming that there is a clear binary between the genders in terms of brain function is worth taking with a sizable grain of salt. Fine warns that "claims of 'essential differences' between the two sexes simply reflect—and give authority to—what I suspect is really a majority opinion."[91] No doubt there are concrete differences in the experience of performing a female or a male gender, but we don't really know if that's because of our brains, our pelvic nerves, our hormones, or simply the effect of living in a society that insists on a gender binary. Fine goes on to say:

> *We can't understand gender differences in female and male minds—the minds that are the source of our thoughts, feelings, abilities, motivations, and behavior— without understanding how psychologically permeable is the skull that separates the mind from the sociocultural context in which it operates.*[92]

---

89   Loeb, Matt. Instagram message to Julie Peters, Sept 19, 2018.
90   Radin, Jeremy. Instagram message to Julie Peters, Sept 17, 2018.
91   Fine, Cordelia. *Delusions of Gender: How Our Minds, Society, and Neurosexism Create Difference.* New York: W.W. Norton and Company (2010): xxv.
92   Ibid, xxvi

We're living in a time with a lot of questions about what gender is and means. It definitely means something, but that meaning seems to be felt inside each of us individually, and the way that it is felt is hardly uniform and not yet predictable by science (and certainly not by our genitals).

So perhaps men's brains are different from women's brains. Maybe lesbian, bisexual, and gay brains are different. Maybe trans men's brains are different from trans women's, and all are different from nonbinary folks. Probably that's true, to some extent. But how much these differences matter might have less to do with physiology and more to do with social differences, and there are probably even more variations within each group than there are between them. Regardless of the problems with Wolf's theory, I'm not going to argue with her that loving, consensual, fun, pleasurable sex is probably empowering—for whoever is enjoying it.

Content warning: some of our collective 'herstory' can make for difficult or triggering reading, including what follows under this next heading.

HUNTING WITCHES

Besides, there is another reason why women might struggle with pleasure in our society that might have nothing to do with our female brains or pelvic nerves: women's sexuality has been specifically and systematically targeted for a really long time. The patriarchal fear of female pleasure was perhaps most salient during the centuries of witch-hunting when mostly women were tortured (often sexually) and killed in brutal ways. The first trials started in the fourteenth century and hit a fever pitch in the sixteenth and seventeenth centuries. Barbara Ehrenreich and Deirdre English put the killings in perspective when they write in their book *Witches, Midwives, and Nurses:*

> *One writer has estimated the number of executions on an average of 600 a year for certain German cities—or two a day, 'leaving out Sundays.' Nine hundred witches were destroyed in a single year in the Wertzberg area, and 1,000 were put to death in a day. In the Bishopric of Trier, in 1585, two villages were left with only one female inhabitant each.*[93]

Men were sometimes accused of witchcraft too, but the authors point out that "women made up some 85 percent of those executed."[94] It's always been so interesting to me that when we hear the phrase "witch hunt" in our cultural lexicon, it's usually coming from a white man feeling persecuted after he got caught abusing his power. Why don't we talk more about the witch hunt era as what it was: a large-scale, wide-reaching historical campaign of terror against women?

---

93   Ehrenreich, Barbara, and Deirdre English, *Witches, Midwives, and Nurses: A History of Women Healers.* New York: The Feminist Press at the City of New York University (2012): 34.
94   Ibid, 35.

There's no evidence witchcraft existed as an organized religion prior to twentieth century Wicca, though as a young teen who would light candles and try to cast spells while blasting the angsty strains of Alanis Morissette, I still can't help but yearn for a ritualistic practice that could literally give women power. Magic wasn't really what was being hunted, though: it was any form of power that could belong to a woman, especially if it related to her reproductive abilities. Before the witch hunts, women were bakers, ale-makers, schoolteachers, doctors, and surgeons. Gynecology was a mostly female profession, with C-sections being performed almost exclusively by women in the fourteenth century, until male-only universities started popping up to certify men and push the midwives and lay healers out of a job. The lay healers were mostly women who would provide counsel and a few herbs, while, by the 1800s, men were getting certified to perform superstitious rituals like bloodletting and treating leprosy with "a broth made of the flesh of a black snake caught in a dry land among stones."[95] As Ehrenreich and English point out, a patient would be likelier to die by the hands of a certified male doctor's bravura than with the "undoubtedly safer" gentle attentions of a female lay healer.[96]

Women were especially targeted if they had any medical knowledge about reproduction or contraception. In her book *Caliban and the Witch*, Silvia Federici argues that the witch hunts were a necessary strategy to transition from feudalism into the capitalist era. Women's bodies were needed to create more laborers for the new economy, so reproduction had to be carefully monitored. "The criminalization of women's control over procreation is a phenomenon whose importance cannot be overemphasized," Federici writes, "both from the viewpoint of its effects on women and its consequences for the capitalist organization of work."[97] And as far as Wolf's argument that targeting women sexually is an age-old strategy of war, the witch hunts were no exception. "In community after community," Wolf writes, "the women identified by inquisitors or by their fellow villagers as 'witches' were often those who were seen as too sexual, or too free. And forms of torture were focused on their sexuality," such as with devices placed in the vagina or with vaginal mutilation.[98] When women were shamed for their sexuality and even tortured at their genital source, the theory goes, they would indeed be willing to step back and relinquish their rights. It is interesting, however, that this subjugation and control of women in the service of capitalism took almost four hundred years. We obviously haven't been *that* easy to subjugate.

Echoes of this sexual suppression and torture continue today in communities where girl's clitorises are cut out or burned, ostensibly for religious reasons. Clitoridectomies are hardly an invention of some other land, however, lest we think we Westerners are somehow more civilized. In 1858, the English doctor Isaac Baker Brown introduced the practice that, Wolf explains, made him "famous and sought after for his 'cure,'

---

95   Ibid, 52.
96   Ibid, 68.
97   Federici, Silvia. *Caliban and the Witch: Women, the Body and Primitive Accumulation.* New York: Autonomedia (2014): 92.
98   Wolf, Naomi. *Vagina: A New Biography.* New York, Ecco: An Imprint of Harper Collins Publishers (2013): 136.

which took argumentative, fiery girls, and, after he had excised their clitorises, returned them to their families in a state of docility, meekness, and obedience."[99] Even Western doctors, it seems, understood that damaging a girl's clitoris would somehow amputate her will to rebel.

PSYCHOANALYZING SEXUALITY

Then, of course, there's our old buddy Sigmund Freud. The (in)famous founder of psychoanalysis has a hidden story that is, in my reading, about his betrayal of womankind. In the last decades of the nineteenth century, Freud and his contemporaries were greatly interested in hysteria—which was, basically, a catchall term for women's psychological problems vaguely associated with the uterus (*hystera* in Greek). In his earnest attempt to understand this common affliction, Freud sat down with women and listened to them. Jean-Martin Charcot and Joseph Breuer, Freud's contemporaries, were similarly focused on the problem. In her book *Trauma and Recovery*, Judith Herman points out that "For a brief decade, men of science listened to women with a devotion and a respect unparalleled before or since."[100] All this listening bore fruit for Freud, at least at first. He discovered that women suffering from hysteria pretty much always had a history of childhood sexual abuse. Freud wrote a triumphant paper called *The Aetiology of Hysteria* clearly explaining the root of the problem.

Instead of being lauded for his discovery, however, he was met with the academic version of an uncomfortable silence. "Hysteria was so common among women," Herman explains,

> *that if his patient's stories were true, and if his theory were correct, he would be forced to conclude that what he called 'perverted acts against children' were endemic, not only among the proletariat of Paris, where he had first studied hysteria, but also among the respectable bourgeois families of Vienna, where he had established his practice.[101]*

That meant that sexual abuse was a systemic issue, a problem of violence against girl children that defied class. Freud's society was not ready to consider such an earth-shattering possibility, so his theory was rejected. In order to maintain his prestigious position in society, he recanted. Herman continues:

> *By the first decade of the twentieth century, without ever offering any clinical documentation of false complaints, Freud had concluded that his hysterical patients' accounts of childhood sexual abuse were untrue: 'I was at last obliged*

99   Ibid, 149.
100   Herman, Judith. *Trauma and Recovery: The Aftermath of Violence—from Domestic Abuse to Political Terror.* New York: Basic Books (1997): 11–12
101   Ibid, 14.

to recognize that these scenes of seduction have never taken place, and that they were only fantasies which my patients had made up.[102]

Betrayal! Freud's psychoanalysis went on to create a theory of neurosis that did not match women's actual experience of reality. He insisted that women lie often and that their fantasies were the source of their problems. He came up with the concept of penis envy, that old canard that little girls hate their mothers forever for not giving them a penis. Not to mention his insulting (and evidence-free) idea that women who can't achieve orgasms from penetration alone are somehow immature, a concept that caused sexual insecurity and an epidemic of sexually frustrated women that still persists to this day. Freud essentially set the precedent for not believing women.

Women have inherited quite a history of sexual shame, terror, and torture from our ancestral grandmothers, even if we have no history of it in our own lives. It's no wonder feeling sexual pleasure is so fraught in our time—not only have we not always felt the right to experience pleasure in the ways that work for us (thanks, Freud!), but we have echoes of intergenerational trauma from a history of being tortured, murdered, and violated, at worst, and silenced, at best.

For these reasons and more, feeling pleasure isn't just a little thing we should try to make more time for in our busy lives because it's fun. It's a radical act of resistance against a history of suppression and pain. Taking pleasure, whether by enjoying great sex, going to see the Superdogs, or simply having a hot cup of tea on a cool day, is an act of self-determination and choice. Our pleasure is a tool of resistance against our own oppression and suppression. Our pleasure matters.

SELF-PLEASURE

As nice as a cup of tea is, let's be honest, it's doesn't come close to masturbation when it comes to pleasure. When I was in high school, I remember so clearly that masturbation was an absolute taboo—until suddenly it wasn't. One year we were making fun of the awkward girl at the back of the class, whispering *I heard she touches herself* with the knowing looks only teenage girls who know nothing can give, and then we were back from another summer break comparing vibrators. Say what you will about the show *Sex and the City*, it made masturbation cool for a generation of high school girls over the course of a TV season.

Masturbation is the ultimate form of self-pleasure. It's still steeped in plenty of shame (*Sex and the City* or not) and is associated with a kind of selfish internal focus that excludes anyone else's needs or wants. Pretentious films, overlong books, and political speeches have all been called masturbatory. But it's also the only place where you can be completely in control of your own sexual experience. It is a zone where you *can* be selfish, where you can focus on your own needs without worrying about anyone else. Small wonder that women, who have been socialized to put everyone else's needs before

---

102   Ibid.

their own, might feel that there is a taboo on their own masturbatory delights. Sexual self-pleasure is rebellious, not to mention an incredibly important practice for healing from sexual assault. Here we are in Step Five exploring the empowering possibilities of self-pleasure. Yup: that means masturbation.

Before my assault, I was a pretty sexual person. I went through a joyful phase in college where I was having one-night stands just for the thrill of it, man (and sometimes woman)-hunting in the clubs of Montreal, picking and choosing, deciding what I wanted to do and not do, naming all my own terms. I was exploring my own sexual power and what that meant. It wasn't all sunshine and roses, don't get me wrong, and I probably wouldn't do it again, but it definitely gives me a little nostalgic wince to think about how courageous I was at that time, how unafraid of exploring my own pleasure. What an innocent little slut I was, truly.

After the assault, I lost my playfulness. I lost my sense of adventure along with my desire. This is a pretty common effect for survivors. Of course, some of us go to the other extreme—seeking out risky sexual experiences, as if to prove that the perpetrator hasn't stolen our right to fuck however we want. Sometimes we swing from one extreme to the other in a matter of months. In any case, sexual problems of some kind are unquestionably a thing if you've been sexually violated. At the time, I wanted to know how to get my desire back, and the best advice anyone seemed to have for me was to wait to have sex until I felt like it again. Uh, okay, but how was I supposed to start feeling like it again?

Well, one way is to masturbate. It's an obvious place to start to explore sexual pleasure again safely and on our own terms. There is some bad news, though: after violation (at least at first), masturbation can feel impossible. Trauma, assault, and abuse can cause stress to kind of hang out in the body like a toxic friend trying to protect us from inevitable harm while also preventing us from having any fun. Stress isn't great for sexual desire or responsiveness. In her book *Come as You Are*, Emily Nagoski explains the current science on sexuality, and specifically how stress can mess with our sexual desire and pleasure. For some of us, stress can be a bit of a turn-on, making us want to chase a little tail, but even in that case, the romps tend to be less fun: "Stress reduces sexual interest in 80–90 percent of people and reduces sexual pleasure for everyone— even the 10–20 percent of people for whom it increases interest," Nagoski explains.[103] Because pleasure requires presence and masturbation involves the physical body, even thinking about touching ourselves can cause a flood of shame, guilt, fear, intrusive memories and all kinds of stuff that is *not* conducive to having a nice safe orgasm by ourselves. It's like having an argument with our genitals.

Every now and again in our lives, our private bits take on a life of their own. I am a strong believer that the vagina speaks—at least, mine does. It has its own perspective and a language worth learning. If you keep getting urinary tract infections or yeast infections with a new partner, for example, that might be because your vagina doesn't like that new

---

103   Nagoski, Emily. *Come as You Are: The Surprising New Science That Will Transform Your Sex Life.* New York: Simon and Schuster (2015): 149.

partner. If you feel butterflies in your vagina like Cardi B when you think about starting a new project at work, your vagina is into that project. If it clams up when you think about moving to a new city, your vagina does not want to move to that city. If you try to touch your vulva and it dries up like that houseplant in the corner you haven't watered in weeks, that's because it probably has some things to say that you haven't been hearing. The vagina (and, presumably, the penis) speaks for the erotic drive that guides us on a physical and subconscious level. It's not always about sex.

Of course, having a genital response to something isn't enough information to go on when we're trying to make a choice. Sometimes a vaginal pulse is a little thrill about something we actually don't want to do. Sometimes we clam up down there because we're nervous about trying something new that we really *do* want to do. It's incredibly common (and much more common than men like to admit) that the first time that many men have sex with someone they *really* like, their penises will not cooperate—even if they usually jump to attention with ease when the men don't care so much about their sex partners. Vaginas will often lubricate and penises will get hard when there is sexually relevant information in the room, but that doesn't always indicate that it's something we want or like. That's a known phenomenon called sexual non-concordance, and it basically means that sometimes your genitals respond without your brain and vice versa, and this is totally normal. Our genital responses don't tell us what's going on in our minds; all they tell us is what's going on in our genitals. It's so important to listen to the information coming from our bodies, but also to understand that information as limited. We must also use our big fancy brains now and again.

Our bodies hold our emotions and memories in them differently from the way our minds do. Psychological help, while essential, has limits in terms of how much it alone can help us. The body experiences everything we experience. Our feelings are called feelings because we feel them, physically. The nervous system takes in information and stores it away for future reference. If we don't approach the body at the source of the wound, there will always be an echo of that wound that affects our day-to-day lives, no matter how many hours we've logged talking about it in therapy. We may understand our violation on a mental level and have created a narrative about it that makes sense. We may have made choices to move on with our lives and let go of the past. We may have even taken steps toward justice and seen our perpetrator face consequences. Doesn't matter to the vagina. The vagina does not forget.

I think the most useful thing about my yoga practice is the way it helps me stretch my tissues and release whatever my body has been carrying that day. I've had sudden, inexplicable tears (and sometimes full-body sobs) in hip openers, backbends, and the simple lying-down-resting pose called *savasana*. I know I'm not the only one—I see tears and the telltale shaking sobs in one or another of my yoga students at least once a month (I swear I'm not hurting them! We weren't in plank pose *that* long). We don't always know why we're crying, but something seems to have let go in our bodies at those moments, and we almost always feel better afterwards. It's like doing emotional laundry. The problem is, there aren't many yoga poses you can do with your vagina.

There are, however, other things you can do with your vagina (and your vulva, more correctly, or your penis, if that's what you have) in the privacy of your own home, in whatever way you like. Just as your hips and shoulders can carry a memory, so can your most sensitive sexual bits. Getting into a sexual zone with yourself means allowing your mind to enter the vulnerability of sense memory. It means opening up to the possibility that painful memories might come up alongside the sensations. One of the things we must understand about pleasure is that if we're going to feel it genuinely, we have to learn to allow other emotions to be present at the same time too. We have to learn to breathe through anger, shame, guilt, and old memories in order to let the pleasure stay present. When we try to escape or avoid these emotions, we have to push the pleasure away, too. We can't separate out pleasure from other emotions.

For me, the physical experience of self-pleasure after the assault was less of a simple, fun stress reliever and more like a challenging, emotional yoga class. If I was going to do it, I realized, I had to be able to face the uncomfortable stuff that was going to come up. I had to learn to breathe with my feelings, even to let them become a part of the flow of sensation and pleasure in my body. I did not try to separate anything out—anytime I tried, I'd have to stop altogether. Sometimes I stopped anyway (it's important to stop if you want to stop). Healing self-pleasure isn't about climax, it's about breathing, feeling, and connecting in whatever way is possible for you that day.

No one ever talked to me about this after my sexual assault. No one explained that masturbation was going to become such a minefield of pain and possibility. No one told me how I'd need my mindfulness skills every time I touched myself, but that if I could use them, I'd have an incredible tool for healing right at my fingertips (literally!). No one explained about masturbation as meditation. I had to figure it out on my own. So now I'll explain it to you.

When I meditate, I try to relax my body and breathe. I allow my mind to wander and just see what's going on in there. The key is to turn on the observing mind, to watch what's happening without getting too involved, using the focus on the breath as an anchor. I try to keep my awareness in my body and relax, but I stay aware of my thoughts, too. All kinds of thoughts come up—about what I'm doing that day, the grocery list, a conversation I had with a friend. Thoughts come and go. I let them come, but I let them go again, too, doing my best not to get hooked into any particular one—but being gentle with myself when that inevitably happens. The secret is to be friendly with whatever is happening, however painful, and try not to judge, fix, or change anything. I do my best to continually allow the sensations and thoughts to flow without trying to direct or control them. In this daily practice, I learn that all my emotional and mental states are temporary and okay, and that if I relax and let them do their thing, they move freely, on their own terms, and generally don't get stuck to me for too long.

Masturbation meditation involves essentially the same technique. I focus on my breath and the sensations in my body. I try to breathe low into my belly and relax my muscles. I don't use porn or high stimulation vibrators most of the time, because they can override the intimacy I'm trying to create with my own flesh and blood. When uncomfortable emotions arise, I don't obsess about them or attach to them; I notice that they are there and allow myself to breathe with them. I let them be a part of the experience, and often they flow in and out just like any other thoughts or sensations. I've learned to notice when I'm avoiding a particular thought or emotion—if I'm doing that, I've tensed up on some level, and the pleasure won't come. If I relax into what I'm feeling, my body can respond to my touch. In part, it's a practice of being honest with myself. If the emotions become too much, I stop, but part of what I'm doing is practicing allowing myself to be present with the truth that there is pain and trauma in my body. There is fear. There are memories. These things are a part of who I am right now. My radical acceptance of my body, my history, and my pleasure means I have to make friends with all of it. Sounds fun, right?

It's not. Well—it's interesting. Sometimes it's beautiful. Sometimes it's painful. Sometimes it makes me cry. But it works. After a while, the bad memories and emotions start to fade. The thoughts and emotions that pop up are more like little windows into how I'm feeling and what my body is holding that day. Rather than being shocked and appalled at what my mind throws at me, I can get friendly with it and see if it will make its way through my cell memory in the cleansing experience of orgasm. Cleansing is really the best word I have for it—it feels like things are coming up to the surface from the murky depths of my emotional body so that breath and (if possible) orgasm can skim them off the surface. Emotions that have been stuck in me for years have an opportunity to move.

And they do move. Those old emotions don't need to come up all the time anymore. Most of the time now, self-pleasure is a simple joy I can create for myself out of nothing (as it should be). Emotions still arise, but they are more mundane now, related to what's happening currently in my life, rather than any old memories from the sexual assault. It tends to be more fun and easy when my life is more fun and easy, and it can get more intense around difficult periods of my life. But even in that way, masturbation meditation is a friend, a tool to help me process my emotions about whatever's going on now.

Masturbation meditation was a huge part of how I reconnected with my own sexuality. I've come to understand that some of my feelings are physiological. They pop up from somewhere in my nervous system for any reason at all, and they may not be related to what's going on in my life. It doesn't always matter why, and it doesn't always need any more attention than just a quick hello and let it go. I don't need to talk to my therapist about every emotion I feel. I certainly don't need to believe everything I think. Sometimes I just need to move or breathe or pleasure it along. I'm doing so much better now, but I'll never stop needing to do my emotional laundry.

There are lots of ways I've worked through my healing since the sexual assault, but I think this one, this vaginal yoga, if you will, has been instrumental in allowing certain things to move through and then out of my body. The bad memories and painful emotions kept me away from sexual self-pleasure for a while, of course. But when I started reentering that zone on my own terms, when I felt safe, when I wanted to, I started practicing the sort of radical self-compassion—yes, even selfishness—that is necessary to heal from a sexual wound. It wasn't always easy, but it helped a lot, and the practice became far easier over time. Now it's mostly just really fun.

Masturbation Meditation

Here are a few things to keep in mind if you'd like to try masturbation as a meditation practice:

⊕ Take your sexual self-pleasure seriously. Give yourself time and space to do it so it's not a quick, shameful, get-it-over-with kind of practice. Plan for it.

⊕ Set the mood. Some people need environmental cues of safety more than others do, and this is apparently even more the case for women than men. This could be soft lingerie, candles, nice music, or simply a locked door: whatever helps you feel calm and relaxed.

⊕ Treat your body with kindness. Don't rush in. Spend time exploring your body, and not just at the genital level—all sorts of places on your body can be erotic, and gentle self-touch can help you calm down and get you in the mood.

⊕ Focus on body sensations. Thoughts will be present, too, but try to stay with what you feel. This could include the sensation of emotions that rise and fall. Stay in your body.

⊕ Relax. It's very important to relax your belly muscles and breathe deeply right down into your pelvis. It's easy to hold muscular tension here, and that tension often relates to avoiding certain feeling states. A lot of us tense our bellies when we feel sexual arousal, but relaxing instead can make the sensations and orgasms far more intense. Relaxing this area can make a huge difference in terms of the pleasurable sensations that you feel and allowing your emotions to flow.

⊕ Breathe. The breath is the key to letting the emotions flow. Consciously take long deep breaths, allowing your belly to expand and relax. Imagine breathing directly into your genital region. If you tense up, come back to this breathing, which helps you stay present in the body and the heart. Let the breath change as you go, but do your best not to hold your breath.

⊕ Stay present. Do *not* focus on your sexual assault or actively try to bring up images or memories. This is not a practice of desensitization, and obsessing about what happened can be retraumatizing. If stuff from the experience arises, stay with the emotions you feel, not the details or the story of what happened. Don't push it away, but there is no need to call it in, either. If it doesn't come up, it isn't ready to come up. It may never come up, and that's just fine too.

⊕ Take consent into account. I know it might sound weird to think about consent with yourself, but remember: the vagina speaks! I have no doubt penises do, too. As you gently explore your body, see if it responds to your touch or tenses up. Don't go in if your body is resisting you. Teach your vagina (or penis) that what it says matters.

⊕ Meditate. Stress reduces sexual desire for most of us and reduces sexual pleasure for everyone. Try meditating for five minutes before your self-pleasure time to focus and calm down. Meditate again for five minutes afterwards so you can acknowledge how you feel. This could be seated or lying down. Imagine breathing and relaxing into your genital region.

⊕ Use your hands (at least sometimes). Porn and vibrators can speed up the process and prevent your mind from wandering to uncomfortable places. At least some of the time, put these tools away and see what happens when you are actually alone with yourself (though lube can be helpful). If they give you pleasure, however, make sure you're making time to enjoy them, too.

⊕ Touch whatever you want to touch. There might be different memories held at the vulva (clitoris and labia) or the vagina (the internal tunnel leading to the cervix). Same idea for the head of a penis, the shaft, the testicles, and the perineum. Everyone is wired differently in terms of what feels good for them, so figure out what that means for you. There's no right or wrong way. Explore whatever you like according to your curiosity and comfort level.

⊕ Fantasize. it's fine to use fantasies, and they can be anything. Let whatever needs to come up emerge, and notice what thoughts or images your body is responding to that day. Don't judge the fantasies and don't get too attached to the images. These fantasies may shift and change constantly, or it might be one thing for a while. Let it be whatever it is as long as you are staying present in your body and not using the fantasy to dissociate.

⊕ Don't force orgasm. Don't get too attached to coming. You might or might not. Show up to experiencing pleasure and see how it goes. Stop if you need to.

⊕ Stay with it. If you do orgasm, keep your hands on your body for a little while, don't rush to get out of there. You could keep your hand on your genitals or rest one or both on your stomach or heart. Breathe with the post-orgasm sensations—a whole new set of emotions might arise afterwards. Stay present.

PORN

I don't like to watch porn when I'm doing this kind of mindful sexual self-pleasure. That's partly because it can be too overstimulating to allow me to actually focus on my emotions, but it's also because porn is honestly a little scary. Any sort of Internet search related to porn can bring up images that are as likely to be hugely triggering as titillating, and then you just can't un-see them. It's not that I wouldn't enjoy watching consenting adults having fun, pleasurable sex, it's just that getting to those images requires a fair amount of sifting. And minimal clicking will get all kinds of shit thrown your way— sometimes literally.

Porn might also be addictive. It is so stimulating that it can desensitize us to such mundane sexual stimulation as our beloved standing naked before us. It might send our dopamine into overdrive, creating a sort of chemical dependency. In her book *Vagina*, Naomi Wolf warns that all this overstimulation can actually make us less sexually connected and harder to turn on. She writes:

> *a nation of masturbating people who are looking at screens rather than at one another—who are consuming sex like any other product and who are rewiring their brains to find less and less abandon and joy in one another' arms, and to bond more and more with pixels—is a subjugated, not a liberated, population.*[104]

Vibrators may pose a similar problem. Sex toys can be fun and helpful, but they can be so effective that our bodies get accustomed to them and start to depend on them. If our brains associate orgasm with only one type of sensation, then loving touch from a partner can't do anything for us (human beings don't vibrate, after all!). The question really comes down to whether these sexual aids are improving our connection with pleasure, our bodies, our internally felt states, and our partners or shutting those connections down. If they help, definitely use them. If they hinder, try something else once in a while.

When I was an undergrad student, I was taking a course on human sexuality and we did a segment on porn. We discussed, among other things, the point of view of feminists like Catharine MacKinnon and Andrea Dworkin, who argued that pornography is fundamentally oppressive to women. Dworkin has written, "The fact is that rape and prostitution caused and continue to cause pornography. Politically, culturally, socially, sexually, and economically, rape and prostitution generated pornography; and pornography depends for its continued existence on the rape and prostitution of women."[105] MacKinnon has argued that because of widespread male dominance in general, it is hard to tell the difference between consensual sex and rape. She has written:

---

104   Wolf, Naomi. *Vagina: A New Biography*. New York, Ecco: An Imprint of Harper Collins Publishers (2013): 234.
105   Dworkin, Andrea. *Letters From a War Zone*. New York: Lawrence Hill Books (1993): 230.

Perhaps the wrong of rape has proven so difficult to articulate because the unquestionable starting point has been that rape is definable as distinct from intercourse, when for women it is difficult to distinguish them under conditions of male dominance.[106]

I can see how MacKinnon got there—consent is confused by all kinds of power, not just physical dominance and force. People can agree to sex they don't really want because the person asking has social influence, financial power, or some other kind of interpersonal dominance over them. How likely is it that with a man and a woman in a room, the man has more money, power, and influence? Real likely. Still, though, there is a difference between sex and rape. Maybe the line isn't always super bright, thick, and clear, but it's important that we understand that not all sex is rape.

On porn, MacKinnon has made the strong claim that "Empirically, all pornography is made under conditions of inequality based on sex, overwhelmingly by poor, desperate, homeless, pimped women who were sexually abused as children."[107] Um—whoa there. I don't know how many sex workers MacKinnon knew, but that is a strong and offensive claim against them. Certainly the porn industry has historically taken advantage of some women, and some women are sex workers of one type or another because they felt coerced or didn't feel they had any other choice. Surely some sex workers have been abused as children, considering that, according to the National Center for Victims of Crime, 20 percent of all women have been.[108] It's not exactly uncommon. But plenty of sex workers—including several I know personally—do what they do because their sexuality is an empowering creative outlet that they love to explore in their work. Lola Frost is a stripper and burlesque dancer who celebrates her sexuality on Instagram with the hashtag #yesastripper. Stoya is a writer and pornographic actor who has written about ethical contracts, fair pay, and feminism in the porn industry. A good friend of mine spent a few years as an escort making a ton of money to get her through school. She doesn't do it anymore but still misses it every now and then, partly because of how much it helped her financially and partly because of the empowerment and independence it afforded her. I'm not going to say that sex work is universally empowering to women, but it's not universally disempowering, either.

In my undergraduate class, we were asked to write an essay on all these fascinating topics, so I decided to do some research. I'm dating myself here, but this was in the heady days of the Internet before Google and its careful filters, so I just sat down at my computer and searched for "porn." It was a mixed bag of nuts (pun intended). There were a few images I found sexy, but there were plenty that were downright terrifying: women being beaten and tied up, forced to give blow jobs while someone held them by their hair. I'm sure these things can be sexy in the right context when consent is clear and the objective is playful, but it's hard to tell when you're looking at these kinds of

---

106   MacKinnon, Catharine. "Feminism, Marxism, Method, and the State: Toward Feminist Jurisprudence." *Signs* Vol. 8, No. 4 (1983): 647.
107   MacKinnon, Catharine. *Only Words*. Cambridge, Harvard University Press (1996): 20.
108   "Child Sexual Abuse Statistics." National Center for Victims of Crime. Dec 2018. http://victimsofcrime. org/media/reporting-on-child-sexual-abuse/child-sexual-abuse-statistics

fast and furious images. I actually remember feeling all my pelvic muscles tightening up when I saw these images. They definitely stressed me out, and stress is not the best for one's sense of sexual connection. I agreed in that moment with MacKinnon's point that there was something awful about pornography.

Someone in my dorm had gotten ahold of a copy of one of the endless versions of *Debbie Does Dallas*, a porn film (on VHS!), so a few of my fellow students got involved in my research project, and we gathered around to watch. The film centers on a woman, Debbie, who likes a guy, Dallas, and everyone else she meets along the way, including several female friends. Everyone in the movie, especially the women, are clearly having fun, and the film itself was silly and playful. I wasn't expecting so many jokes. The images found in my random Internet search were serious, intense, aggressive, even violent. But the *Debbie* movie was shot in a mood I prefer for sex itself: playful, exploratory, and totally unserious. Stress and pressure are major reasons sexual desire might go into hiding, and there's nothing like a bad pun to lighten the mood. I liked this weird, silly VHS porn movie, and I think my dorm mates liked it too. Perhaps we've lost something in an era where porn has been whittled down from VHS films that had narratives to an extremely easy to access plethora of short, constantly looping GIFs. I sat down to write my paper and argued that the problem with porn isn't porn, it's that it is an industry that's far too male-dominated. If more women became consumers, directors, and producers, unquestionably porn would become friendlier to women, and then maybe it would be more fun for all of us.

It turns out (and I love saying this) I was right. More women than ever are involved in all levels of pornography. The popular video site Pornhub saw a 1,400 percent increase in the search term "porn for women" in the year 2017.[109] Responding like good capitalists, Pornhub set up a system where women could enter the details of their menstrual cycles and get free porn on their period. They called the campaign, charmingly, "Fuck Your Period"—considering that, of course, orgasms are great for cramps.[110] How thoughtful! Tumblr is a popular blogging site that was, for a time, very popular with people who wanted to be able to access feminist and queer porn that wouldn't assault you with violent images or subject you to a constantly shifting roster of people who all look the same. Tumblr was the place to go for feminist, queer, alternative porn with a diversity of acts and actors. Many of my female friends had a secret account they would use to access what they liked using the hashtag #feministporn. As I write this, however, Tumblr is in the process of shutting down all of its accounts with a connection to sex and sexuality, which has left many of its users despondent at the loss, leaving a gap that someone will likely (hopefully) quickly fill to meet the high demand for friendly alternative porn.[111]

109   "Pornhub 2017 Year in Review." Pornhub Insights. Jan 9, 2018. https://www.pornhub.com/insights/2017-year-in-review

110   "Fuck Your Period." Pornhub. Dec 2018. https://www.pornhub.com/fuckyourperiod

111   Mufson, Beckett. "Sex Bloggers Say Tumblr Is 'as Good as Gone' After Porn Ban." VICE. Dec 4, 2018. https://www.vice.com/en_ca/article/ev3ayk/sex-bloggers-say-tumblr-is-as-good-as-gone-after-porn-ban

One of the reasons for this huge jump in porn use for women might be because of a little something called responsive desire. We have this idea that our sexual desire is a drive, like hunger, something that works to continually satisfy a need. This is a dangerous concept, because if we believe sex is like hunger or thirst, we believe we are entitled to get it and that the longer we go without it, the more we "need" it—the more we'll suffer. Not only do some predators use the sex drive myth as a rationale for hurting people to get what they want, it puts a lot of pressure on our partners and adds a layer of anxiety to the single life. Sex is fun and has a lot of benefits, but no one ever died from not having enough sex. As it turns out, our sexual desire isn't a drive, it's responsive—we respond to sexually relevant stimuli, and if we are not too stressed and feel relatively safe, we might want to engage in some sexual contact. If we go without it for a while, we don't suffer: many of us simply stop wanting it as much. It's not a survival need, it's a response to our internal and external environments.

Some people are more sensitive to sexually relevant stimulation, so their desire seems more spontaneous—it seems to come out of nowhere. Men are more likely to have desire like this—they can be sensitive to all kinds of possible sexual situations and able to feel their desire pretty much anytime, anywhere. But as Emily Nagoski points out in her book *Come as You Are,* for 5 percent of men and a whopping 30 percent of women, sexual desire is generally pretty quiet until some really obvious sexually relevant stimuli—like the right kind of porn—shows up in the right (safe) context.[112] We're just not thinking about it until it's right in front of us. There is nothing wrong with having a desire pattern like this, it's normal and healthy. When women have access to porn that is not scary and stress-inducing, it might help them access their desire and get them in the mood to enjoy sex. It might give their responsive desire something to respond to.

If porn turns you on, makes you feel good, and helps you connect to your body, your mind, and your partners, then it can be a beautiful part of your pleasure practice. But if it's triggering, stress-inducing, or numbing, then it might be having an adverse effect on your healing. It's worth considering what kinds of images we are consuming and how they make us feel. There's nothing inherently wrong with porn, sex work, sex toys, or any kind of (consensual) sexual expression. What makes the difference is whether those expressions make us feel more or less connected.

FANTASIES

If we are practicing mindful sexual self-pleasure, we try, at least some of the time, to go without porn or sex toys. Ideally, we're focusing on our body sensations, but our brain is, after all, our biggest sex organ. That means we're left alone with our imaginations: marooned on fantasy island. Sexual fantasies may be the most private types of thoughts we have. They can be scary or disturbing, and this is especially common if we've been sexually violated. A woman who has been raped might have rape fantasies. Kind,

---

112   Nagoski, Emily. *Come as You Are: The Surprising New Science That Will Transform Your Sex Life.* New York: Simon and Schuster (2015): 225.

generous souls might have fantasies about whips and chains. Die-hard feminists might imagine being objectified and used. Many of these fantasies will stay on the island, never to manifest in real life.

If we do want to act out a fantasy, however, we generally do it in the service of consensual pleasure, even if it doesn't look like that on the surface. If someone wanted to act out a fantasy of being raped, for example, it would be explicit that she is actually in complete control and can stop the play instantly with a word. Ironically, the submissive partner in consensual sex play is actually the person who has the power. Generally, fantasy rape is about surrendering, experiencing pleasure, and possibly working out old traumas in a safe environment. It is not anything like real rape.

In her book *Anatomy of Masochism*, June Rathbone explores the phenomenon of sadomasochism in sexual play. She argues that in some cases, couples are working out anxieties about power and control, whether that's about a past trauma or simply about living in an ambiently hierarchical and power-obsessed culture. S&M is for some people a zone of potential healing. Rathbone explains that those she interviewed engage in "the reenactment of situations, long past, in which they were helpless but which they now master."[113] Sadomasochistic scenarios often have much more explicit consent structures (such as having a "safe word") than regular old sex, where no one even knows how to ask how it's going. Playing out S&M scenarios or rape fantasies require a lot of trust and communication and can give a survivor a strategy to take their power back—to say, in effect, "I'm in charge now!"[114]

Our fantasies have a relationship with how we currently feel in our bodies, what's happening in our relationships, what lives in our sexual past, and what we've learned from our culture. In my masturbation meditation practice, I've noticed that my fantasies tend to shift depending on what's going on in my life. I might think about a current partner or not. I might feel powerful and in control or might be in a state of surrender. Specific images and scenarios come and go. There was a long period during my healing where my fantasies only ever featured women. I am attracted to women and date them sometimes, but, at that time, I think it was a way to create safety in an imagined sexual world when I was, on a certain level, terrified of men. I remember when I briefly dated a rich man, I noticed my fantasies started centering around things like buying a house. Apparently, the real estate market is so prohibitive in Vancouver, BC, that the forbidden act of shopping for a house has taken on a shade of the erotic.

In this way, sexual fantasies are a bit like dreams. Dreams aren't literal representations of our lives, they are metaphorical expressions of our emotions. Dreams are always about how we feel in them, not their literal content. Fantasies metaphorically express what's happening for us on the erotic level, that semiconscious place where the nervous system meets up with our desire, our deepest feelings, our anxieties about intimacy, and our cultural conditioning. Sometimes a rape fantasy is really about being held, being taken care of, having our needs being met without having to ask, or that ultimate dream—

---

113   Rathbone, June. *Anatomy of Masochism*. New York, Kluwer (2001): 261.
114   Ibid

letting go of control. Imagining whipping or tying someone else up might be about a desire to be *in* control. Fantasizing about having sex with someone you never would do it with in real life might be about the thrill of novelty. Exhibitionism and getting caught could express a desire to be seen, appreciated, and validated. Stranger sex could be about feeling so safe and carefree that anything is possible. These things probably wouldn't *feel* like that if we did them in real life—at least not without a fair amount of preparation and communication with our consenting partners and collaborators.

A lot of the time, we hide our fantasies away, feeling they are shameful, and are afraid not only to talk about them but even to acknowledge them to ourselves. When we can approach them with mindfulness and compassion rather than shame and judgment, they may have something to teach us about how we feel, what we want, and what we need. Sex therapist Ian Kerner points out:

> **What this boils down to is that fantasies, much like dreams, free your brain to explore secret, extraordinary realms without the compunction of practicality, morality, or logic. Flooded by a barrage of images, memories, and thoughts, your body can basically kick back and enjoy the show.**[115]

Besides, fantasies might be really helpful when we are having a hard time being present in our bodies and relaxing into what's happening, especially when intrusive thoughts start coming up. People (apparently especially women) need to be able to let go of control and quiet the mind in order to enjoy a sexual experience, and fantasies may help with that. Kerner goes on, "Fantasy also helps your mind shut down, an important component of the female orgasm."[116]

Our culture so inextricably links power and sexuality that even if you've had nothing but great sexual experiences, power is probably going to play a part in your sexual life. At least, unless and until you carefully unlearn these inherited power dynamics in exchange for loving, equal relationships. In her book on sex and addiction, Charlotte Davis Kasl writes, "If we lived in a country where women were never sexually abused, had equal rights, and were never portrayed as sex objects, I do not believe we would associate passive fantasies of being tied up or abused with sexual arousal."[117] Fair enough, but of course it's impossible to know what life would be like if we lived in that world—we don't. There's nothing wrong with us if we do have fantasies of being tied up or abused. There's enough shame going around out there, there's no reason to shame ourselves for our fantasies, too.

That being said, sometimes we can use fantasies as a way to numb our feelings, avoid ourselves, or even punish ourselves for some piece of guilt or shame left over in our nervous systems. Fantasies are a tool, just like porn, food, alcohol, or gambling, that can be fun but can also be potentially dangerous. Pleasure means feeling more present in

---

115   Kerner, Ian. Passionista: The Empowered Woman's Guide to Pleasuring a Man. New York: Collins (2008): 69.

116   Ibid.

117   Kasl, Charlotte Davis. Women, Sex, and Addiction: A Search for Love and Power. New York: Harper & Row Perennial Library (1990): 65.

our bodies and more connected to our emotions. If these behaviors are causing us to
feel numb, guilty, shameful, or self-hating, they are not giving us genuine pleasure.

Sometimes the only problem with a certain fantasy is that we feel guilty about having
it. Again, most fantasies are never going to manifest in reality—they are useful as what
they are: fantasies and imaginative leaps. There's no such thing as a wrong thought or
feeling—what matters is what we do about what we think and feel. Our behaviors matter
a lot—including in terms of how we treat ourselves. But aside from that, fantasies
are an expression of our imaginations, and our imaginations can be wild and intense.
Sometimes all we need to do is go ahead and fantasize about whatever it is that turns
us on and stop feeling like a bad feminist/partner/person simply because of what we're
dreaming up in our heads.

The key with fantasies, then, is not to overfocus on *what* comes up unbidden in our
minds but rather to put some energy and intention into *how* we work with these
thoughts and images. The content matters a lot less than how what you're thinking
makes you feel. Besides, trying to push a certain thought away only makes it stronger.
A fantasy is purely imaginative, and the fact that we fantasize about something does not
necessarily mean we want to do it or will do it in life. But if a certain fantasy makes us
feel like crap, it is already doing damage to our bodies, our hearts, and our relationship
with ourselves.

So what do we do if we've got a few fantasies that leave us cold when it's all over? Use
our imaginations, of course. Try out different scenarios in our minds and see if they
make us feel more or less connected. This doesn't mean the old fantasies won't still pop
up—they will, but focusing on the ones that give us genuine pleasure and make us feel
good about ourselves rather than the ones that give us a momentary high and then a
crash will help us keep working on that loving relationship with our own sexuality. Over
time, we will have more fantasies to play with and more space in our imaginations for
sexual scenarios that feel good to us. We must mindfully consume our own fantasies
just as we mindfully consume porn, feeding ourselves nourishing and healthy sexual
food rather than junk food that tastes good in the moment but leaves us hungover in
the morning.

CRAVING VS. DESIRE

Sexual violation (not to mention all the other difficult realities of being a human) can
make us suppress, repress, and avoid our feelings. Pleasure can help us be present,
but we can also use it to check out. Many trauma survivors know this one well, but
we all have the capacity to reach for whatever will let us tune out the second we get
uncomfortable. One drink is pleasurable and delightful, but, after four or five, we're on
another planet. Shopping is soothing until we accidentally max out our credit cards in
a daze. Comfort food is comforting until we black out, eat all of it, and come to with
a stomachache. Too much of a good thing can overload our systems so that we switch

from pleasure and presence to numbness and dissociation. Even though the overload doesn't actually feel pleasurable, we keep going for more because it distracts us from the demons trying to crawl out our throats.

Our clear, authentic desires point us toward those relationships and life pursuits that will give us a sense of meaning, allow us to grow as people, and help us evolve in our lives. The pleasure that follows this kind of desire often includes discomfort, because, without it, growth is impossible. Craving, on the other hand, masquerades as desire. Craving pushes us toward something, but with the intention of making everything but the craved object go silent. Craving actually prevents us from accessing our true desires because it is focused only on itself. Craving doesn't want growth or evolution. Desire wants us to move. Craving wants us to stay where we are.

Craving is also a mechanism that shuts down our willingness to fight back against oppression. When we're too busy satisfying our need for TV, food, booze, porn, or even excessive work, we don't pause to think about bigger concepts like how we'd want to change our lives or the world around us. Our revolutionary instincts dampen when we're too busy chasing our cravings all day to think about change. This is the meaning of the cliché about bread and circuses—the Roman government provided its people with free food and exciting distracting spectacles with the explicit purpose of keeping their minds off resistance. Keep the people fed and entertained, and they'll never bother resisting their own oppression. Our cravings are like an internal Roman government: they keep us fixated on a short-term high so we can't access our deeper desire for meaning, connection, or change—all things that involve both genuine pleasure and a measure of discomfort. We never reach for the powerful beauty of the bittersweet.

In his book *In the Realm of Hungry Ghosts: Close Encounters with Addiction*, Dr. Gabor Maté points out that it's sometimes hard to tell from the outside whether someone is engaging with a life-giving desire, which he calls passion, or a mind-numbing craving, here understood as addiction. Maté writes:

> *The difference between passion and addiction is that between a divine spark and a flame that incinerates. [...] Passion is generous because it's not ego-driven; addiction is self-centered. Passion gives and enriches; addiction is a thief. Passion is a source of truth and enlightenment; addictive behaviors lead you into darkness. You're more alive when you are passionate, and you triumph whether or not you attain your goal. But an addiction requires a specific outcome that feeds the ego; without that outcome, the ego feels empty and deprived. A consuming passion that you are helpless to resist, no matter what the consequences, is an addiction.*[118]

When we are connected with our generative desire, we are connected with passion and the erotic drive that pushes us toward growth. We are brave, willing to be vulnerable, and able to make a mess and keep following what feels most true for us in our hearts. We are fully present in our minds and bodies (and vaginas). We are in contact with our

---

118   Maté, Gabor. *In the Realm of Hungry Ghosts: Close Encounters with Addiction.* Berkeley, North Atlantic Books (2010): 116.

deepest unacknowledged emotions. Craving shows up because we're too afraid to feel these disruptive desires. Craving protects us from change. That can be a lifeline when facing the truth is too painful.

Addiction is painful and destructive, to be sure, but it's important to remember that it's also a survival strategy. Whether or not we identify them as addictive, our cravings help us focus on something other than our unaddressed pain. They protect us by keeping us from contact with our truest feelings—with the suffering that comes with generative desire and our capacity to heal ourselves. Our cravings can help us slow down our stress responses, but they don't heal us either. Stress hangs out in our bodies until it finds a way out. When we numb our feelings, it's like applying anesthetic to something that is going to have to wake up eventually. We get a break, but we've only hit pause on the painful healing that needs to happen one way or another. We have to be able to allow genuine pleasure and passion to exist alongside pain, loss, fear, shame, guilt, and all the rest. When we let pleasure be an aspect of our healing, we become less afraid of our painful emotions and memories, and with time, in my experience, anyway, the pain fades, the pleasure gets stronger, and we get better at tapping into our life-giving passions.

PLEASURE PRACTICE

Pleasure, like self-love, is not a given. It's a practice. Especially when we've been mired in loss, heartbreak, or trauma for a long time, we can be habituated to feeling like garbage and forget that there's another way of being in the world. We focus on our stress and pain and forget to see the tiny happy moments that show up on the daily. Our brains are wired to focus more on negative information than positive. This is a good survival strategy: it's more useful to remember where the tiger popped out of the bushes than the last time you shared a nice meal with friends. Our brains will tend to filter out pleasure information in order to focus on survival information, especially when we're stressed. The brain is not looking out for a good spot to sip tea in the sun (let alone sexually relevant information); it is too busy looking for tigers. The good news is that we can help the brain get out of this habit and rewire our neural pathways to get better at noticing, appreciating, and experiencing pleasure. Pleasure is like anything else—you have to practice it, and if you keep at it, you get better over time.

I know that gratitude practices are useful for a lot of people. There is plenty of evidence that keeping a journal of all the things you're grateful for, for example, helps people feel happier and more relaxed. It never worked for me. I don't like being told to feel something I don't feel. You can't just will yourself to feel gratitude when you're full of frustration and exhaustion. Besides, I felt like an asshole sitting there at the end of the day counting all the ways my life was better than someone else's. I'm grateful I have a roof over my head. I'm grateful I have somewhere to sleep. Yeah, and, there are tons of people out there who don't have that! Then I'd start feeling guilty and get stressed out, and it did not make me feel happy and relaxed. The other flaw with the gratitude practices for me is that they generally happen at the end of the day, after the nice parts of your day have come and gone. It's not a presence practice.

Pleasure practice, on the other hand, is about noticing little moments of sweetness while they are happening. It's not a practice of trying to will yourself to feel something you don't feel, it's a practice of shifting your attention to pleasurable experiences that are already happening so you can cultivate them and make them stronger. You hunt down any little joyful thing, from the taste of your first cup of coffee in the morning to the hilarious butt wiggle of a dog that's happy to see you. When we get better at noticing these little moments and try to stay present with them rather than immediately grabbing our phones to document whatever is happening on social media, we get better at feeling the enjoyment that comes with these moments. They are so easy to blow past, but we have to put a little work into really letting ourselves have them.

I remember when I first started doing this I was going through a pretty soul-crushing breakup. It overshadowed everything in my life, and I could barely think about anything else. I was walking my dog and looked down while he sniffed around for a good place to pee, and there were these huge, perfect, autumn leaves on the ground that were encrusted with a diamond-like frost glittering in the morning light. It was so beautiful. I stopped to admire the sight and took a breath, trying to feel my body in the presence of this sudden small beauty. I started to collect moments like this, just noticing when they were happening and trying to stop and be present with them in my body. I had to remember that they were not a betrayal of my grief. I could be heartbroken and fully present with a moment of beauty at the same time. Sometimes the moments of pleasure would bring up the grief; I might wish, for example, that I could share this with the person I was missing, and I let that be there, too. Over time, the moments of sweetness became sweeter and more common, and the painful emotions ebbed a little more than they flowed. It occurred to me that all happiness means is having a pretty good number of sweet moments in your boring everyday life. Happiness isn't about having all the things you want. It's about hunting down whatever sweetness is on offer, giving yourself permission to feel it, and just really being with that.

Pleasure Practice

Here are some tips for practicing pleasure with daily moments of sweetness:

Be on the lookout for tiny pleasurable things. They don't have to be big and dramatic: look for a song you like on the radio while you're sitting in traffic, a delicious bite of food, a cute photo of a dog on Instagram, or a hot shower. Don't blow past these moments; slow down, if you can, take a breath, and feel how your body responds to them. This makes it easier for you to notice when something nice is happening, and it teaches your brain to pay more attention to the sweet things than the bitter (though bitter is okay, too!).

Prioritize your pleasure. It matters. Sit with the discomfort and guilt that will probably come up when you put your pleasure above the things you think you *should* be doing instead.

Include more tiny pleasurable things in your life and take them seriously. Set up routines of pleasure—you might already have a few of these. What is your morning routine like? Do you have little rituals you do when you get to work or take an afternoon break? See if there's a way you can add more pleasure to these little routines. Wake up five minutes earlier to give yourself a few minutes of peace before the kids wake up. Or set the alarm a little earlier so you can hit snooze, because those extra snooze minutes are always the best. Walk the extra few blocks on your break to sit at the nice cafe that has the prettiest tea. Turn your daily moisturizing routine or shave into a ritual—take your time, massage your skin, focus on the pleasurable feeling you can give yourself.

Be honest with yourself about your craving behaviors. You might not even realize you have them. Social media is an example of something that we often crave, but then when we start scrolling, we don't actually feel any pleasure. Consider implementing more boundaries around these kinds of craving activities that don't give you genuine pleasure.

Create a pleasure challenge for yourself. Every day for forty days (or whatever timeline makes sense for you) do one thing that gives you genuine pleasure. It could be the same thing every day, like carving out thirty minutes to work on that short story you've been wanting to write, or you could choose a new thing every day, like trying a new recipe or going go-karting. Write about the experience in a journal and note down the sensations that you felt while you were doing the pleasurable thing (including whether uncomfortable emotions came up).

If you do the challenge, remember to differentiate satisfying a craving, which is a numbing relief, and pleasure, which requires full presence with whatever your body has going on that day. You might mix them up as you go, and that's totally okay; sometimes it takes a while to learn the difference for ourselves in our own lives. That's part of the practice.

Pleasure isn't guilty. Excise the words "guilty pleasure" from your vocabulary. If reading trashy novels, watching reality TV shows about wedding dresses, or eating spoonfuls of peanut butter coated in chocolate chips gives you delight, then do that. Let these things bring you into your body, fill up your soul, and nourish your healing. Pleasure isn't shameful, and it's not something you have to earn or deserve. Genuine pleasure is the food of desire. It asks a lot of us, and certainly we have to get better at holding it alongside the reasonable grief and pain we feel from time to time as human beings with skin. The tiniest moments of sweetness can accumulate over time to reduce our stress, encourage our resilience, and maybe even put a little bit of fight into us. Healing starts in your body, and you must give it pleasure, every single day. You have to take your own joy seriously. Tough homework, I know, but I believe in you.

EAT

I always know something is wrong when I find myself under the bright lights of the grocery store, putting Kraft Dinner into my basket. It's an omen: I don't always know cognitively that I'm sick or sad, but something is definitely about to hit me when that little blue box with its hard white macaronis and neon orange cheese comes home with me. Inevitably I end up with a bowl of the stuff in front of some bad TV, sniffling either from tears or a head cold. It's a Kraft Dinner premonition.

Neon orange pasta is level one. I'm eating crap, but with a sort of hopefulness and an attempt to comfort myself. Level two is popcorn for dinner. I somehow convince myself it stands in for a meal and get away with barely eating. Level three is "accidentally" skipping lunch. This one usually comes along with another bad habit—overscheduling. I overlap appointments all day and somehow forget the part where I'm supposed to sit down and refuel. I haven't hit level four in a long time—that's when I don't even try to eat. I won't admit it to myself at the time, but it gives me a gleeful sense of control when I don't put real food inside of my body. I get high on hunger and stress.

I've had this tendency since I was a young teenager, when life was scary and my need to control something—anything—bloomed into full-scale anorexia. I ate nothing but the piece of toast my mom would anxiously put in front of me in the mornings for about a year. At my skinniest (and my sickly proudest), I weighed 102 pounds at a height of five feet eight. That's a BMI of 15.51, just on the edge between severely underweight and *very* severely underweight. Under 15 is the lowest the scale goes—they stop counting after that. I really (almost) accomplished something there, huh.

At the time, I got nothing but compliments on my bony frame. There's a photo of me from back then at a school dance, draped in an old dress, my feet poking out like flippers, huge under my toothpick calves. I thought I looked great. At least, that's what all my teenage girlfriends told me. But I wasn't really intending to lose weight to look better. I was trying to find some sense of order in an unpredictable world. Most of all, I think, I was trying to protect myself from becoming a sexual woman. I had been getting catcalled on the street since I was maybe nine, and it was only escalating as puberty loomed. I could feel the way my body was turning into an object for strange men's eyes. I felt the pressure to date boys, to make out, to have sex. I could feel the inevitable flood of changes coming on with puberty, and, subconsciously, I wanted it all to fucking stop. Not eating is a great way to shut down your body's sexual systems (plus it's culturally sanctioned by every women's magazine). It worked—I didn't get my period until I was almost fifteen, at the beginning of my food recovery.

In her book *Women, Sex, and Addiction*, Charlotte Davis Kasl names what I was doing: "Self-starvation may also be a child's unconscious defense against covert sexual energy [...] the child literally shrinks from becoming a woman."[119] For me, not eating is an addiction. It was then, and it is now. Kasl indicates that I may not be alone here:

> *Part of a woman's deepest programming is the belief that she has no control over her consumption of food and participation in sex. This, in turn, leads to obsession, because we form obsessions with things we can't control. An obsession with food drains energy and distracts a woman from the deeper issues of her life.*[120]

It is incredibly common for sexual issues to show up alongside food issues. It's been a long time since I've been actively anorexic, but I still tend to restrict food when I feel threatened or out of control (or when, I don't know, someone sexually assaults me).

In a society that is quite sexually threatening a lot of the time, food has played a sometimes helpful and sometimes harmful part in helping me feel safer and more in control in my own body. In my recovery from sexual assault and anorexia, I've learned that I can practice safety, consent, pleasure, and desire within my relationship with food. Food *is* relationship at a very fundamental level and most especially represents my relationship with my own self. Healing my feelings about food sparked a very real healing in my body and my heart. That's why Step Six on our journey to heal from sexual assault is Eat. And yes, Kraft Dinner is allowed.

FOOD AND RELATIONSHIPS

Food and love are inextricably linked. The association is old: when we are babies, food almost always comes alongside touch, with the closeness of a caregiver. Most babies quickly learn that when they cry, they generally get milk. We learn early on that food soothes. When we get older, food can become a replacement for love. As Kasl points out, "For many people, food is the most reliable source of pleasure. You can't always count on sex or other people, but you can always count on chocolate."[121]

Food represents relationship on quite a literal level. In order to physically survive, we have to put food—living material from a plant or animal being that is not us—inside of our bodies. We have to physically connect with other beings, to draw them in and let scores of little bacterial beings that live in us (but are not us) digest them. We have to let the food crawl into our most intimate places until it *becomes* us. I know it's an intense metaphor, but eating is a form of penetration. We have to literally take it inside. I tried for a long time to refuse that vulnerability, to exist as a self alone, to not need anyone or anything. I wasn't just rejecting the threat of those strange men catcalling at me on the street, I was rejecting relationship of any kind. But a human body needs connection

---

119   Kasl, Charlotte Davis. *Women, Sex, and Addiction: A Search for Love and Power.* New York: Harper & Row Perennial Library (1990): 184.
120   Ibid, 187.
121   Ibid, 183.

to other living things: to our first caregiver's bodies (whether through the breast or the bottle-hand), to animals that produce meat and dairy products, and/or to the living plants that grow out of the ground, nourished by sun and water. These living beings transform inside of us in order for us to survive. A piece of food is a part of our bodies that hasn't been integrated yet. Our bodies are made out of food; without these other living beings we are nothing. We are what we eat—we are in relationship with all that we eat.

We also need relationships with other human beings in order to get the food we put in our bodies. We need a connection to those who hunt, gather, grow, package, and prepare our food. Sharing food has been an aspect of our survival since our species began. Food has always been a collaborative effort. Relationships are woven into eating both physically and socially: we have to eat other plant or animal beings that have generally been caught, grown, prepared, or offered by a community of other human beings. Healing our relationship with food means healing our relationship with—well, relationships.

We all want to be nourished, both in our hearts and in our bellies. We all have a few relationship patterns we tend to repeat over and over, especially if we have a history of sexual abuse, stress in our families, or any number of things that can happen to us in an unhealthy society. We keep trying to repair some original hurt, and we take it out on our food and on our people, for better or for worse. These relationship patterns probably won't change unless we can go to the source: our relationship with ourselves. Therapy, communicating with our partners, and journaling about our daddy issues can all be helpful, but if we keep teaching our nervous systems that we don't deserve nourishing food in a calm environment, that we can't have food when we're hungry, or that we'll keep stuffing our faces when our bodies say to stop, our nervous systems will not believe in the possibility of a truly nourishing love. That doesn't mean we won't have love or successful relationships, of course, but we might be making it a lot harder on ourselves than we need to. Feeding ourselves is a fundamental way of loving ourselves.

Food is generally easier to control than other people. Most of us have some choice about what and how we eat, but other human beings are unpredictable. Sexual violation makes us feel on a deep, unconscious level that we are not safe and that we can't protect ourselves from something unwanted entering into our bodies. Relearning to eat consciously with a loving intention can help teach our nervous systems that we do still have choices about what happens to our bodies. We can show our bodies through food that there are zones of safety that we do have some control over. We can practice boundaries, desire, pleasure, and presence every day by working on our relationship with what we put in our mouths. We can heal by playing with our food.

Love as Nourishment

Consider an intimate relationship. This could be a past or present romantic partner or someone else in your life who you are close with. If we consider that we learned to associate food and love as little children, how do our love/nourishment patterns manifest in our adult relationships? Does the way we eat mirror the way we love? Journal or reflect on the following questions:

⊕   How do you consume love in your life? Do you nibble at it all day without really paying attention? Do you push it away? Hide it in cupboards and under the bed without eating it and then cling onto it until it withers in your white-knuckle grip? Do you gorge on junk, not really believing you can access the kind of nourishment that would feed you in the long term?

⊕   Do you feel nourished by your relationships? When you are hungry for attention, affection, or connection, do you trust you will be fed?

⊕   Can you access your love when you need it, or do you have to starve until your other feels like offering it?

⊕   Do you feel you can say no to your other, or are you force-fed time, attention, affection, sex?

⊕   Can you feed yourself with the love and connection you need outside of your primary relationship, or do you rely on your other alone to feed you?

⊕   Is love shared and enjoyed, or is it a game of give-and-take-away?

⊕   Does your other know how to feed themselves, or do they rely on you to meet their needs?

⊕   Do you feel abundant, full of love, time, and energy to offer to your special person, or do you feel starving and exhausted, unable to share what you have?

⊕   What could you do to feed yourself more outside your primary relationship so you have more to give inside it?

SEXUAL ASSAULT AND DISORDERED EATING

Like any other addiction, eating disorders are dangerous and have negative consequences, but they are also a tool for survival. They are a function of the nervous system trying to protect itself. Disordered eating was already a part of my toolbox when I was assaulted, and eating issues are sneaky because you can't quit food like you can quit drinking (no matter how hard you try). Food was an enemy that I unconsciously associated with sexuality, my body image, and being seen as sexual prey, so in order to heal from sexual assault, I had to make friends with food.

Women are much likelier than men to have some form of an eating disorder like anorexia, bulimia, or binge eating disorder, but that doesn't mean men don't suffer from them: one in every three people affected by an eating disorder is male.[122] No one knows exactly why it's so prevalent in women, but the common theory is that it's because women have more pressure to be thin. I know for myself, though, that anorexia wasn't really about trying to be thin. You don't resist your fundamental survival urges just because you want to fit into your skinny jeans. What I wanted was to be safe. At least one study on the topic has found that the occurrence of bulimia, the binge-and-purge cycle of eating, was 2.5 times higher for girls who had one incident of childhood sexual abuse and 4.9 times higher for girls who had experienced one or more episodes of abuse.[123] The pressure to diet might just help a woman find a way to make her threatening and scary sexuality disappear, especially if she's already been assaulted.

In my life and those of many of my friends who have experienced eating disorders, there is always some relationship between trying to control our food and trying to control our sexuality. It's not always about some specific moment of sexual violence. Often, it's about protecting our bodies from the ambiently threatening sexuality that infuses our culture, as in, I don't know, perfume ads that show a woman who looks kind of dead strapped to the hood of a car. Some of us try to disappear by not eating enough. Some of us try to disappear underneath a protective layer of fat. Some of us binge, desperately trying to fill the void, and then, consumed with guilt and nausea, purge the shame right back out. Some of us do cleanses where we consume nothing but lemon juice and cayenne pepper—the ol' shit-yourself-thin diet. This one makes us feel pure and empty, and, as a friend of mine who did it has jokingly phrased it, as if "no one will be able to see my bowels!" We refuse the violation of food entering our vulnerable bodies, or we try to stuff ourselves with comfort, and then, panicked, eject it back out. Kasl writes, "Many women, unable to say 'no, I don't want to be sexual, I'm hurting inside, I'm afraid, I'm sad, I need to change my life,' use food as a language for their feelings."[124] We know somehow that our voices don't matter, so we communicate silently to the only one that we know will listen: our food.

FEED AND FUCK

Food has a very close relationship with stress. Stress essentially means going into our sympathetic nervous systems: into fight, flight, freeze, or possibly tend and befriend. It's panic mode. A hallmark of stress is that the digestive and reproductive systems shut down in order to provide energy to the limbs and brain to handle the stressor, whatever it is. If there's a tiger chasing us, we're not wasting time thinking about our next meal.

122   "Eating Disorders in Men and Boys." National Eating Disorder Association. Dec 2018. https://www.nationaleatingdisorders.org/learn/general-information/research-on-males

123   Sanci, Lena, Carolyn Coffey, Craig Olsson, Sophie Reid, John B. Carlin and George Patton. "Childhood Sexual Abuse and Eating Disorders in Females: Findings From the Victorian Adolescent Health Cohort Study." Archives of Pediatrics and Adolescent Medicine, Volume 162, No. 3 (2008): 261–267.

124   Kasl, Charlotte Davis. Women, Sex, and Addiction: A Search for Love and Power. New York: Harper & Row Perennial Library (1990): 183.

Once the stressor has gone and we know we're safe again, we can complete the stress cycle: we might sigh or cry; many animals physically shake the stress off, signaling that the danger has passed. The body resumes its parasympathetic functioning, waking the digestion and the reproductive functions back up. The tigers are gone, so we can get hungry, eat, snuggle, and/or make love. This is the relaxed parasympathetic state called rest and digest, or, more pointedly, feed and fuck.

The problem with sexual violence is that it's stressful—real stressful. PTSD, which happens to about 90 percent of rape survivors,[125] is (as the name indicates) a disorder that has to do with stress—the stress cycle doesn't complete and we never return to the calm, relaxed, healing parasympathetic state. The stressor has gone, but not the stress: the body still feels under threat. That makes it hard to properly feed and fuck.

When I was hit by a car while riding my bike, I remember first being in shock and trying to get back on my bike and keep going to work. When I saw how mangled my bike was and that it was completely unrideable, I realized what had happened and I started to cry uncontrollably. When I got home, I sat on the back stairs and sobbed and sobbed. My body was shaking off the excess adrenaline so that I could return to my baseline and let the stress go. It worked pretty well—I had some healing to do, and I didn't want to get back on my bike for a while, but I wasn't really traumatized by that experience. I understood that it was an accident that fit pretty neatly into my understanding of the general risks of the road. But being assaulted by my best friend was a different kind of experience. It wasn't quite like being hit by a four-thousand-pound vehicle, but it made me realize that I had no idea how safe I was in any sexual situation. I did not have a good sense of the risks of this road. It was so confusing that I didn't want to believe it, I tried to pretend it hadn't happened. I never cried, I never shook it off, I never completed the stress cycle. The difference between the mild-mannered hipster who assaulted me and a tiger was no longer clear. Suddenly the tigers were everywhere, walking down the street, showing up at parties with my friends, riding the bus. I had to stay vigilant: the stress cycle could never end because, as far as I knew, I was constantly surrounded by tigers in hipster's clothing.

Sexual violence may damage the pelvic nerves and interrupt the dopamine flow to the brain, which is one kind of problem. But sexual violence also damages our social relationships. Because our culture so rarely protects and believes people who go through this experience, a whole bunch of shame and anxiety get piled on top of the sexual assault. It's hard enough to shake off the feeling of being dirty and unfixably broken after violation, but now we feel we will be outcast from a community that didn't protect us and doesn't believe us. We feel on an instinctual level that we're being exiled to the forest full of tigers. It's not always the fact of physical sexual violence that causes us problems, especially when it's one of those ambiguous manipulative sexual coercion situations that doesn't involve a lot of force. The problem is that we lose our sense

---

125   "Victims of Sexual Violence: Statistics." RAINN.org. Dec 2018. https://www.rainn.org/statistics/victims-sexual-violence

of safety, our belief that people respect our autonomy, and our sense that our "no" matters. Sexual assault is, among other things, a stress problem.

Chronic stress often transforms into anxiety and/or depression, which can have a major effect on our digestive systems. Anxiety is a form of fight-or-flight response. It wants to do something to try to protect us. The brain and muscles snatch as much energy as they can from the digestive system in order to run away from or fight the tiger, so the nervous system instructs the gut to get rid of whatever it's been working on so we can focus: cue the stress-puking and diarrhea. When there's no tiger to flee or fight, however, all that energy and adrenaline just keeps swimming around in the body waiting for a fight that never comes. So we end up micromanaging dinner parties, working sixteen hours a day, or booking appointments with ten different kinds of alternative healers trying to manage all the weird physical symptoms that come up when it's impossible to be still or relax. Anxiety, as they say, is just depression that hasn't given up yet.

Depression, on the other hand, is a form of the freeze response. The tiger is way bigger and faster than we are, so we freeze, hoping it either doesn't see us or at the very least eats us quickly. Depression is a problem of helplessness and despair. It's the nervous system deciding there's nothing that can be done. In this case, digestion just stops. It shuts down. Everybody goes home for the day; no point doing any more work if we're about to be eaten by a tiger. Food just sits there not being digested. Neither we nor our bowels feel like getting out of bed and doing anything: cue constipation. Anxiety and depression are opposite sides of the same problem, but that doesn't mean they are mutually exclusive. Plenty of us swing from one extreme to the other, sometimes in the course of a single day. Whether we have one, the other, or both at the same time, these chronic stress conditions can put our guts through the ringer.

Nausea, stress-puking, and diarrhea make food seem poisonous because the body keeps rejecting it, so food restriction is a common stress-management technique for people with anxiety. It's not the food that's toxic, however, it's the nonexistent but ever-present tiger. In a way, the system is trying to cleanse itself of the toxin that entered the body, not with the food, but with the perpetrator. When depression and constipation are a part of the equation, it can feel like nothing will ever change, like it's impossible to ever be anything other than the person who was assaulted. It's common for depression to come along with binge eating, which can be a subconscious attempt to bury that toxic energy with food. Part of the shame survivors feel can be their sense that they are carrying some poison with them that was implanted by the person who violated them. It feels like some trace of the perpetrator is still with us, inside of our bodies. In her book about women's sexual stories called *Aphrodite's Daughters*, Jalaja Bonheim writes:

> *No matter how we describe it, the fact is that the abuser's energy penetrates the victim and takes up residence within her. When a woman connects with the darkness that has penetrated her flesh, she often experiences nausea and vomiting, along with the desperate desire to expel the toxicity that has been ingested. Darkness threatens to engulf her not only from without, but even more*

insidiously from within her own psyche. Deep despair arises as she faces the fact
that all her attempts to repress the abuse or leave it behind have failed. The
revolting, slimy creature still sits in her belly and has no intention of leaving.[126]

We don't avoid being alone with our own thoughts after sexual trauma simply because it was a bad experience we don't like remembering. We avoid being alone with ourselves because, on some level, we feel that the perpetrator has claimed us, brought us into their world, impregnated us with some evil. Being alone with our bodies in the quiet, sober and able to feel our feelings, means being alone with the trace the perpetrator left in us. The perpetrator doesn't leave our bodies even long after they have left the room.

We try to get rid of this undigested clump of shame and fear by throwing up, refusing to eat, or stuffing our faces in an attempt to suffocate it or swallow it down. It won't go anywhere, no matter how much we try to barf it out. The only choice, Bonheim insists, is to digest this perpetrator energy:

Since all her attempts at spitting and sweating and cursing the evil out have
failed, she will have to digest it. She will have to stop treating it as a foreign object
and claim it as hers to transform. Instead of insisting, "They did it to me. They
are guilty and I am innocent," she must take the next step of saying, "I and they
are one. Their darkness now lives within me. This is my wound, which only I can
transform and heal."[127]

This is that moment that we dread where we have to start doing the work of actively processing what happened to us. If we recall Tracy Lindberg's owl returning home to find a wolf has peed all over the floor, this is the moment when we decide to stop flying around like crazy trying to find some other roost to sleep in, go home, and pick up that goddamned mop. We have to claim our own healing process. It's unfair, it's painful, and it can be hard, but it's the only way through. We can't reject this piece of ourselves anymore. We have to digest it. With food.

FEELING FAT

Food is complicated for lots of reasons, and one of them is the way our culture teaches us to hate and fear our bodies, and specifically our fat. A lot of this anxiety has been channeled into the phenomenon of feeling fat—even though, you know, fat is not an emotion. Every woman I know (and several of the men) feels fat from time to time. This is true across size, shape, and weight. This has never in my experience been something I could see with my eyes—I've never looked at someone feeling fat and thought, "Oh, yeah, I can see that extra five pounds right there in your face!" Fat in this context really is a feeling, an internally felt sense, not a measurable reflection of reality. As far as I can tell, it has to do with how powerful we feel in our bodies and our lives, and how closely

126   Bonheim, Jalaja. *Aphrodite's Daughters: Women's Sexual Stories and the Journey of the Soul.* New York: Fireside (1997): 310.
127   Ibid.

we feel we are matching society's standards of what we should look like and feel like in our lives. I've learned that when I start feeling fat—that is, when I start to feel sensitive around my belly and those little loops of flesh on my haunches and hear a really critical voice every time I look in the mirror—it means I'm feeling out of control. For me, the high of not eating and seeing myself disappear a little bit more every time I got on the scale was the way I felt I was conquering myself, my baser instincts, my shame and fear, my disgusting unpredictable weak female body. It made me feel powerful. Now that I'm healthier, my weight fluctuates like anyone else's, but feeling fat doesn't have anything to do with what I actually weigh. I can be physically bigger and feel great—strong, healthy, and sexy. If anything, I've noticed I'm often at my lower weight range when I feel fat, because for me, feeling fat means I'm feeling anxious, which means I'm probably not eating properly.

Our society tells us that only one type of body (never yours!) is the right type of body. We're trained to scrutinize every curve, wrinkle, scar, and stretch mark we have, to feel shame about everything from a knobby big toe to a dry looking elbow. Lots of this stuff is internalized, but plenty of it is externalized, too. People judge fatness harshly and publicly (especially in Internet comment sections). The world is physically set up for a narrow range of people (sometimes literally, at least when it comes to airplane seats), and being bigger can make day-to-day life a lot more annoying than it should be. We're taught to be fat-phobic from a young age, so we turn against each other and our own bodies with judgment and cruelty, sometimes even when we're actively trying to be body positive. I remember the mixed feelings I had when I started recovering from my anorexia. Every time I saw the numbers on the scale go up, I both felt that I was doing well and also that I was losing at some existential game I'd been playing—which I would have had to die in order to win. Feeling fat isn't about being fat. It's a symptom of feeling powerless in a fat-phobic culture.

We need to unlearn our cultural fear of fat. People can be healthy in a huge range of physical sizes, and, if anything, it's safer healthwise to be significantly overweight than even just a tiny bit underweight. Our fat cells store energy, hormones, and vitamins. They keep us warm and pad our bones and vital organs. Fat is a vilified food source that, in the right forms, is vital for our brain and joint function and can help us regulate blood sugar. When we don't have enough fat, our bodies are essentially in survival mode, which means sex is probably off the table. We stop menstruating when we don't have enough fat to support our reproductive functions. We need fat to be able to access our sexual desire. We need fat to be sexy. We need fat to survive.

As I've gotten older, I've gotten much better at ignoring the fat-phobic alarm bell inside that pokes my soft flesh when I'm feeling out of control, but now I've got a great new way to criticize myself: feeling old. Our society tells women, especially, that their only power is sexual, and that sexual power starts to fade when we cross the line of age twenty-five or so. Every year after that, we're told, we lose a little bit more of our value. If we "keep it tight" with antiaging serums and exercise routines, we're okay, but if we let our wrinkles spread and our hair turn gray, we might as well retire to the land of unwanted space wasters. While I enjoyed seeing fiftysomethings Sandra Bullock and Cate Blanchett looking super hot and fashionable in the 2018 film *Ocean's Eight*, I also noticed that their faces do not move. I'm all for having more older women in awesome movie roles, but if I'm going to look like that when I'm in my fifties, it's going to cost a lot more dollars in injectables than I have or want to spend.

The antiaging, anti-fat, anti-ugliness, anti-human-beings-with-skin industry makes a lot of money on all this feeling bad about ourselves. Women spend an unfair amount of time and money on makeup, diets, antiaging serums, and elbow rejuvenators. A SkinStore survey found that women spend on average eight dollars per day on makeup, including around sixteen products every single morning.[128] That's almost three thousand dollars per year—just on makeup. That doesn't include hair products, salon visits, diet supplements, and all the other nonsense we're coerced into buying. Men don't have to spend money on all this crap, and they make on average of ten thousand dollars more than we do every year.[129] When I think about how egregiously unfair this is, it makes me want to throw every beauty product I own out the window (and hope they hit some rich dude on the way down).

I can say this as a white woman, too, who already has the light skin and straight hair that our culture mostly deems acceptable. Many black people have had experiences of being told either outright or by implication that their natural black hairstyles, like afros or dreadlocks, are "unprofessional" and that they should get an expensive weave in order to "fit in."[130] So while I might feel unattractive when my hair falls flat, a black woman who hasn't spent hours in a salon relaxing her hair has to grapple with feeling *unemployable* as well. According to a Nielsen report, black consumers spend nine times more on beauty products than non-black consumers—and these products tend to be more toxic than the ones marketed to white people.[131] Loving our bodies and accepting ourselves as we are is a radical act in a society that wants to keep us small (and take all our money) by never allowing us to feel good enough—or even firing us if we step out of bounds. Getting out of the cycle of beauty routines and fad diets would free up a lot of our energy. And how powerful could we be with all that time, money, and energy on our side?

Quite powerful. Our desire, remember, is a force. Truly believing we're enough can help us access the erotic energy in our bodies that can push toward growth and change—and maybe even resistance. Makeup and hair products should be fun and playful, and we should have every right to use them when and if we feel like it (and every gender should have that same right, too). But when we think that leaving the house without makeup or

---

128   Gerstein, Julie. "Here's What The Average Woman In The US Spends On Makeup—And It's A Lot." Buzzfeed, March 2017. https://www.buzzfeed.com/juliegerstein/heres-what-the-average-american-woman-spends-on-makeup-and?utm_term=.ih7j3xAeN).anx9qPnyo

129   Sheth, Sonam, Shayanne Gal and Skye Gould. "6 charts show how much more men make than women." Business Insider. August 2018, https://www.businessinsider.com/gender-wage-pay-gap-charts-2017-3

130   "Ever Been Made to Feel That Your Afro Is Unprofessional?." Vice. Nov 2012. https://www.vice.com/en_ca/article/znqkv5/ever-been-made-to-feel-that-your-afro-is-unprofessional

131   Harmon, Stephenetta (isis). "Black Consumers Spend Nine Times More in Hair and Beauty: Report." HypeHair.com. https://www.hypehair.com/86642/black-consumers-continue-to-spend-nine-times-more-in-beauty-report/

with our roots showing is shameful—or worse, when an employer tells us to weave up or get out—we're caught in a (very expensive) trap. If we could figure out how to get out of it, we could spend that three thousand dollars getting out of debt, paying for a night course on French cooking, or, I don't know, going to Vegas. If we loved ourselves for who we already are, we could be more powerful, more inventive, and more courageous (though we might have to deal with being out of a job). Maybe we'd even fight back against the powers that be who keep telling us to buy stuff because we're so old, ugly, and fat—or at least stop giving them so much money. We could, at the very least, be having better sex.

BODY IMAGE AND SEX

In her book *Come as You Are*, Emily Nagoski explains that our sexual response system has an accelerator, which points to things that "make you all sticky and eager,"[132] and brakes, which hit your "neurological 'off' signals."[133] The accelerator is your sexual excitation system (SES), a function of your central nervous system that notices sexually relevant information and tells the body to turn on. Your SES is your internal sexual "yes." The brakes are your sexual inhibition system (SIS), which notices potential threats and tells the sexual system to shut off. Your SIS essentially lets you know there are more important things to think about than sex right now—it's your internal sexual "no." Everyone is different in terms of the sensitivity of their accelerator and brakes. You know that thing that happens sometimes when you want to have sex and you're into it but then you start obsessing about whether or not you'll come or what your partner will think about your performance or your lackluster elbows, and you want to do it but you just kind of can't? That's a fun thing when your accelerator and brakes are going at the same time.

If there's a "yes" coming from the SES and the SIS is quiet enough, three separate things ideally come together—expecting, eagerness, and enjoyment.[134] Expecting means we're aware that there's something sexually relevant in the room—this is where vaginas tend to lubricate and penises tend to get erect. This doesn't necessarily lead to eagerness and/or enjoyment; it may not have anything to do with whether we like what we see or want more of it. When our bodies respond but we're not into it (or we're into it but the body doesn't respond), that's called sexual non-concordance. Sexual non-concordance is a very common thing for everyone, including assault survivors. We may have lubricated or had an erection during an assault because the body was responding to sexually relevant information, but that does not mean we liked it, wanted more of it, or consented to it—at all.

---

132   Nagoski, Emily. *Come as You Are: The Surprising New Science That Will Transform Your Sex Life.* New York: Simon and Schuster (2015): 58.

133   Ibid, 49.

134   Ibid, 84.

Enjoyment is exactly what it sounds like—enjoying the sexual stimuli. Pleasure tends to make us want more pleasure, so enjoyment itself can encourage the accelerator. If our sexual experiences have lately been lacking in enjoyment, on the other hand, or if we associate sex with pain, boredom, or pressure to perform, that hits the brakes. Expecting might come along with dread rather than eagerness.

For most of us, any kind of stress, whether or not it's related to the sexual context, hits the brakes. For 10–20 percent of us, stress accelerates our expecting and eagerness responses, which sounds like a pretty good deal, but it dampens our enjoyment. So in order to be fully in the three layers of our internal sexual "yes," for all the systems to say "go" and bring on expecting, enjoying, and eagerness, the brakes have to be at least mostly off—which means removing as much stress as possible. When a stressor has gone and we feel safe, we can enter the parasympathetic feed-and-fuck mode. No tigers, the nervous system says. Let's get busy.

Stress can come in many different forms, and could be anything: worrying about the baby, having a deadline at work, not having exercised in a while, having a history of sexual trauma, conflict in a relationship, worries about performance, fears about pregnancy or STIs, or feeling fat/old/ugly/stupid. One reason women notoriously have a harder time with sexual desire could be because our culture has taught us to hate ourselves so much. When seeing a new wrinkle or gaining a couple of pounds makes us feel powerless and panicked, it's a lot harder to relax and enjoy fun sexy times with a partner, no matter how much they tell us we're beautiful with no makeup on and morning breath. Self-hatred is a form of stress that's not doing anything for us between the sheets.

Taking Your Foot off the Brake

Constant, low-level stress, whether or not it has anything to do with sexual assault, can dampen sexual desire. If you want to be having sex with your partner but just don't feel like it very often, here are some things you can try:

⌗   Make an intimacy date. Set aside an hour or three to focus on intimacy with each other. It's very important that there be no pressure on either partner to have sex. The point is just to hang out. No movies, no food, no phones, no distractions, just focus on each other alone in a private space. If this works for you, schedule it in regularly—once a week or once a month, whatever is reasonable for you both.

⌗   If sex has become a zone of stress in your partnership, make a rule for these intimacy dates—no sex allowed (and you might want to define what that means together). This creates a completely pressure-free zone to reconnect in nonsexual ways that could include affection, which may paradoxically help you get back into a sexual mood.

⊕   Set the mood. An environment that's conducive to sex will mean different
     things for different people, but it generally means a space relatively free
     of stressors. A locked door, a quiet room with no phones or screens, dim
     lighting, candles, nice music playing, a private dungeon—whatever works
     for you.

⊕   Touch. Start with nonsexual touch, and again, there should be no pressure
     for this touch to become sexual unless both partners want it. Massage
     each other, stroke arms, play with each other's hair, cuddle. Affection can
     help complete the stress cycle, letting your nervous system know you are
     safe and all the tigers are gone.

⊕   Accept your body as it is. I know this is by far easier said than done, but
     there's nothing like self-criticism to hit the brakes. See the next box for
     tips on improving your body image.

Sex is a form of unstructured adult play. It's at its best when we can relax and go with
the flow. Creativity is one of the manifestations of the erotic drive that flows through
us when we are in contact with our deepest emotions—and constant self-judgment
can really gum up that flow. In her book on female sexuality called *Vagina*, Naomi Wolf
argues that the right kinds of sexual experiences can improve the way we think. She
writes, "Sexual pleasure for women (and a society that lets women respect their own
desire) is indeed connected to women's ability to access certain kinds of creativity—
and to do less pedestrian thinking in general."[135] This could be because the right kind
of sexual stimulation quiets the cortex: that area of the brain responsible for judging,
counting, and self-criticism. During sexual arousal and orgasm, the self-conscious cortex
takes a little nap—just as it does when we are in a state of play or creative flow. When
dancing, writing, painting, or playing music, we focus in on what we're doing, our sense
of time disappears, and the boundaries between categories of things can soften, opening
up the possibility of new perspectives. Women's learned obsessions about beauty, Wolf
theorizes, prevent them from fully accessing their creative power:

> *Ever since I had looked at what I saw as the negative effect on women's minds*
> *of such mundane "tracking" activities as calorie counting, I had sensed that the*
> *reason so many tasks women are expected to do in society involve this kind of*
> *thinking (e.g. scanning, list making, judging themselves critically, "measuring*
> *up") had something to do with the suppressive effect this kind of thinking has on*
> *other, bolder kinds of intellectual or emotional leaps.*[136]

One of the things that makes me angriest about feeling fat (and its fun new corollary,
feeling old) is that I know it's a conditioned response related to not feeling good enough
and it distracts me from all sorts of more interesting things I could be thinking about. It
forces my attention to things like when I'm going to get to the gym next and how guilty
I should feel about eating cheese. It is mentally, emotionally, creatively, and financially

135   Wolf, Naomi. *Vagina: A New Biography*. New York, Ecco: An Imprint of Harper Collins Publishers (2013):
30.
136   Ibid.

oppressive. It makes me tired, poor, and boring. There are way more fun things to think about than all the ways I'm not good enough.

THE BEAUTY OF UGLINESS

It's easy enough to understand that we are taught to feel insecure so that companies can get rich off our anxieties. It's not so easy to turn it off, though. I admit it—I put three different creams on my face before I even get to the makeup (I'm in that delightful anti-aging/ anti-acne stage of my life). I'm working on it, though. Just as we need to practice pleasure, we need to practice self-love, no matter how much we weigh or how many wrinkles we have. Shifting a perspective isn't easy, but it's definitely possible.

Have you ever noticed those little signs that get put up on public bathroom mirrors that say, "You are beautiful"? I hate those. Firstly, because when we tell someone they are beautiful, we tend to mean that they fit into a very narrow set of characteristics: generally young, thin, white, and performing their gender in a way that is considered "appropriate." Secondly, the passive-aggressive bathroom mirror message insisting that (sight unseen) you're beautiful implies that if you weren't it wouldn't be okay.

I've often suspected that the impossibly narrow understanding of beauty in our culture comes at the expense of our deeper aesthetic instincts. We don't just have "types" that we tend to be attracted to, we are taught to eroticize the attributes our culture has decided are the right ones. Fashion magazines and advertising sell us images of ideal beauty that keep changing depending on what's for sale. Movies and TV shows teach us that sexiness exists only in rugged white men who don't express their feelings and young, big-breasted white women who don't have their own opinions.

This plays out in disturbing ways in the modern tendency to date—sometimes exclusively—online. Apps like Tinder and Bumble can help us meet people we otherwise wouldn't, and plenty of people find success with them. They also, however, exacerbate our tendency to objectify each other as we make quick judgments and either swipe right or left, indicating our interest or rejection based on a single photo. We treat online dating like online shopping, judging human beings based on just a few qualities, constantly looking for an upgrade, and simply discarding people when we become bored. People are shuffled into categories according to their erotic capital, which is made up of superficial things like facial symmetry, body size, height, and skin color. When we no longer feel like putting any work in, we simply stop responding to messages and never explain why, which is a phenomenon called "ghosting."

Racist undercurrents become blatant on online dating services, some of which allow users to filter their matches according to race. Statistically, Asian men are at the bottom of the list for users who date men, and black women are at the bottom for users who date women.[137] Asian women are at the top of the swipeable pile, but that comes

---

137 "Race and Attraction, 2009–2014." OkCupid. Sept 2014. https://theblog.okcupid.com/race-and-attraction-2009-2014-107dcbb4f060

with its own issues, as Asian women are often sexualized and infantilized, and it doesn't feel very good to be pursued simply because you're someone's fetish. The vast majority of online dating users probably aren't explicitly racist, but we live in a racist culture that subconsciously teaches us who to find attractive. We haven't been exposed to a wide variety of Asian guys starring as complex romantic leads or black women as cherished love interests in our most popular Hollywood movies. This is improving, but if you watch almost any movie from the '90s, which is the decade many of today's daters grew up with, it's kind of shocking that the number of people of color in these films hovers between zero and one, and if there is one, they tend to be loitering in the background, playing the role of the white romantic lead's sassy sidekick.

I don't think things have to be like that. I think human beings are actually quite good at seeing each other as human beings we might want to connect to. Sexiness and attraction are so much more than "types" and physical "preferences"—phrases that can act as euphemisms for racialized dating practices. I think we would all do well to let go of the idea that we have certain physical types, anyway. Life could be so much richer if we practiced seeing each other as whole, interesting, and attractive with all our differences and similarities. We might just have to get past treating online dating like online shopping and start swiping with a little bit more openmindedness or, you know, meeting people in person, where we will have a chance to get to know them before we judge them.

We have the capacity to see lots of different kinds of body types, skin colors, hair textures, and so on as attractive, especially when we like the human being in front of us. I'm aware that this is probably significantly easier for me to say than it might be for someone else, as I do fit a lot of our culture's beauty standards as a slim white woman. I do know, though, that people naturally become more attractive when we get to know them and find them interesting, sweet, kind, or funny. Even when we don't, though, there are so many ways a person can be delightful to look at even when they don't fit into our narrow cultural definition of "beautiful." I have always loved the look of an older woman with long, white hair. Whenever I see a woman in her thirties or forties sporting some cute haircut full of salt and pepper, she looks confident and clear about who she is, and those are incredibly attractive qualities. When I'm in my sixties and seventies, I want to emulate the older women I see who own their bright white hair. White hair should be seen as so much cooler than how it is generally seen, because you can't fake it—you have to earn your status as a silver fox. I started getting quite a few gray hairs in the stressful first years of running my business, and I'm proud of them. I worked hard for those little white strands! I don't want to cover them up. They are my wisdom highlights. Despite the time I admit I do spend scrutinizing my own, I like wrinkles, too. Crow's feet are my favorite. My friends who have them seem to smile more deeply and genuinely when the crinkles highlight their eyes. I also love birthmarks, crooked teeth, and when people have a chunk missing out of one eyebrow. These little quirks make them seem special in a sea of people all trying to look the same.

Another thing I've loved since I was a kid is stretch marks. When I tell other women this, they look at me like I'm crazy, but before I internalized all the crap out there about how women's bodies should be nothing but a flawless sheen, I always stared at stretch marks when I could see them and thought they looked like the coolest tattoos—like tiger stripes. I didn't know it when I was a little kid staring at my mom's thighs in admiration, but stretch marks are literally marks of growth. They are the scars that come with having a living human body, and every little kid knows scars are badass. They are literally proof we've grown. Our marks, wrinkles, and scars are awesome, no matter what the magazines say we need to buy to cover them up.

Now to be clear, I'm not trying to do the bathroom mirror thing where I convince you that everyone is beautiful no matter what they look like. I'm not. Ugliness is a thing, and if you feel that your stretch marks are ugly, I'm not going to tell you your feelings are wrong. You have every right to want to lose weight, wear a different shade of lipstick every day, or put Botox in your forehead. It's your body. The problem is that we've learned that being ugly is not okay—that as women, if we show signs of ugliness (especially related to age or fat), that means we have less value. We've learned that if our bodies dare to show that we've been through some shit, we are less worthy as people. That's the piece we have to work on. Body acceptance isn't about forcing yourself to see every aspect of yourself that you hate as beautiful. It's about seeing your ugliness for what it is and still believing that you are a human being worthy of love and respect.

Improving Body Image

Accepting and loving your body as it is doesn't happen overnight. It's a practice that takes time and patience and some willful ignorance of the external world, which is constantly trying to tell you you're not good enough. Here are a few tips:

⊞ Focus on your health, not your appearance. Exercise often, doing something you genuinely enjoy (walking, dancing, running, yoga, martial arts, whatever), and eat reasonably well. If you feel good on the inside, it's much less likely the negative thoughts will crop up about your outside.

⊞ When you look in the mirror and find yourself scrutinizing things you don't like, see if you can find one or two things you do like. Name those and focus on them. They can exist alongside the flaws.

⊞ Limit your consumption of products, environments, TV shows, and people that exacerbate negative feelings about your body. Women's magazines are major culprits, as are many TV shows—especially the commercial breaks. Refuse to talk about diet and weight with your friends. If they bring it up, change the subject. If you go to a gym or yoga studio with a lot of focus on image and losing weight, consider finding a more body positive spot to work out.

⊕   Curate your social media feeds to include more body positive material
and happy, interesting, and authentic people who look like you. There
are plenty of Instagram accounts, for example, that focus on body
acceptance, health at every size, and older women who love fashion.

⊕   Seek out movies and TV shows that star a diversity of bodies, skin colors,
and so on. There might not be a lot out there, but the more love you give
these projects, the bigger audience they will have, and the likelier more
will get made.

⊕   Limit your negative self-talk, at least out loud. It's hard to stop your
thoughts, but if you spend a lot of time talking about your diet or weight
or wrinkles, quit it. Shut your mouth and leave space to talk about other
more interesting things. Consider a verbal cleanse—no negative self-talk
(out loud) for a week or a month.

⊕   Compliment other people. Focus on the good qualities you see in your
friends, and make sure they know it—just don't get dragged into a cycle
where they complain about how ugly they are and you try to convince
them they are wrong. Tell them one true thing about their appearance
or personality, and then change the subject if they try to twist it around.

⊕   Consider honestly how much time and money you spend on beauty
routines. If they make you feel calm, relaxed, and confident, that's
great. But if they cause anxiety or insecurity, or if they cut into the time
and money that could be spent on more interesting pursuits, consider
cutting down.

⊕   Notice your thoughts about other people's bodies. Do you scrutinize your
partners or friends, looking for every flaw? If you do, it's likely you do it to
yourself. If you don't, keep that in mind when you worry about whether
or not your partners or friends are scrutinizing you. Work on seeing other
people as whole, including their flaws and ugliness, and it may become
easier to see yourself that way, too.

HUNGER AND FULLNESS AS A CONSENT PRACTICE

Hunger is a form of physical desire. It is something that we feel in our bodies, and when
we're healthy it's unambiguous. We can feel it right there in our stomachs. Fullness is
a physically felt aversion, an internally felt "no" or "stop" signal. Feeling and following
our hunger and fullness signals is a powerful way to practice consent within our own
bodies, to teach our nervous systems that our desires and our limits matter. If you've
been assaulted, though, these signals can get a little scrambled. For me, there is only
a subtle difference between nausea and hunger; I feel them in exactly the same place.
Sensations in the stomach might be hunger, or if there's stress it could be nervous
butterflies caused by the blood and energy leaving the digestive system in preparation

for fight or flight. In a way, hunger *is* a kind of anxiety. It's a low-level signal that we need to put food in our bodies *or we'll die*. Hunger has a relationship with survival. When we associate stomach sensations with fear, we get mixed up about hunger. My strategy is to avoid food in order to control the nausea/anxiety. Others eat and eat to keep the nauseous/anxious demons at bay. Both strategies are unconscious attempts to avoid discomfort at a physical and existential level. Food restriction and binge eating are opposite sides of the same coin.

For someone with anorexic tendencies, the work is to identify and feed genuine hunger. For someone with binging tendencies, the work is to identify and honor fullness signals. Food restricters need to work on their "yes." Bingers need to work on their "no." Most of us need a little of both. Honoring these internal signals is vitally important because sexual violation generally teaches us that our "yes" and "no" don't matter. Regardless of what we think about it consciously, our nervous systems don't forget. They don't believe our brains when we try to tell them we're safe and that it matters what we want and don't want. Honoring hunger and fullness signals is the most visceral way—literally, at the level of our viscera—to teach our nervous systems that our "yes" and "no" *do* matter. Eating can be a way to practice consent with ourselves.

Hunger, our internal "yes" to food, is controlled by the hormone ghrelin. Ghrelin gives you that empty feeling in your stomach, indicating that you need to fuel up. This hormone also prepares your body for digestion, so if you eat when you're hungry, the food tends to be better absorbed than if you eat when you're not. Leptin, the fullness hormone, lets us know that we've had enough and it's time to stop eating. It slows down the digestive processes so that any food we eat when we're already full won't be as easily digested. Sounds easy enough, right? Eat when you're hungry, stop when you're full. No problemo—at least not for those of us who have a clean, easy, anxiety-free relationship with food. Anyone here have that? Hello? Anyone?

In an ideal world, we'd all have access to plenty of healthy food and eat according to our internal signals. We'd all probably be at a healthy weight for our bodies (barring other medical issues), though our sizes would undoubtedly be quite varied—healthy weight can mean a lot of different things, and it's natural for there to be fluctuations at different times in our lives. In that same ideal world, we wouldn't push a particular body shape onto everyone and make them feel bad for deviating from that one shape. We'd eat just enough of our plentiful healthy food and dance around with glee in the diversity of our nourished, energetic, happy bodies.

Of course, that's not the world we live in. There are a lot of reasons our hunger and fullness signals can get mixed up. Overweight people tend to have a bit more leptin, the fullness hormone, in their systems as a natural way to try to rebalance. But leptin can be inhibited by lack of exercise or—you guessed it—stress. Underweight people tend to have more ghrelin in their systems, the hunger hormone, signaling that they need more calories. The body believes there is a shortage (which there might be), so it insists that we stay on the hunt until we find food. Unless, of course, we override the hunger signal with cigarettes, booze, anxiety, or sheer denial.

Unfortunately for dieters, losing weight too quickly tends to instigate increases in levels of the hunger hormone, because the body likes the status quo. Certain types of diets can backfire because they cause an overload of hunger signals, which exacerbates stress and the panic to find food, overriding fullness signals. Starving is stressful. I have a friend who was going through some extreme dieting practices for a while for health reasons, including short-term fasting, where she could only eat within a short window during the day. "My body doesn't trust me anymore," she told me. "It doesn't believe I'll feed it enough, so it never tells me to stop eating." She'd end up binging on forbidden grapes, one of the few "treats" her medical diet allowed, at eight in the evening, long after her eating window had closed. The fullness signal would never come no matter how many grapes she put in her mouth, because when you're starving and the only thing on the menu is grapes, then it will be as many grapes as your desperate maw can hold. Our bodies do not like to be denied when we are hungry. Resisting hunger, especially when we do actually have access to nutritious food, means resisting one of our basest survival instincts. It's not just that diets don't work, it's that when they insist on keeping us hungry, they become a mechanism of cruelty against our own instincts. Willpower doesn't stand a chance against the drive to survive.

Plenty of us have a long history of ignoring our hunger and fullness signals. When we ignore them long enough, they start ignoring us back—and fair enough. It's a bad sign when we stop feeling hungry altogether. It means we've taught our bodies that there's no point talking to us. It's pretty hard to feel safe when our own bodies can't trust us to feed them. The best and worst thing about our relationship with our own body, of course, is that we can never leave it, no matter how hard we try. This is one of those relationships we're going to have to work on, for better or for worse. The good news is that when we start implementing consistent, loving, consensual, nonjudgmental practices for encouraging the body to trust us and talk to us again, these signals can come back.

Coaxing Hunger and Fullness Signals

The digestive system needs food some of the time and rest some of the time. Digesting requires a lot of energy, and eating constantly can stress our systems because it redirects energy from other places (like our brains) to constantly deal with the incoming food. If for whatever reason your hunger and fullness signals don't talk to you, eating more mechanically for a while is vital. When the body understands that there will be nourishing food on a regular schedule, it can start trusting you again. Inviting your internal "yes" and "no" signals back can be a powerful form of healing. Everyone is different, and you may need to play around a little bit with what works for you, but here are some suggestions:

⊕   Eat breakfast, lunch, and dinner around the same times every day.

　　⊕　Snack moderately, if at all. Eat enough healthy whole foods at meals that you don't need to snack, but if you are hungry, eat something. Have healthy snacks with you if possible.

　　⊕　Leave four to five hours between meals so your system can rest, and try not to eat too late at night. There's a whole sweeping mechanism your stomach and intestines do to clear out larger particles and cleanse everything in your gut called the migrating motor complex (MMC). The gut needs a few hours with no calories incoming (water is fine) to perform this function properly, and if food is constantly coming in that function can become impaired and lead to bacterial imbalances and other issues.

　　⊕　Don't eat too close to bedtime. It's harder to sleep when your body is busy trying to digest, and the MMC prefers ten to twelve hours overnight to do its best work.

　　⊕　Watch out for processed sugar. It can make you crash and feel hungrier than you normally would.

　　⊕　Protein, fiber, and healthy fats tend to keep you full longer.

　　⊕　Be aware of portion control. It takes time for the body to acknowledge the food that's coming in, so try not to eat too fast. Wait ten minutes or so after you finish a meal to go back for more food. The fullness signal might come in that window.

　　⊕　Pay attention to how you feel as you go through this process. You may sometimes need to eat when you don't feel hungry or stop eating when you don't feel full because life happens. If you do get a strong hunger or fullness signal, follow it. Everyone is different, and it takes some time to get to know your body and its unique language. Trust your gut. With time, it will start to trust you, too.

THE GUT/BRAIN CONNECTION

Whether or not we're aware of it, our guts are already in an intimate relationship with our brains. It might be loving, contentious, or full-out dysfunctional, but it's intimate all the same. Our digestive tract has its own nervous system. The enteric nervous system is populated by fifty to a hundred million nerve cells—as many as your spinal cord. Your gut manufactures most of your body's supply of serotonin, which balances your mood as well as your gut function. Your gut and brain talk to each other, generally through the vagus nerve, creating what's known as the gut/brain axis. Some brain information moves down to the gut, but 90 percent of it goes the other way, up from the gut to the brain.[138] Mood disorders and gut problems are so frequently linked that doctors and researchers

---

138　　Mayer, Emeran. *The Mind-Gut Connection: How the Hidden Conversation Within Our Bodies Impacts our Mood, Our Choices, and Our Overall Health.* New York: Harperwave (2016): 66.

are now exploring using diet instead of or in addition to medication to treat conditions like anxiety and depression. In some cases, these mood disorders aren't psychological, they are caused by some imbalance in the digestive system. With the prevalence of the unhealthy Western diet, digestive imbalances are incredibly common: a 2013 survey revealed that 74 percent of US adults suffer from some form of digestive ailment lasting longer than six months.[139]

Our guts are certainly emotional beasts. They reflect everything we feel, manifesting each emotion with a kind of intestinal theatricality. Dr. Emeran Mayer explains in his book *The Mind-Gut Connection* that the last time you were angry, for example,

> *your intestines twisted and spit mucus and other digestive juices. A similar yet distinct pattern happens when you're anxious or upset. When you're depressed, your intestines hardly move at all. In fact, we now know that your gut mirrors every emotion that arises in your brain.[140]*

We do indeed literally have gut reactions. When something is going on that makes us feel we have to run from or fight a tiger, the intestines spasm and contract in an attempt to clear out whatever's in there. When we feel helpless against the tiger, the gut shuts down in a kind of Victorian swoon. Our brains interpret our external circumstances, which can cause our guts to react. Sometimes, however, the gut reacts to something internal, like poor diet or a bacterial imbalance, and that tells our brains something is wrong even when everything is fine. We might have digestive problems because we're anxious, or we might be anxious because we have digestive problems, and each issue may be exacerbating the other. There is a constant ongoing conversation between the gut and the brain.

My gut talks to me all the time. It has all sorts of opinions about which people I should be spending time with, whether a relationship is working, and which work environments are the right ones for me. It tells me right away when I've been pushing too hard or not resting enough, or when things feel out of my control. I'm a big believer in gut intuition, but only in the sense that my gut can tell me something about how I feel. It is absolutely not always in touch with reality. Having a sensitive anxiety response also means sometimes I feel unsafe when everything is just fine. In fact, sometimes I get nauseous when I'm excited or experiencing pleasure, which tells me that happiness makes me feel vulnerable. Doing anything out of my ordinary routine tends to make my anxiety spike—and if I let that stop me, I would live a very boring life.

I've also noticed that my gut sensitivity and anxiety levels are at their worst when I'm trying to change. Saying no, getting angry, standing up for my needs, pushing someone away who is hurting me—these things are extra hard because my anxiety-reducing strategies have always been to put my needs last and people-please until it kills me. The

139   "New Survey Reveals More than Half of Americans are Living with Gastrointestinal Symptoms and Not Seeking Care from a Doctor." Abbvie. Nov 6, 2013. https://news.abbvie.com/news/new-survey-reveals-more-than-half-americans-are-living-with-gastrointestinal-symptoms-and-not-seeking-care-from-doctor.htm
140   Mayer, Emeran. *The Mind-Gut Connection: How the Hidden Conversation Within Our Bodies Impacts our Mood, Our Choices, and Our Overall Health.* New York: Harperwave (2016): 31.

tiger, in this case, is the fear of being abandoned. Standing up for myself is scary, and when I do it my gut asks me why I'm trying to get myself eaten when I am inevitably abandoned in the forest full of tigers. Those are the moments when I have to thank my body for trying to protect me and then do what I'm going to do anyway. Breaking relationship patterns is incredibly hard because those patterns are usually there, at least on some level, in order to ease anxiety. The nervous system will fight change all the way—at least, until the benefits are clearly felt in the body and we continue to not get abandoned in the forest full of tigers.

Writing this book has made all my old symptoms flare—the nausea, the anxiety, the sensitive startle response, the ebb and flow of depression. Remembering and processing all these old stories and what they mean has triggered the alarm in my nervous system even though everything is okay right now. I know that telling my story might make me vulnerable to judgment. Talking about what happened breaks a stubborn code of silence around sexual violation. I might indeed be criticized, ignored, dismissed, or abandoned. I've been writing while feeling nauseated and with tears in my eyes, but also with the thrill of finally letting my story out of my body. I'm digesting what happened to me. The nausea tells me that I'm breaking a pattern and it's scary, but I know it's the right thing for me, whatever happens on the other side. Thank you, body, for trying to protect me. I'm going to do this anyway.

I used to think if I got good enough at understanding my gut's language, I could read minds or predict the future. I thought I had a crystal ball in my gut. Unfortunately, it does not work like that. I'm far too often awkward at parties to read minds, and if I could tell the future I'd certainly be richer than I am right now. No one has that kind of crystal ball, and it only exacerbates our anxiety to think we do. Besides, my intuition let me down when someone I completely trusted sexually assaulted me. Unquestionably part of my anxiety came from learning firsthand that the world is unpredictable and trusting someone doesn't prevent them from betraying you. I can't always tell whether the fire alarms in my stomach are useful intuitions, echoes from trauma, or signals that I'm actually moving toward positive change. All I can do is work on a loving relationship with the babble in my belly and keep using my brain as well as my gut to make the best choices I can as I go.

LOVING OUR GUT BUGS

All this internal intestinal gesticulation seems to be at least in part orchestrated by the community of tiny beasts that live inside our bodies, which is collectively called the microbiome. Taken together, all the little bugs that live on our skin, in our hair, and inside our digestive tracts make up about 90 percent of our DNA. Mayer writes:

> *This means only 10 percent of the cells in or on a human being are actually human. (If you include the body's red blood cells, this, number may be closer to 50 percent). If you put all your gut microbes together and shaped them into an*

organ, it would weigh between 2 and 6 pounds—on par with the brain, which weighs in at 2.6 pounds. Based on this comparison, some people have referred to the gut microbiota as a "forgotten organ."[141]

So when I talk about working on our relationship with food and our relationship with ourselves, part of what I mean is developing a loving, healthy relationship with all the little dudes lining our digestive tracts. When we feed them the food they like and not too much of the food they don't, when we garden our microbiome, taking care of the weeds and nourishing the good seeds, the garden bears fruit. When we starve our gut bugs or glut them on sugar and processed crap, they can make us anxious or depressed—even if nothing else is wrong in our lives. We have to understand that this interaction is a relationship—like any other relationship, it needs loving communication and patience. When there is a power dynamic, like when our so-called superior brain tries to will our gut to feel something other than what it feels, the gut will strike back as if to say, "Don't tell me what to do!"

We are not completely in control of our guts. We have to honor and care for them, talk to them, and treat them with kindness. Therapy is super helpful in dealing with our psychological disorders, but many of our mental problems originate in our nervous systems or hide in some spasmodic corner of our colons. The brain already knows we're safe, but the gut doesn't speak English. We need to explain to our bodies that we are okay in a language they can understand. The gut's language is food.

When we eat, we might think on a vaguely abstract level about how we are treating our bodies. But if we consider that our microbiome is a living, breathing, reproducing, dying, nonhuman "forgotten organ" inside of us, then maybe we should be thinking about how we eat as the only language we have to communicate with this friendly alien internal self.

Our microbiomes are as different as our fingerprints. They are shaped by whatever we first contacted as we burst through our mother's vagina or belly, how much dirt we ate as kids, how many times we've taken antibiotics in our lives, and what we eat on a daily basis. Our early emotional environments seem to also have an impact on our microbiomes. Now that we know that stress inhibits digestion, it makes sense that if every time you sat down at the dinner table, your parents were actively fighting or coldly ignoring each other, it would affect the way your nervous system relates to food. We might have really, really old patterns in our bellies for how food is received or rejected.

There is no one-size-fits-all diet that's going to work best for any one person. I know we all want a magic bullet, but it just is not a thing. Intermittent fasting, veganism, the Mediterranean diet, raw food, Atkins—there are millions of diets that exist out there for you to lose weight and live a long life, but no single one of them is guaranteed to work for any individual microbiome. If you find something that works, stick with it. But as far

141   Ibid, 17.

as the recent science is concerned, plain old common sense seems to hold court over nutritional best practices for the microbiome.

Eating healthy food on a regular schedule is a great idea, but it's not always possible when we're suffering. Binging, purging, and/or starvation might be the only way we can get through the day when we're having a flare-up. There's no need to feel shame about that—we've already talked about how helpful shame is for healing (that is, not helpful). Sometimes we have to acknowledge that we are in a bit of a pit and just do the best we can to eat reasonably well, get some kind of exercise, and keep surviving. Knowing something is good for us doesn't make it easy to do.

Still, though, developing healthy habits when we're feeling okay goes a long way toward preventing bad episodes and getting through them a little more easily when they hit. Basic self-care is both incredibly hard and absolutely vital when we're anxious or depressed. Just like we sometimes have to eat mechanically, sometimes we have to go through the motions of taking care of ourselves when we don't really want to. The best time to start working on our diet (and everything else) is when we're feeling good, so that when the inevitable stresses of life slam us, the kitchen will be full of healthy food and we'll have some good habits on autopilot. It takes a lot of energy to be in the pits, so it's a good idea to hand over some of the work to that autopilot.

In general, our forgotten organ likes diversity, fermented foods, and lots of plant fibers. It does not like a lot of sugar, fat, simple carbohydrates, or too much meat. This doesn't mean we have to cut these things out of our diet altogether—meat and dairy, so often vilified in health-nut circles, contain mood stabilizing vitamins and minerals that help some people. Cheese has actually been found to have morphine-like compounds called casomorphins in them that can actually reduce pain. Cheese is unquestionably a comfort food for me, and now I know why!

The Western diet is much too reliant on meat, however, and there are so many unethical and environmentally unsound practices in the meat and dairy industry that reducing our consumption of animal products is important for health and ethical reasons. The other thing about meat is that it tends to be expensive—especially the ethically sourced kind. Diet is in part a question of class. Not too long ago I bought a ridiculously priced two-dollar apple, and I noticed on my way home that a fast-food chain was offering an entire meal (which might as well be made of plastic) for less than that. It's much cheaper to eat crap, which means that people with fewer resources, especially if they already have mental health challenges, can't access the sort of food that might help them feel stronger and more capable of handling those challenges. It's no wonder we have a health crisis in North America: only the rich can afford to eat the food that will keep them well.

Feeding Your Gut Bugs

Everyone is different, and you may have to experiment for a while to find the right diet for your microbiome and your wallet. My mama always taught me that if you're going to spend money on anything, spend it on good food, and I agree with her. A healthy diet can go a long way toward reducing stress and improving mood, along with other benefits. Here are some general tips for feeding your microbiome.

- ⊕ Fiber: Your healthy gut bugs love plant fiber more than anything else. It's easy to add chia seeds, flaxseeds, wheat bran, etc. to your breakfast meal. They are easier to digest if they are ground. Add these things slowly—too much at once might overwhelm your system. Start with a sprinkle and slowly work your way up to a tablespoon or so. Beans have been associated with longer life, probably because of their fiber content. Slowly incorporate more of them into your diet. You can't eat too much fiber in general, but you can eat too much fiber all at once.

- ⊕ Soluble vs. insoluble fiber: Soluble fiber such as oats and psyllium can bulk up your intestinal contents and help the food stay in your body longer so you can actually digest it. Insoluble fiber, such as that found in wheat bran, vegetables, and whole grains, encourages food to move through your digestive tract, which is helpful if you tend toward constipation. Flaxseeds and chia seeds are great because they have both types of fiber, and most people benefit from a balance of both.

- ⊕ Water: drink lots of it, especially if you are upping your fiber. Add lemon and drink it before a meal to improve your stomach acid production and help you digest better.

- ⊕ Probiotic foods: Kefir, yogurt, kombucha, kimchi, and sauerkraut are probiotic foods which encourage healthy gut bugs. You can also take probiotic supplements, but diversity is important, so try to vary supplements with different probiotic whole foods.

- ⊕ Bacterial imbalances: Sometimes there's something deeper going on than just an imbalanced diet. If you have a lot of problems with digestion, you could have a condition like small intestine bacterial overgrowth, where healthy bacteria that are supposed to stay in the large intestine are in the small intestine instead. This condition is exacerbated by sugar, soluble fiber, and probiotic foods. Exocrine pancreatic insufficiency is a disorder of the pancreas that prevents proper digestion of fats, proteins, and carbohydrates. Many people don't talk to their doctors about these issues, and some doctors don't think to test for these conditions. If you have a lot of digestive problems, ask your doctor to test you for these and/or find a good naturopath to help you sort out what's going on.

⊕   Plant foods: Eat your fruits and vegetables, just like your mama told you—at every sitting if possible. There are so many ways to prepare them, there will be at least a couple of ways that you'll like them. Go for color: dark leafy greens, purple cabbage, bright orange butternut squash: they look great and tend to be full of vitamins and fiber.

⊕   Processed sugar: processed sugar might actually inhibit the healthy diversity of your microbiome. Again, you don't have to cut it out altogether, but reduce it if you eat it a lot. Try naturally occurring sweet snacks like dried fruit, which have the added benefit of being full of fiber and vitamin C.

⊕   Raw vs. cooked: Cooked food is easier to digest in general, but the cooking process can kill some nutrients. Cooking is like a form of external digestion, and our brains almost certainly wouldn't be as big as they are without the invention of cooking. Raw food takes more chewing and more work from the system to break down, but is likely to have more probiotic qualities. If you fry something to within an inch of its life, there won't be much left to nourish you with. Lightly steaming a vegetable is a great way to break down the food enough that it's easy to digest without losing its benefits. Play around with the ratio of raw to cooked in your diet and see what works for you.

⊕   Vegetarian/vegan diets: There are many reasons to reduce the meat, dairy, and eggs in your diet. If you make the switch, do your research: you will need to replace vital minerals and vitamins (especially iron and vitamin B12) that you'd normally get from animal products with alternative food sources and supplements.

INTUITIVE EATING

A little while ago, I was out with a friend at a local diner, looking at the menu. It had a lot of options and my friend didn't know what to get. "Well, ask your gut what it wants," I said. He looked at me like I was nuts.

"Um. What?"

"Yeah, just, like, look at the menu item, imagine the food, and then see if your gut says yes or no," I explained. I do this all the time. My gut is usually uncompromising with me and extremely clear on the yes/no signal when I offer up a menu image. Chicken salad? Nope, it's a little twinge of nausea. Soup and a vegetarian sandwich? Yup—salivation and nudge of hunger. "It's easy," I told my friend. "Just get what you want. Trust that your body knows what you need." This is intuitive eating.

"Okay then," he said, and paused for half a beat. "Chili fries it is." Chili fries it was. Sure enough, they were totally gross, and my friend started feeling sick before he could even finish eating them. So much for intuitive eating!

I blame the chili fries in this scenario (and my friend 100 percent blames me), but it wasn't the fault of intuitive eating. In the right context, listening to your body's natural cravings is a delicious way to tune in and trust your intuition. Part of it is about eating when we are hungry and stopping when we are full, but I do believe our bodies mostly know what we need and that we can follow our guts to good nutrition. Food cravings have gotten a bad rap: half the magazine covers at the grocery store give advice on how to stop them. I think there's a reason, though, that our guts send images to our brains of exactly which foods they want on certain days. In the right balance, food cravings can actually help us figure out what a healthy diet might look like for our unique bodies.

Here's my theory—and please keep in mind that I am not a scientist, so you have already been served your grain of salt (with the chili fries). Cravings are based on associations. Sugar, chocolate, fat, simple carbohydrates, and cheese, with its delicious casomorphins, make us feel good. They give us an immediate little spike of energy, pleasure, or a little mini morphine-like high. Food in general can calm our nervous systems because of its association with the feed-and-fuck/rest-and-digest state, so we may associate eating with feeling relaxed. If, on the other hand, we associate food with vulnerability, nausea, or stress, we might restrict food to manage anxiety. But these associations are all about what happens immediately after we eat. We don't often think to associate what we ate an hour ago with the sluggishness we're feeling now. Sugar highs usually come with a crash. High fat and carbohydrate foods can make us bloated and lethargic. Overeating to calm anxiety can make us feel sick and guilty later, and, in my experience, restricting food only exacerbates my anxiety in the long term (not to mention, you know, hair falling out, shutting down menstruation, and dying from starvation or whatever). So we have to practice associating our food choices and behaviors with how they affect us more holistically. We have to taste not only with our tongues, but with our guts, our brains, and our whole bodies.

If you start eating intuitively—eating whatever you want, whenever you want, in whatever quantity pleases you—the first thing you'll probably go for is sugar. Sugar, salt, and fat have addictive tendencies, and sugar, at least for me, is particularly insidious. My body does not do well when I eat a lot of sugar. It makes me feel sick, and then it makes me crave more and more sugar. Like the rest of our bodies, the microbiome will habituate to whatever we do. If we eat a lot of sugar, we're feeding the gut bugs that like sugar—including Candida albicans, a naturally occurring fungus that can overgrow, causing yeast infections and other problems. Just like in any other ecosystem, the organisms that have lots of food will tend to stay healthy, live longer, and produce more babies. Take away a food source, and you threaten the species that relies on that food. Consistently feeding your internal ecosystem with plant fibers, whole grains, and other healthy stuff will encourage the growth of the microorganisms that love those foods and reduce the population of the dudes that want to have a yeast party. Then the healthy bugs will get stronger and more populous and eventually start clamoring for kale and walnuts.

Even if you don't sit in front of a menu like I do and offer images of the food to your gut, you already eat intuitively to a degree. You know how sometimes you feel like spicy, rich food and sometimes you *really* don't? That's intuitive eating. When you ask someone, "What do you feel like having for lunch?" you're asking an intuitive eating question. Our cravings are there to keep our bodies in balance according to the ecosystem that's thriving in there. Humans need a huge diversity of vitamins and minerals to stay in optimal health. Eating the exact same thing every day, no matter how healthy, isn't ideal for a human body—that's why if you had tuna for lunch, you probably won't feel like eating tuna for dinner. Our guts are healthiest when we have a range of different kinds of bacteria that can digest a range of different kinds of foods. I crave red meat about once a month, usually right around my period, because my body needs to replenish my iron stores. If I eat red meat when I'm not craving it, on the other hand, I don't digest it very well. I crave yogurt if I haven't eaten it for a day because my body really needs those probiotics. I know I'm probably fighting the beginnings of a cold when I crave oranges because I need a little boost of vitamin C. And I crave cheese because, you know cheese. I think my body is very smart and it knows a lot about what I need in my diet.

The Language of Cravings

One way to get your cravings on your side is to try to feed your body what it really wants, thereby adjusting the dial on your cravings in a healthier direction. Here's what to do with the following cravings:

⊞   Sugar: Sugar gives you an immediate boost, so sugar cravings could mean that you are tired, sad, or just hungry—you might have low blood sugar. It might also be a cry from overabundant sugar-loving gut bugs. If you are hungry, eating anything will probably help. Taking a probiotic food like plain kefir, yogurt, or kombucha can help improve the balance between the sugar bugs and the others. If it's a what-should-I-do-with-my-hands craving, try a cup of coffee or tea instead—I find Earl Grey always hits my sweet tooth without actually being sweet.

⊞   Meat: Craving meat, especially red meat, probably means you need iron and/or vitamin B. If you don't eat meat, you can get iron from pumpkin seeds and dark leafy greens. The iron will be better absorbed if it's paired with a little vitamin C, so add a tomato or some bell pepper to the dish or drink a little lemon water on the side. Nutritional yeast is my favorite source for vitamin B: it has a mild but cheesy taste that you can add to almost anything. I like to put it on popcorn with a little butter.

⊕   Bread: Craving carbs is sometimes a call for comfort and sometimes means you need to fill yourself up in that stick-to-your-ribs kind of way. That usually means you need fiber. Whole grain bread is better than white, and you can also add a few chia seeds to whatever you're having as a snack. Carb cravings can also be related to mood, especially low serotonin. Whole grains, fish oil, and exercise can help with that.

⊕   Chocolate: Chocolate is delicious, but it is also rich in magnesium, which we can lose when we're under stress. Yogurt, bananas, nuts, seeds, avocados, and whole grains also have magnesium. It's common for many women to crave chocolate on their periods, which might be because periods are uncomfortable and chocolate tastes good. You might need a hug more than a bite of chocolate, but there is some evidence that chocolate can be good for you in small amounts—just watch the sugar content.

Intuitive eating works really well for me and makes me feel really good, unless I'm stressed. I know I'm anxious or depressed (or both) when I offer my gut menu items and it gives me nothing, like a little kid sulking with arms crossed in the corner. Hunger doesn't rise up until it's sudden, desperate, and a little nauseous. I wait too long to eat, so my body panics and then doesn't give me fullness signals because it doesn't know when its next meal is coming. Everything goes haywire. My gut is convinced there is a tiger in the room, and it is *not* interested in perusing the menu. I can't convince it otherwise. I need to find a way to feed myself while still honoring my internal "yes" and "no" signals when they come.

So I have to be gentle. I try to focus on healthy food prepared in a way that gives me pleasure. Reminding my body of the pleasure of eating food is one of the best ways to get me out of my restrictive eating spirals—so there are steamed greens, but you better believe they are buttered. The food is usually warm, which is more comforting and calming for me than, for example, cold raw salads. I lean on smoothies when I'm in this kind of mood, because I know I can throw some healthy things in there, but drinking my food is not as confronting as eating whole foods I have to look at and, you know, chew.

Do I sound neurotic yet? Well, I can't hide it from you. And I suspect I'm not alone. In fact, I'm pretty sure most of those crazy fad diets and cleanses out there provide a way for us to channel our neurotic disordered eating into socially acceptable avenues. There's nothing wrong with adjusting our diets with small, sustainable changes over time, but crash diets are just another way to punish ourselves for having a shameful human body. There might be benefits to some of these diets, especially if they help reset sugar cravings, for example, but for the most part they make us obsess about rules and calories to distract us from our existential pain. Diets that tell us some foods are "good" and others "evil"—as if food had some sort of moral intention—are a recipe (pun intended) for shame. And guess what shame does? It spikes our anxiety and makes us act out in even more extreme, guilt-ridden, and unhealthy ways. Add that to a culturally learned hatred of our bodies, and we become so busy and exhausted we can't lift a finger to change our lives in any positive way. Following the strict rules of a diet is basically just another way to try to please daddy, and daddy will *never be pleased.*

HOW TO EAT

All my old anxieties about love, trust, and relationships that came up after the sexual assault manifested themselves in my relationship to food. As I've gone through my recovery process and found ways to practice being in a kinder and gentler relationship with my body, the way I approach my food has changed a lot. Food used to be the place where I would put all my unconscious anger and anxiety, where I would punish myself without fully acknowledging that's what I was doing. As we've learned, the brain can talk to the nervous system, but the nervous system can also talk to the brain. Working on my food practices has been a fundamental way of healing my relationship with myself. I've found that my ability to digest and metabolize my food has a lot more to do with *how* I'm eating than what I'm eating.

I try not to restrict any specific thing in my diet unless I know it makes me sick or I have an allergy—and even this, I now know, can sometimes change with time. I do my best to try new things when I can and be open to new flavors and experiences with food, though this can certainly be a challenge to my anxiety and my desire to control absolutely everything in my environment. Knowing what I do about how strongly the gut reacts to emotional states, I've started to cultivate meal times as relaxing experiences. I try to put away my phone, I make sure I have enough time to eat, and I chew slowly enough to be able to taste my food. I am learning to respect my food and the gut bugs inside me that will be transforming that food into my body. I'm learning to cook more, and I've been having a lot of fun experimenting on my friends. The deal is that I'll feed them if they are kind to me as they taste the food I'm learning to cook. Oh, and they have to bring me wine.

I've been noticing lately that the toddlers in my life eat really differently from the adults. Give an adult a chocolate chip cookie, and it's gone in seconds. Give it to a toddler, and they take a bite and chew contemplatively, looking off into the distance as they experience the texture and flavor of this miraculous thing that's in their mouths. They want more, for sure, but they don't rush to swallow the whole thing. They stay with the experience of tasting and enjoying each bite before they reach for the next one. I'm trying to do that more, to chew like a contemplative toddler tasting for the first time (though I don't then throw the food on the floor as some of these little eaters like to do), and I eat far more slowly than I used to. I've also started making sure I have space between meals for my body to digest and for my system to do its internal cleansing mechanism, the migrating motor complex, before I snack for no reason. It feels good to let my system rest between meals so the rest of my body and my brain can do whatever they need to do. Taking that time gives me a chance to get hungry and then feed my desires.

For me, honoring my hunger and fullness cues is deeply related to my healing from sexual assault. I'm practicing consent with myself. I want to cultivate my body's ability to tell me what it wants and when and at what point I should stop. This isn't always obvious, and I don't always get it right, but it's a practice that I'm getting better at all the time. The more I cultivate relaxing routines with meals, the easier it is for my body to associate eating with calm and pleasure instead of anxiety and nausea. I'm aware of how lucky I am to be able to afford healthy food and a comfortable place in which to eat it, and I'm not going to take that for granted anymore. I'm learning to honor food and digestion not only as necessarily survival mechanisms, but as opportunities to experience desire and pleasure. Every meal is a chance to work on my relationship with myself.

Food Rules

There are plenty of food rules out there that I think are stupid or even dangerous, but there are four that I do follow religiously. They are:

- ⌗ Sit down. If there is food in your mouth, you're sitting down. It doesn't matter if it's a fancy meal or a handful of chips. Sit down and show that food some respect. It is literally about to become you. That food is a part of your body that hasn't been integrated yet: show yourself some respect.

- ⌗ Chew. Digestion starts in the mouth. Your stomach is powerful, but it doesn't have teeth. Saliva starts breaking down the food so your stomach can handle it. Enjoy your food. Give your brain's reward centers a chance to light up. Give your stomach time to know whether or not it's full so it can tell you when to stop eating. Put your utensils down between bites, chew, and taste your food.

- ⌗ Relax your belly. Lean back. Slow down. Soften your belly so it can receive the food you're giving it. Repattern the experience of eating into a stress-relieving ritual rather than something you're trying to quickly finish.

- ⌗ Forgive yourself when you break these rules. New habits are hard. Do the best you can, and be kind to yourself when life happens and you need to scarf an energy bar on the way to a meeting. The three preceding rules should help you relax and enjoy your food, so if they are causing you stress when you can't do them, let them go. We don't need shame in our food rules.

Intuitive eating, tasting with our whole bodies, improving our diets, sitting down and chewing—these are great practices, but they're not exactly easy. They require that we be present in our bodies, and that can make us feel our feelings. Our hunger and fullness signals may be buried pretty deep, but practicing kindness and slowness around food might help coax them back. When the body begins to trust us again, when eating becomes an opportunity for pleasure and listening to our internal signals rather than numbing out, we can teach the body that we care what it wants and doesn't want. We can change the way the nervous system responds to nourishment, pleasure, and maybe even love. We're cultivating safety in that most fundamental relationship—the one we have with ourselves.

Feeding ourselves is a fundamental survival skill, but it also means that we are able to take care of ourselves, to show ourselves love, to be kind to ourselves, no matter who we happen to be today. Developing kinder practices, including compassion for our binge/purge/restrict moments, helps us feel calmer, more self-sufficient, more able to nourish ourselves. When we can treat our food with respect, we treat ourselves with respect. We don't need to rely solely on our love relationships for care, validation, or security. We don't need to blame our others for starving us out, either. Filling our own love-starved bellies makes us feel that we have more time, energy, attention, and food to share with our others. Practice with food first—because the next step is sex. With another person. You'll need your calories.

SEX

It had been a bit of a rough summer. I was exploring the wild world of online dating, which was, predictably, a mess. One guy was bright on the first date and then drunk and morose while professing his undying love to me on the second. Another, a philosophy student according to his profile, confessed in person that he'd been kicked out of the program for beating someone up—oh, and that he had recently become homeless. One guy snapped at me at the end of a date to finish my drink because he wanted to go home. Plus, you never know when a dick pic is going to slide into your message folder and make you want to throw your phone across the room.

I started seeing one guy for a little while who seemed pretty normal. I had been trying out my new skills with him, of being honest about what I needed and asking for what I wanted, and encouraging him to do the same. After a couple of months of this, he disclosed that he had been sleeping with someone else without my knowledge. He explained that this new girl he was seeing was "softer" than me and that he felt more comfortable with her, so he wanted to end things with me. I mewled, "Oh, okay, I understand, no big deal." I hung up the phone with a stone in my stomach and hopped on my bike. About halfway to work, I started crying uncontrollably, pedaling like my life depended on it, my tears streaming into the wind. As usual, my anger took a little while to show up, but then there it was, ready to explain to me how my boundaries had been crossed.

Two things pissed me off (and neither of them were that I wanted to keep seeing him). Firstly, this dude had compromised my consent. I was sleeping with him under a certain set of expectations that we had clearly laid out together, and this made a difference as far as the form of birth control we were using, if not so much to the exclusivity clause. He'd had a million opportunities to tell me he was sleeping with other people but had neglected to mention anything until after he'd already put me at risk. He took away the choice I could have had to decide whether or not to keep sleeping with him while he was also with other people. I might have even said yes, but he took the option away. I imagine this is part of the reason infidelity can be so traumatic: you are with your partner under a given set of information and agreements, and when that person is with someone else without your knowledge, they put you at physical and emotional risk without your consent. It can impact your health, even your life. This part was massively triggering. This part was why I was struggling to pull myself together and slap a smile on my puffy red face before work.

The second thing that pissed me off was the implication that my practice of speaking up for my needs and inviting communication made me somehow hard or scary and that this "softer" woman was more suited to what he wanted. Many times I've been told some version of this by the men I was dating—that I was too smart, too ambitious, worked too hard, talked too much, that I needed to be quieter and smaller if I wanted to make a man feel like a man. I'll be honest with you—being present, intelligent, vulnerable, and willing to speak up does make it harder to get a date, at least if you're a woman who likes to date men. Society wants women to act a certain way, and a huge part of my healing has been about unlearning those lessons and insisting on being who I actually am. Our culture dehumanizes women, so people don't always like it when we act like we have human thoughts and feelings. It ain't easy in a world that wants women to be meek, quiet, and "soft."

Not long after that incident (fresh from my STI test, which came out clear), I was out with a friend at my local bar's trivia night. I was feeling extremely single, and I noticed a couple sitting near us, a reasonably attractive guy with a very pretty girl with about an inch of makeup on her face and a massive diamond ring on her finger. She was completely silent during the entire game of trivia until the question: "What's the main fruit ingredient in a Bellini?" She piped up in a kittenish baby voice, "Strawberries!" Her man patted her on the back and said, "Good guess, honey!" The right answer is peaches.

I stared at this girl out of the corner of my eye. I suspected she was a lot smarter than she seemed, playing the role she'd been given and doing it really well. And of course, if she wasn't, that's fine too. I'm sure she was lovely. Let me tell you, I was jealous. I turned to my friend and said, "See? That's what guys want. They don't want someone like me. They want someone who can't answer trivia questions and won't leave the house without seven layers of mascara. I'm never going to be like that girl." My friend commiserated but had no words of comfort for me. We'd both been rejected by men who felt threatened by our accomplishments and ability to answer trivia questions.

I was working on accepting this truth about life and the possibility that I would always be single when an old boyfriend showed up in town for a few days. We met up, had a few drinks, and felt the ten-year-old spark that was apparently still there. He loved hearing my stories and wistfully called me "the smartest woman I've ever dated"—something I was coming to believe was a liability. We spent the night together not only making love but cuddling, talking, and experiencing the kind of intimacy I had forgotten was possible in the deadlands of dating that year. In the morning, we went out for breakfast, and I was so nauseous I couldn't eat my bagel. The night before had been so fun and unexpected I hadn't had time to get nervous, but in the bright morning light, possibility and expectation weighed on me, complete with the specter of another soul-crushing relationship that would inevitably break my heart. I excused myself to barf, rinsed out my mouth, and then hugged him goodbye, trying not to ralph all over his jacket. The second he walked away, my stomach settled and I felt completely fine.

Ladies, gentlemen, and gender non-conforming individuals: let me introduce you to a little something called Dating Related Anxiety Illness, or DRAI (pronounced "*dry*," which is what your love life will be if you have it). This is not a real diagnosis but something my friend Emilee and I decided needed a name, because though it is not in the Diagnostic and Statistical Manual, it is most certainly a thing. Dating is scary enough on its own, but if you've been sexually assaulted, abused, cheated on, manipulated, or otherwise scarred by a past partner, physical and emotional intimacy is pretty much an entire forest full of hungry tigers. The brain understands there is a life-endangering threat (dating!) and tells the digestive system to eject its contents in preparation to fight or run away, which, as we learned in the last chapter, can cause stress barfing and diarrhea. Later, when I told this story to my French-Canadian friend, she pointed out that in French nausea is referred to as *mal au coeur*: heart-sickness. My heart was sick all right—sick in the back of a bagel shop bathroom.

The NPR show *Invisibilia* validated DRAI when they told the story of twenty-six-year-old Amelia, who was so plagued with anxieties on her dates that she'd throw up—once barely missing her date's shoes.[142] She traced the root of this affliction back to her first relationship with a woman who hated talking about feelings. Amelia learned to keep her emotions to herself, so all her anxieties would kind of get stuck inside her body until they were physically ejected. Similar romance-related stress-barfing stories have been told by men and women in *Cosmopolitan*,[143] the *Washington Post*,[144] Buzzfeed,[145] and countless message boards. Think of Stan on the show *South Park*, who upchucks every time the girl he likes walks into a room. DRAI is a thing.

Amelia discovered that if she spoke up about her emotions right away while on a date with a new woman, she'd be able to get words out instead of vomit. I've found a similar thing is true for me—the roiling in my stomach will usually settle if I say my fears out loud. This isn't always appropriate or a good idea—not everyone wants to talk about feelings, let alone sexual assault, on a third date. This might be one of the reasons some guys feel more comfortable with girls who are "softer," more baggage-free, and know how to keep their mouths shut (except to say, "Strawberries!" at the opportune moment).

It's okay that some people turn away from an honest expression of vulnerability. Knowing how I'm feeling and speaking up are essential practices for me to feel powerful in my life, and it is a fantastic way to weed out the wrong guys. I don't really want to be with someone who freezes at the sight of a feeling. I want a man who is secure enough in his masculinity to be willing to meet that vulnerability, and our culture doesn't teach guys to do that super well. For me, intimacy comes along with a willingness to be a bit uncomfortable in the service of growth. I want to be around people who are genuine, ethical, and able to think critically about their own reactions. I want, in the pit of my

142   *Invisibilia*. "High Voltage (Emotions Part Two)." NPR, June 1, 2017. https://www.npr.org/2017/06/01/530936928/emotions-part-two

143   Sepulveres, Danielle. "My Anxiety Makes Me Want to Throw Up on Dates." *Cosmopolitan*, August 21, 2017. https://www.cosmopolitan.com/sex-love/a12028878/anxiety-dating-stomach-issues-dating/

144   Possanza, Amelia. "I really like you. Now how do I keep myself from throwing up?" The Washington Post. Feb 3, 2017. https://www.washingtonpost.com/news/soloish/wp/2017/02/03/i-really-like-you-now-how-do-i-keep-myself-from-throwing-up/?noredirect=on&utm_term=.4b5e52a11654

145   Kassel, Matthew. "The Revolting Truth Of Dating Anxiety." Buzzfeed News. June 22, 2015.

stomach, to be able to face the uncomfortable brightness of true love with another person who is also committed to growth. I feel safer with people who can understand the existential nausea that comes with being a human being with tender organs. I'd much prefer intimacy and honesty to a huge diamond ring on my finger. Except, of course, that intimacy and honesty also sometimes make me want to barf.

So why do it? Why bother dating and having sex? It's all so scary, and, if you have DRAI, kind of disgusting. I've wondered this many times and have frequently taken myself out of the running to enjoy evenings alone with my dog. My dog is great. Intimacy is scary. But sex is also fun, and is in my opinion a really important step for healing from sexual assault.

Erotic energy (whether it's expressed physically or not) is a source of our internally felt power. At its heart, sexual assault makes us feel powerless, and that can close us off from the ability to access what Audre Lorde calls the erotic force, the ability to be in contact with our deepest feelings. We've learned to understand sex as an expression of "power over" in this culture, and that's certainly what it is in a context of assault. We do it to express domination over someone or to trade for something else, like security or validation. Being willing to experience sex as an expression of tenderness, pleasure, and intimacy requires that everyone involved feels powerful enough within themselves that they don't need to steal that power from anyone else. We can't control what other people do. We cannot protect ourselves from every dick pic headed our way. But we can cultivate our own inner strength enough so that we can authentically connect with another human being at the level of our own erotic force, which has the power to heal, protect, and empower us. Welcome to Step Seven: Sex.

SACRED SEXUAL ENERGY

Have you ever heard the joke about how sex is like pizza—when it's good, it's great, and when it's bad, it's still pretty good? It's a bad joke. There is a huge difference between good sex and bad sex. Bad sex, as you probably know from your own experience, can fuck your whole life up. Good sex, on the other hand, can heal the damage from all that bad sex (if you can keep the vomiting under control). We can try to convince ourselves all day that sex is fine and comfortable and easy, but our bodies will not believe us until they can have that experience in real time. The body does not forget—but it can learn new information.

After healing from sexual assault, sex has to change. Whatever your experience of sex before the assault and however it has affected your life, sex can never be the same again. Here's the good news: it can be *way better*.

As Audre Lorde argues, our sexual energy is related to a larger erotic energy in our lives. For Lorde, this erotic energy imbues every aspect of our lives, and when we are connected to it it makes us more powerful. Lorde warns, "Of course, women so empowered are dangerous. So we are taught to separate the erotic from most vital areas of our lives other than sex."[146] We don't have to channel this erotic energy toward sex if we don't want to. Celibacy can be a powerful and erotic expression of commitment to the self or some spiritual goal. There are phases in our lives where we are not having sex, and phases where we are not even remotely interested in sex. That doesn't mean our erotic energy has to go underground, it simply means we can channel it into another place, like caring for children, creating stuff, focusing on our work, spending time in nature, or even working on nonsexual intimacy with ourselves and our loved ones. This is the energy you can see in the interns on the TV show *Grey's Anatomy*. They put everything they had into long hours learning to become surgeons because that's where their passion was. They would drop anything to get into an operating room, and, when they left one, they would be feeling high, fulfilled, and so excited to do it again. Erotic energy isn't necessarily about sex. But if you do want to do it, sex can be a pretty direct way of tapping into this passionate life energy.

At its best, sex is playful, fun, and pleasurable. The people involved can relax, be themselves, and let sensation take over. Orgasm is the ultimate expression of surrender, of total abandon. We need to feel powerful enough in our lives and in our relationships that we can surrender into the experience of sex. Even if we haven't been sexually assaulted, many of us are so busy worrying about what we look like and how we're performing, it's a wonder any of us can relax enough to come at all, let alone have full-body, heart-shaking orgasms.

The way many of us have sex in this culture does not feed our erotic energy. Lorde sees our sex lives as having been pornified, by which she means disconnected from true emotional expression. She writes:

> **The erotic has often been misnamed by men and used against women. It has been made into the confused, the trivial, the psychotic, and plasticized sensation. For this reason, we have turned away from the exploration and consideration of the erotic as a source of power and information, confusing it with the pornographic. But pornography is a direct denial of the power of the erotic, for it represents the suppression of true feeling. Pornography emphasizes sensation without feeling.[147]**

Lorde's argument is, in part, based on the idea that the erotic is a resource within women that has been suppressed and repressed by men. And while I think that makes sense, I believe that men and other genders have also been cut off from this energy, and that we all have the same right to access it within ourselves. Sex has been pornified for all of us. It takes some work to reconnect to our own erotic power as an expression of our deepest, truest selves.

It's worth working toward something more. When we can relax and enjoy the sex we're having, our minds can open to more than just climax. In his book *O: An Intimate History of Orgasm*, Jonathan Margolis points out that during orgasm, "Both sexes may experience a burst of creative thought since orgasm produces a near lightning storm in

---

146   Lorde, Audre. *Sister Outsider: Essays and Speeches*. Berkeley: Crossing Press (2007): 55.
147   Ibid, 54.

the right, creative-thinking, side of the brain."[148] Vancouver sex and relationship coach Kim Anami adds that sexual flow is related not only to creativity but to financial power as well. She writes, "If you are feeling financially stuck, chances are that you are sexually stuck. Sexual energy is life force energy."[149] As mystical as this may sound, I do think it makes sense that when we're sexually connected, that probably means we're not overly stressed or in denial about anything in particular, which makes it a lot easier to come up with new ideas and focus on new avenues for our work. When we're traumatized, stressed, and/or exhausted, we're not going to have much at the end of the day for going deeper into our sexuality and our creativity or pushing for that promotion. Sex is so often cordoned off to a separate (shameful, silent) place in our society that we don't talk about the ways it relates to everything else, including our body image, our connectedness to nature, our art, each other, and even the ways we make money.

For many sexual assault survivors, sex is off the table. The constant stress created by the trauma keeps our brakes on all the time and prevents us from wanting to engage in an activity that requires us to let go. We must remain vigilant, and vigilance is not a friend to orgasm. Plenty of us avoid sex, mentally check out while we're doing it, or fake orgasms to get it over with. Some of us—perhaps the 10–20 percent of people for whom stress activates sexual desire—seek out sex, chasing after inappropriate partners or risky situations in a misplaced search for power. The orgasms that come from this kind of desperate desire tend to be shallow and plasticized, to paraphrase Audre Lorde. Even if we're in safe, committed partnerships and are able to come most of the time, we may still be miles away from the deep connection and surrender that our erotic energy could bring us. When we get into sex routines with our partners that are reasonably functional but lack deeper connection, sex therapist Ian Kerner points out, our orgasms can become "emotionally and creatively hollow, no better in qualitative terms than the sexual release each partner could have had on their own."[150] This kind of sex doesn't bring us closer to our own authentic feelings or help us access our erotic power. Whether or not stress ramps up desire, it always dampens pleasure. It makes it harder for us to feel. This kind of sex is about power, pleasing a partner, or getting it over with, not about surrender, intimacy, or connection. This, Kerner says, "is the world of the lonely orgasm."[151]

When we are sexually violated, our power is taken away. We don't feel we are in control of our own sexual field or anything else, and that can be a real turnoff. Sex researcher Lori Brotto points out that women are much likelier to have sexual problems if they are unemployed, didn't graduate from high school, or suffer from low mood, especially depression.[152] Populations that have limited access to things like high quality education and well-paid work are likely to feel less powerful in general. In a capitalist society, money is related to power, and knowing you can support yourself makes you feel

148   Margolis, Jonathan. *O: The Intimate History of the Orgasm.* New York: Grove Press (2004): 14.
149   Anami, Kim. "Sexual Flow = Financial Flow." kimanami.com. July 2012. https://kimanami.com/sexual-flow-financial-flow/
150   Kerner, Ian. *Passionista: The Empowered Woman's Guide to Pleasuring a Man.* New York: Collins (2008): 28.
151   Ibid.
152   Brotto, Lori. *Better Sex Through Mindfulness.* Vancouver, Greystone Books (2018): 20.

stronger, safer, and more effective in your life. Money stress is one of the central sources of instinctively experienced survival stress in our capitalist society. Great sex may improve our bank accounts, as Kim Anami conjectures, but perhaps we should reverse her logic: when we have enough money to feel we've conquered the capitalist tigers, we can relax enough to get turned on.

In general, men have more social power than women or other marginalized groups (and they usually have more money), but they are messed up in their own special ways. Psychologist Steve Bearman argues in his essay "Why Men Are So Obsessed with Sex" that in a patriarchal society that prevents men from fully accessing their vulnerability, sex becomes more important than perhaps it otherwise would be. Little boys are comforted and cuddled less than little girls, and then they are socialized to "take it like a man" and told that "boys don't cry." They are encouraged into ritualized competitive violence with their fellows in sports, which teaches them to disconnect from their bodies and harden themselves against physical pain so they can push harder. All this social training leaves men isolated and susceptible to sexual obsession. Bearman writes,

> *Directly and indirectly, we are handed sexuality as the one vehicle through which it might still be possible to express and experience essential aspects of our humanness that have been slowly and systematically conditioned out of us. Sex was, and is, presented as the road to real intimacy, complete closeness, as the arena in which it is okay to openly love, to be tender and vulnerable and yet remain safe, to not feel so deeply alone. Sex is the one place sensuality seems to be permissible, where we can be gentle with our own bodies and allow ourselves our overflowing passion. [...] This is why men are so obsessed with sex.[153]*

Heterosexual couples, then, can involve a woman who feels powerless and thus desireless, and a man who desperately wants sexual connection because he isn't allowed to feel his feelings anywhere else. He desperately craves it; she needs to know she can say no to it. Men are taught to pursue and push; women are taught their "no" doesn't matter. We are set up for sexual violence along gendered lines from the get-go. And still, straight women are hardly the only ones who are assaulted. Gay men and women and plenty of transgendered and nonbinary people have been through this, too, in many cases in even higher numbers. No wonder so many of us struggle with sexual issues. Sex is a minefield.

Don't barf; I have good news. Unlearning these cultural lessons can go a long way toward recovering the delightful healing possibilities of sexual intimacy. There are plenty of ways to empower ourselves and create the space for loving (sexy) intimacy with each other, whatever our gender or sexual orientation. That's why Sex is one of the last steps in our recovery journey—the previous steps have pretty much all been about finding ways to listen to our bodies, trust ourselves, and be brave in the face of our most uncomfortable feels. That makes us powerful within ourselves. When we feel powerful,

153   Bearman, Steve. "Why Men are So Obsessed with Sex." Interchange Counseling Institute. Feb 13, 2013. http://www.interchangecounseling.com/blog/why-men-are-so-obsessed-with-sex/

we can be sexually vulnerable. When we're not afraid to be vulnerable, we don't have to depend on sex to feel powerful.

SCHOOLS OF LOVE

Most of us don't start out with a great template for a healthy sexuality. Our fear and compartmentalization of sexuality is something we learn when we are very little kids. Our society places a great taboo on children's sexuality, which is likely motivated by our collective desire to protect our children from sexual violence. Fair enough—but shaming kids for having sexuality doesn't do anything to protect them from abusers. Children do have sexuality, and that's normal. It's not a mature sexuality in the sense that they want to have sex with another person, but in that they can feel their genitals and can experience weird pleasurable sensations "down there" that make them curious. It's natural for a kid to want to explore those sensations in their body, but when they are caught with their hands down their pants, some parents gasp in shock and immediately teach the child that "down there" is not a safe place for them to go. All that fear and anxiety hasn't stopped one in five girls and one in twenty boys from experiencing sexual violence in childhood.[154] That figure doesn't even include the many incidents that go unreported.

The fact that children have individual experiences of their own sexuality is an important thing to acknowledge because it's vital to maintain appropriate sexual boundaries with them. They need to know that no one has a right to their sexual bodies but them. Kids have excellent intuition about what kind of touch is good and what kind of touch is bad, and this is something a lot of us lose when we're taught to feel nothing but shame about our sexuality. When a child's sexual boundaries are violated by a caregiver, even when there's no overt sexual contact, children are not given a chance to take ownership over their own sexual bodies. They learn that boundary-crossing by adults is normal. They are taught to doubt their own intuitions. Teaching kids shame doesn't stop adults from taking advantage of them, but it might prevent the kids from getting help if something *is* wrong. Right out of the gate, many of us learn that sex is scary and unsafe, and it's pretty hard for us to figure out our relationship with our own sexual boundaries.

Even if we don't have any history of sexual abuse in childhood, most of us picked up some weird lessons about sex as kids—that is, if we talked about it at all. Then, freshly through the gates of puberty, we're supposed to somehow instinctively understand what we're supposed to do, how to be safe, how to treat each other, and how to communicate about what we want. Our only guidance comes from our equally confused peers, our awkward parents, the paltry sex education given in school, magazines, porn, or the wild world of the Internet. Needless to say, these schools of love tend to be somewhat lacking in useful information. If we're lucky, we learn a thing or two about condoms, but it's rare to be taught where the clitoris is on a vulva (or, ahem, what a vulva is). We

154   "Child Sexual Abuse Statistics." The National Center for Victims of Crime. Dec 2018. http://victimsofcrime.org/media/reporting-on-child-sexual-abuse/child-sexual-abuse-statistics

rarely learn anything about pleasure except vaguely that the penis goes in the vagina and everyone is supposed to like that. It's shocking how little the average adult knows about female anatomy. The full anatomical structure of the clitoris, which wraps around the vagina and extends deep into the body, was only discovered in 1998. I couldn't find an actual statistic on how many people out there think women pee out of their vaginas, but I can tell you that a quick Google search resulted in fourteen separate articles explaining that no, honey, women don't pee out of their vaginas. There's a whole separate hole for that.

Thanks to our good buddy Freud and his assertion that only immature women need clitoral stimulation to orgasm, there have been generations of heterosexual couples containing one unsatisfied woman and one very confused man. Our society has been much harder on homosexual people in general, of course, but they may have one advantage over their hetero neighbors: they are probably having better sex. When your sex life is not completely dominated by some cultural script of what sex is supposed to look like and how it's supposed to feel, you are free to play and actually enjoy the experience. In an interview with *HuffPost Live*, sex columnist Dan Savage points out that gay people may have better sex than straight people, because without a script telling them how it's supposed to go they have to actually communicate. When a straight couple goes to bed, everyone knows what's going to happen: once consent is obtained (ideally), penis enters vagina. "When two dudes go to bed together," Savage explains, "they get to yes, they get to consent, and that's the *beginning* of the conversation." Considering that 25–30 percent of gay men don't even have anal sex, straight people are confused about what's supposed to happen next. If there's no penetration, what do gay people *do*? "Well," Savage explains to this imaginary straight questioner, "we do all kinds of other fun stuff that you can do too that would really improve your sex life!"[155]

When we are stuck trying to play out a script of what we think sex is supposed to look like, we can miss out on plenty of fun. Even the straightest of us could benefit from queering up our sex a little, at least in terms of our willingness to experiment with a sex life beyond penis-in-vagina. More than one man I know who dates women has confessed to me that he learned all his first lessons about sex from porn, which caused a great deal of difficult unlearning when he finally came into contact with human women. One told me that he memorized a set of moves and simply went through them the first few times he had sex. "I don't think I felt anything those first few times," he explained. He only started to enjoy sex when he learned to let go of that performance, slow down, and actually be present with his partner.

When we can let go of those expectations, worlds can open up. We can touch all over our partner's body: people have many erogenous zones, including the nipples, ears, back of the neck, top of the shoulder, inner thighs, and so on, and everyone's zones are different. Trying to figure out what your partner responds to with a tongue, lips, or hands can be like a treasure hunt for hot spots. Skin to skin contact can feel amazing,

155   "Dan Savage: Why Gays are Better at Sex." HuffPost Live. Dec 2018. https://www.huffingtonpost.ca/entry/dan-savage-why-gays-are-better-at-sex_us_5b509ae5e4b01e373aabf5af

even if it's not genital contact. And genitals can be touched with hands, mouths, even breasts or thighs. Mouths can get so much pleasure from exploring another body, and so can hands. Genital-to-genital contact doesn't always have to be about penetration, either. Vulvas love to be touched in all kinds of ways, and there are many more nerve endings in the outer regions, in the clitoris and entrance of the vagina, than inside it where all that thrusting happens. Penises also have a range of sensitivity, with most of the nerve endings located around the head of the penis. There can be lots of pleasure without any penetration at all. Thrusting madly as they do in porn is not the most creative, nor the most effective, way to enjoy sexual contact with another person. It's certainly not the only way, anyway.

This emphasis on penis-in-vagina sex tyrannizes heterosexual couples who think that's the meaning and goal of sex. It makes me wonder if all those women out there suffering from low sexual desire are actually just having bad sex—especially considering the dearth of useful information straight men get from porn about female sexual response and what works for vaginas and vulvas. A major, large-scale British study called the National Survey of Sexual Attitudes and Lifestyles suggests that low desire affects a third of women (meaning, in this case, people with vaginas who self-identify as women).[156] The vagina doesn't have nearly as many nerve endings as the clitoris, which has around eight thousand—double the nerve endings of your average penis.[157] Science cannot come to an agreement about whether vaginal orgasms (from penetration alone) exist or not, but it seems that at most about 25–30 percent of women are able to achieve them. Some argue that women who do are probably orgasming because of stimulation to the internal branches of the clitoris, which wrap around the vaginal canal.

Penetration is not only the least likely way to make a woman orgasm, but for some of us, it hurts. Hormonal imbalances can cause sensitivity in some women at the introitus, the entrance of the vagina, causing pain and burning with penetration. This can happen to women who are on hormonal birth control, to postmenopausal women, and—you guessed it—to women who have experienced sexual violence.

Pain with penetration is treatable, but having it doesn't mean you have to stop having sex. It may simply mean you have to widen your definition of what "sex" means. People with vaginal pain usually have perfectly healthy clitorises, and if they want sexual intimacy, there are a million places to touch that don't hurt. Still, heterosexual sex is so focused on the act of penetration that anything else that we do involving the clitoris, the sure-thing orgasm generator for most women, is dismissively called "foreplay," as if it's an optional warmup leading to the main event. As sex therapist Ian Kerner puts it, "All of that scrumptious kissing, touching, stripping down, nibbling, teasing, and sucking—that's not foreplay. It's *coreplay*."[158]

It's not a bad idea to stimulate a woman's clitoris, even to give her an orgasm, before penetration occurs, if it's going to. When a woman is sufficiently aroused, her body

156   Brotto, Lori. *Better Sex Through Mindfulness*. Vancouver, Greystone Books (2018): 18.
157   Margolis, Jonathan. *O: The Intimate History of the Orgasm*. New York: Grove Press (2004): 11.
158   Kerner, Ian. *Passionista: The Empowered Woman's Guide to Pleasuring a Man*. New York: Collins (2008): 95–96.

is generally physically ready for penetration: she lubricates, and her vagina lengthens and expands. If she's penetrated before any of that happens, sex won't feel great, and it might even hurt. If sex feels bad or hurts, that creates a bad association and further dampens her interest in sex. Hot, fun orgasms, on the other hand, tend to make you want more hot, fun orgasms. It makes sense that twice as many women have low sexual desire than men, considering our definition of sex means penetration and penetration generally always feels good for a penis and only sometimes for a vagina. So yeah, maybe bad sex is still going to be pretty good if you have a penis. But if every slice of pizza you'd ever had tasted bad and hurt your insides, you'd probably stop ordering the pizza.

Pelvic Floor Breathing

Orgasm usually involves a contraction of the pelvic floor muscles, so it's a rhythmic pulse of tension and release. Tension during most sexual action is not a great sign, and being overly clenched can dampen our pleasure and our orgasms. Understandably, many people who have experienced assault carry a lot of tension in the pelvic floor, which can make it harder to orgasm. If sex is ever painful, it's even more likely that these muscles are overly tight, which can lead to a vicious cycle that exacerbates the pain. If you do have this issue, you may want to see a pelvic floor physiotherapist who can help you figure out exercises that will help.

Learning to breathe with your pelvic floor is a relaxing meditation practice that is calming, and it may help you stay present and relaxed while you are having sex (whatever genitals you have). Bonus—this practice is great for keeping your pelvic organs supported and preventing issues like prolapse or incontinence. It may also make your orgasms stronger, including into older age. You might also like to use this awareness to experiment with relaxing the pelvic floor during orgasm instead of tensing up—some people find this makes orgasm much more intense, and it is the beginning of a Tantric practice that can allow men to orgasm without ejaculating. Try this at home, but check with a doctor first if you have any medical issues, especially genital pain. For some people with tight pelvic floors, engaging these muscles can exacerbate the issue. If you're not sure, focus on the relaxation only, no tightening—and make an appointment with a pelvic floor physiotherapist:

⊕ Lie down on your back in a comfortable position with your knees bent and relax as much as you can. Begin to focus on your breath.

⊕ Your pelvic floor is a net of muscles that runs between your two sitting bones, your pubic bone, and your tailbone surrounding your genitals. It is a little bit like the breathing diaphragm: it expands and is pushed down as you inhale and draw air into your lungs, and it relaxes and moves upward as you exhale, pushing air out of your lungs. See if you can feel this rhythm around your genitals. If you have a lot of tightness or looseness here, you might not feel anything at first. Be patient and keep your awareness here.

⊞   Relax as you inhale, and then as you exhale, squeeze the pelvic floor
     muscles like you are trying to hold in your pee. Relax on the inhale, engage
     on the exhale. Repeat five times.

⊞   Now switch: relax on the exhale and engage these muscles on the inhale.
     Repeat five times.

⊞   Now relax as completely as you can on the inhale and the exhale. Stay for
     ten deep, relaxing breaths, allowing the pelvic floor to move and relax as
     much as possible.

SEXUAL RESPONSIVENESS

For a long time, female sexuality simply wasn't studied, and that's changing, which is a
good thing. Researchers are discovering that female sexuality is quite complex, much
more complex than we used to think. There is a danger here, however: the idea that
women's bodies are mysterious and complex leans into an old misogynist notion that
we're all witches doing nefarious things in secret corners (which...maybe we are!). It also
assumes that male sexuality is much simpler and more straightforward than is probably
true. The stereotype that women tend to have low sex drives and men always want it all
the time may not be anywhere close to true. As Kerner points out,

> *Contrary to cliches, it's been my experience in working with couples with*
> *mismatched libidos that the partner with the lower sex drive is often the guy, so*
> *much so that I would say that low male desire is a silent epidemic, with sex-*
> *starved women often suffering in confusion and silent desperation.*[159]

All humans have to negotiate the sometimes messy relationship between our genitals
and our brains, whatever our gender. Surveys bear out the stereotype that men always
want sex, but we must keep in mind that surveys are subjective and many people lie,
especially when they are asked embarrassing questions. Desire is a pretty subjective
thing to measure. Men may simply not want to admit that they have low desire.

It's important to remember that we are all more similar than we are different. As Emily
Nagoski stresses in her book *Come as You Are*, all humans are made up of the same
parts, we're just organized in different ways. Clitorises are a little like penises. Labia
are formed from the same fetal tissue that becomes testicles. The G-spot is made up
of essentially the same spongy material as the prostate, and stimulation of this area is
generally pretty intense and pleasurable whatever your genitals. We all have complex
brains and fluctuating hormones, and our subjective experiences can change a lot in
different phases of our lives. The information we're about to discuss is mostly based on
studies of cisgendered women (people born with vaginas who self-identify as women),
but plenty of it will carry over to people of any gender. Let's also keep in mind that no

---

159   Ibid, 29.

two individuals are the same, no matter how much they share in terms of genitals or gender identity.

We tend to think of sexual desire as a drive, a need that arises spontaneously that must be met or we'll suffer sexual frustration (or the great mythological blue balls). That's not true. Sex is not a drive nor a need. It doesn't crop up in our systems and make us go insane if we don't get it. We'll be just fine if we don't have sex, and we can live happy fulfilled lives without ever getting it on if we don't want to—though it's completely fair to want to.

Sexual desire may not be spontaneous at all. We may simply feel it in reaction to something sexy that we like as long as there's nothing else distracting us. Dr. Rosemary Basson is a sex researcher who argues that most of us are sitting around in a sexually neutral place, neither turned on nor off, until something about our internal or external environment changes.[160] If our sexual inhibition system (SIS) is activated, there are too many stressors or distractions to allow us to consider sex. The brakes are on. In order for sexual arousal to occur, we need the right context: a space that is relatively free of stressors and distractions. Add some appropriate sexual stimuli to the mix and we'll hit the sexual excitation system (SES): the accelerator.

Appropriate sexual stimulus means different things for different people. It might mean your partner looking sharp in a new outfit, the right kind of touch, or sexually relevant images. This causes arousal, which means your body prepares for sex physiologically, sending blood to the genitals. Penises become erect, and vaginas lubricate and expand (a phenomenon charmingly called "tenting"). If the SIS stays off (with no further stresses or distractions), *then* sexual desire can appear. If your partner is willing and all goes well, sexual contact can begin. If it doesn't, you'll be fine. No one ever died from not having sex.

The idea that our sex "drive" is a need, like hunger, is dangerous little piece of mythology. It implies that if someone wants sex (usually a male someone), they are entitled to get it at any cost. That's part of why we have such a problem with sexualized violence in our culture. Sexual desire matters, it's important and worthy of attention, but no one owes anyone sex. It's not a justification for cheating on a partner if you want sex and your monogamous partner doesn't (though that certainly might be an issue that needs attention in your relationship). It's completely reasonable to pursue sexual contact if you want to, but if you're not getting it, you'll really be okay. In fact, if you feel stressed because you feel like you really *should* want to have sex but you actually don't, maybe instead you could sit back, relax, focus on some other passions, and just be open to desire popping up when and if the right context comes along. Or maybe you're just not into it right now, and that's completely fine and normal. If you don't feel like having sex that much and there's no particular weight sitting on your brakes (if you're not also depressed, anxious, stressed, or have other health concerns), maybe there's nothing to fix. Erotic energy can move in a million ways, and it doesn't ever have to be about sex. It doesn't have to be about making babies, making art, or making money. It

160   Brotto, Lori. *Better Sex Through Mindfulness*. Vancouver, Greystone Books (2018): 98.

doesn't have to be anything in particular at all. Erotic energy isn't just about sex. Sex is not a need.

Connection, however, is a need. Humans need community, if not romantic partners, and intimate conversation and affectionate touch may be a part of that—though no one is entitled to anyone's affection, either. Women sometimes seek sex when what they really want is to be seen, heard, and valued. Many men have learned to channel all of their intimacy and connection needs into the sexual realm and are discouraged from asking for these needs to be met anywhere else. It makes sense that sex, the only zone sanctioned for connection and affection for men, can *feel* like a need. It's not. Rather than coerce someone into sex you think you deserve, maybe do a little therapy instead, okay, guys?

When we're free of the kind of stress that keeps our brakes on, we can hit the accelerator. Sometimes, the right kind of stimuli can take the form of a sort of "good" stress. Arousal can come with the thrill of getting caught, your partner lightly holding down your wrists, or a little bite in the right place. Novelty is a known sexual stimulator. A little danger can be fun when we know we're actually in control. As long as nothing hits the brakes (no sudden fear arising with sexual contact, no distracting thoughts of self-criticism, no worrying about whether you'll have time to pick up the dry cleaning), we will probably have a grand old time. Desire is not a random, spontaneous need that must be met, it's a natural and variable reaction to our internal and external environment.

SEXUAL NON-CONCORDANCE

Sexual desire, then, only happens *after* arousal: in the right context with the right sexual stimuli, the body will usually start to respond, and the mind may or may not follow. Low sexual desire could simply be a combination of too much stress and not enough of the right stimuli. It could also be an issue of communication between the body and the mind—your mind can get turned on while your body sits there quietly as if you're watching paint dry. On the other hand, your body might be gushing with lubrication while there is zero desire in your mind. That's a phenomenon called sexual non-concordance.

Sexual non-concordance basically means the body and the mind are not on the same page. This has been studied in laboratory settings where participants were fitted with a kind of pleasure-o-meter, either around the penis to measure hardness or inside the vagina to measure blood flow and lubrication. They were also given a dial to mark their subjective experience of sexual arousal and then shown a short erotic film. In general, men (people with penises; I don't believe any transgender or intersex people participated in these studies) tended to be more concordant—their penises went up with the dial. Women showed much less concordance, with many of them reporting little or no desire while their vaginal pleasure-o-meter went off the charts. Some have argued that this is because women lie or misinterpret their own experience, but Lori Brotto and Emily Nagoski (among others) agree that it's simply a normal phenomenon of the mind and body disagreeing.

Lori Brotto studies the effects of mindfulness on women's sexuality and has found that improving concordance by strengthening the flow of signals between the brain and the genitals may be a key treatment for low sexual desire. Men may tend to be more concordant because, from their earliest hard-ons, they learned to interpret the signal from their bodies to mean that they were turned on. They tend to associate erections with sexual excitement. It's harder to notice if you're lubricating or if your vagina is tenting—not to mention that many women have been taught to keep quiet about or ignore any sexual desire they do feel.

Brotto has noticed that, unsurprisingly, sexual assault survivors tend to have a high degree of non-concordance, especially if they experienced abuse in childhood. She writes:

> *As a result of previous sexual trauma, some women continue to dissociate during sex to protect themselves both physically and emotionally, as they learned to do during the abuse. Dissociation can continue later in the woman's life, when she is in a safe and consensual encounter, because the brain has "learned" to dissociate in response to sexual triggers.*[161]

Mentally and emotionally, a survivor in a consensual, safe encounter may very much want to be turned on, but her brain and body have learned that sex is scary. The heart is willing, but the nervous system is sitting in the corner with its arms crossed, brakes held to the floor.

For some of us, the opposite happens: the body responds when the mind wants to get the hell out of there. Having a sexual response during a coerced encounter can include lubrication, erection, pleasure, and even orgasm. Lubrication and vaginal tenting may be an instinctive response to sexually relevant information because they can help prevent injury and infection if penetration happens, whether it's wanted or not. Sexual response may be partly a physiological survival instinct.

The stress of a coerced encounter might very well shut down one's ability to feel pleasure, but not always. Pleasure is a physiological response, and the problem with coerced sex isn't just that it's painful or uncomfortable, which it may or may not be, it's that something is happening to a person's body without their consent. Sometimes our bodies betray us in these situations, and having a sexual response in a coerced encounter is a piece of shame that can stick like toilet paper to the bottom of our proverbial shoes.

This is one reason I feel a little frustrated when people try to separate rape from sex. I absolutely get the concept that rape is an act of domination, not an act of love. Sometimes rape is purely painful and terrifying and has nothing in common with the sexual act. For some of us, it might totally make sense to separate the two things. But

---

161   Ibid, 146.

for me, insisting that the one has nothing to do with the other only makes me feel confused and ashamed. So many of us experience rape, coercion, or other forms of assault with someone we trusted, even someone we've had consensual sex with in the past. These encounters may have been forced through emotional manipulation rather than physical force. This kind of rape is very different from a violent encounter brought on by a stranger holding a gun to our heads, but it's still rape—and it sure feels like sex. Implying that sexual violence has nothing to do with sex is unsettling for those of us who feel we were targeted in a sexual place. Sexual abuse is different than other kinds of abuse precisely because it is sexual. It has different effects. Usually it has consequences for the sex we *do* want to have.

Paul Gilmartin, host of the podcast *Mental Illness Happy Hour,* is a survivor of childhood covert incest, a type of abuse that consists of sexually inappropriate behavior from a caregiver that doesn't result in direct, physical sexual contact. Reflecting on his experiences with a sexually intrusive mother, he points out, "Even though the act of abusing a child isn't a sexual act—it's an act of really violence and anger and control—in the child's mind, it feels sexual." It causes a wound in a sexual place and makes it difficult to sexually connect later in life. Gilmartin explains how his patriarchal training played a role in preventing him from getting help:

> **There were so many times in my life where I would be having sex and I would just check out. There was a part of me that didn't want to be there, but I would say *You're a man! Every man wants to get laid!* That's what I would say in my head, and then I would blame myself.[162]**

If our bodies have responded during an assault or violation the way they always do when we have sex—with a physical "yes" while we struggled with an internal mental "no"—we don't just lose trust in potential sexual partners, we lose trust in our own bodies. That's a much more painful, shameful, and devastating betrayal than anything another person could do to us. If it's useful for a survivor to completely separate the abusive act from sex, that's completely fair. But many of us need to sort out a different knot of nuance: it's not that *sex* is wrong, it's that *abuse* is wrong.

If your body responded to a coerced sexual encounter, there is nothing wrong with you. It does not mean the coercion wasn't coercion. If you are dry as a bone or limp as a sock when you really want to be having sex with your partner, there may be something hitting the brake somewhere that needs to be discussed, or it might just be a quirk of your system. Your physical "no" does not mean you don't actually love or desire your partner. You can reach for the lube and/or try non-penetrative ways of being close and sexual with each other. Escape from the tyranny of penetrative sex! If, on the other hand, your partner is telling you that you must be turned on when they approach you because you're hard/lubricating when you're angry, upset, or just want to be left alone to watch *Real Housewives,* sit them down and give them a lecture on sexual non-concordance.

---

162   *I Survivor.* "Covert Affairs." Wondery, Oct 9, 2018. https://wondery.com/shows/i-survivor/

MINDFULNESS FOR BETTER SEX

The good news is that we can work on the relationship between the mind and the genitals just like we'd work on any relationship: with time, patience, and lots of loving communication. Lori Brotto's research shows that teaching survivors mindfulness practices, which largely include paying attention to body sensations, greatly improved their concordance over time. This, in turn, improved their sexual responsiveness.[163] If we understand sexual responsiveness as being—well, responsive, not spontaneous, we understand that mental desire arises only *after* physical arousal has already started happening. When we can get better at feeling our internal signals, we are more likely to notice when there's a little tingle down there, and then, if the context is right, that might help spark the desire for sex.

Mindfulness can help us sit with the vulnerability that sex inevitably brings to the fore. Just like with anger, pleasure, and food, if we want to get better at feeling things, we have to practice feeling them. There is nothing that can bring up emotion more intensely than sex. Sex can be a receptacle for our relationship anxieties, our expressions of love, and our desire to feel connected to our other, but it is also a physical, sensory experience. If we fear opening the floodgates of our feelings, we're not going to be able to be present with the pleasure, vulnerability, and unpredictability of having sex with another human being. We can physically do it, but if we're dissociating, waiting for it to be over with, or desperately fantasizing about anything other than what's actually happening, we're not really present. We're not tapping into our sexual energy as sacred or empowering. We're not really feeling much at all.

Genuine, honest, loving sex after sexual trauma means encountering our deepest emotions at the locus of our wound. The nervous system has sense memories of what happened to us, and sometimes it feels like those memories are just hiding out in our bodies, ready to be unleashed in a sudden rush of tears, shocking that poor unsuspecting one-night-stand. Learning to work with these emotions and sensations with kindness can help us be brave, relax, and stay present with our pleasure.

Mindfulness Meditation

For me, mindfulness is a practice of allowing my mind and body to get friendly with each other. It's like the time you spend with a best friend—you talk about your feelings, get to know each other, learn the ways you're similar, and respect the ways you're different. Mindfulness helps me know when I'm feeling exhausted, sick, angry, or even when I'm overreacting and need to cool down. It helps me sit with my shame and regret and pain and keep being kind to myself anyway. It helps me see myself as valuable and interesting—even when I'm being a pain in the ass.

---

163   Brotto, Lori. *Better Sex Through Mindfulness*. Vancouver, Greystone Books (2018): 147

There are only two main components of mindfulness: 1) Notice what's happening, and 2) Be kind to whatever that is. I practice mindfulness as a formal meditation for a few minutes every morning while the coffee is brewing, but you can do it on the bus, on your walk to work, or while lying down to relax. With time, you'll start applying mindfulness to everything: you'll get better at observing your body and mind and being kind to whatever's going on. Even a minute a day makes a difference. My ideal is ten minutes twice a day; some people do better with twenty. The point isn't how long you meditate, it's that you do it every day in some way that works for you. The meditation practice goes like this:

⊕   Get comfortable and take a few deep breaths. Relax your body.

⊕   Tune in to what you're physically feeling. You can do this by paying attention to the different sensations of inhaling and exhaling, or if you are in a public place, like on the bus, pay attention to how your body is responding to the images, sounds, and smells around you.

⊕   Try to notice the specific location of different sensations in your body, and relax those places if you can.

⊕   If emotions come up, try to feel them physically. If possible, name them in your mind. Don't try to fix or change anything, just relax around the physical sensation.

⊕   Notice if judgment, impatience, boredom, or frustration arise. Those are sensations, too. Notice them, relax around them, watch them change. Remind yourself to be kind—and even to be kind to yourself for being unkind to yourself. It's all okay, it's just where you're at today.

⊕   Thoughts will come and go. Observing your thoughts is a little more advanced than paying attention to body sensations. Don't push them away or hold onto them, just notice that you are thinking them, take a breath, and try to return to your body.

⊕   Your mind will wander to the past and the future and anywhere but here and now. That's normal and natural and totally okay. Just notice that whenever you can, and gently come back to focusing your attention on your breath and/or your body sensations. Keep doing your best to return to your body in the present, which can include thoughts, sensations, and emotions.

Mindfulness can help teach us how to stay present no matter what's going on, which is especially useful if sexual contact triggers dissociation. Dissociation can take the form of spectatoring, a phenomenon in which we watch ourselves having sex from a distance, judging our own cellulite or how squeaky our moans are or whatever instead of actively participating in the sexual contact. It can also take the form of distracting ourselves with the grocery list or a deadline coming up—anything but the here and now. It's helpful to catch ourselves doing this, but sometimes we think, "Shit! I'm spectatoring again! I'm so bad at this!" and then our self-judgment adds more stress, contributing to the cycle of pleasureless sex. When we practice mindfulness daily, we observe how thoughts and emotions come and go, and when we let them in rather than pushing them away, they tend to lose their power and dissolve. With mindfulness, you can notice that you are spectatoring or distracting yourself and just observe it: "Oh, look, I'm slipping out of the room here. That's okay." Take a breath and notice what else is going on. What do you feel in your body? Thoughts and sensations can exist side by side. Remember, you can't change your emotions, but you can choose where to put your attention. You don't have to push anything away, just try to redirect your focus to a sensation that you feel in your body. Relax that part of your body and breathe into it. Gently guide yourself back to the present and what you feel in your body.

For some of us, sexual contact might trigger specific memories, images, or emotions that relate to a sexual trauma. It's natural to want to avoid situations and scenarios that bring up bad memories, but sometimes these bad associations completely overtake our sexual experiences, blocking our enjoyment. Mindfulness can help with this, too. Let's say, for example, you have a bad association with someone touching your nipples in a sexual way, and any time a partner even accidentally brushes your nipples, you're brought right back to that one bad memory. Rather than keeping a Madonna-style cone bra on every time you have sex, you can let the emotion or memory arise. You can acknowledge it, say hello to it, and return to your body, neither holding onto the thought nor pushing it away. Shaming yourself for having the thought and trying to force it down only tends to make it more powerful. Rather, you can say, "Oh, look, there's that same old memory about my nipples. That makes me feel angry and scared and nauseous. That's okay. That's a part of my experience right now." Then you can take a breath and remind yourself that this danger is a past danger, not a present one. You can investigate what else is going on: "I am also taking a deep breath in my belly. I also feel my trusted partner's hand on my arm. That feels nice." Remember that you are in control and can stop if you want to—sex isn't exposure therapy. It's completely okay to let partners know that your nipples (or wherever) are a no-touch zone.

As we discussed in the chapter on pleasure, it's incredibly useful to allow nice sensations to exist alongside really gross ones. When the gross sensations become tolerable, we are able to get curious about what else is happening at the same time. Over time, the brain learns that we do not fear the intrusive memory and may start to associate the nipple touch with positive emotions as well—or at least allow it to become neutral enough that it doesn't interrupt our flow. The good associations can become more powerful than the negative ones over time. When we fear and avoid anything that might bring up our bad memories, those memories are in control of our experience. We don't need to use sex to actively bring up negative emotions or triggers, but if they are happening and affecting our ability to be present, we can work with them rather than avoiding sex altogether. When we let ourselves be fully present with these emotions with courage and kindness (and perhaps also discomfort), they have no more power over us.

This kind of mindfulness practice isn't always easy. It's best to try it first on our own without another person present. Masturbation meditation can teach us to be courageous about our sexual associations before we share our bodies with another person. Sex with another human being is undoubtedly going to bring up new thoughts, images, and associations, of course, so it's very important that we already feel safe enough in our own bodies before we try this with anyone else. It helps to trust a partner enough to be able to stop anytime we want to and for it to be okay if we dissolve in a pile of tears. It's confronting to allow these uncomfortable feelings to come into our sexual worlds, especially if we've been actively trying to keep them out for years or even decades. It might be awkward, scary, or nauseating the first few times, and that's totally okay, too. The key is really just to practice, to keep doing it, to teach the brain to redirect its focus. Don't expect everything to change the first time you try this. We're not going to be expert guitarists the first time we pick up the instrument. We have to practice. Mindfulness teaches us to be kind to ourselves (and capable of taking responsibility) no matter what is happening and no matter how other people react to us. It helps us be brave. When we're brave, we can access our pleasure.

SEXUAL HEALING

If you can get to sexual concordance, stop dissociating, and actually start having consensual sex that feels good, there are a whole bunch of other things that might or might not happen next. In her book *Vagina*, Naomi Wolf points to the way the pelvic nerves are differently organized for people with penises and people with vaginas. When Wolf discovered that a spinal compression was blocking part of her pelvic nerve structure, she found an explanation for why her orgasms had been feeling so different lately. She writes:

> *It still felt really good, but I increasingly did not experience sex as being incredibly emotionally meaningful. I wanted it physically—it was a hunger and a repletion—but I no longer experienced it in a poetic dimension; I no longer felt it as being vitally connected to everything else in my life. I had lost the rush of seeing the connections between things; instead, things seemed discrete and unrelated to me in a way that was atypical for me; and colors were just colors—they did not seem heightened after lovemaking any longer.*[164]

There isn't a lot of science on which branches of the pelvic nerve structures might give you poetic feelings, of course, but the pelvic nerves are important to sexual response, and they are different for everyone. They branch out from your sacrum and lower back vertebrae and connect into your clitoris, vagina, and cervix. Wolf's theory is that these nerves create a direct line from the pelvis to the parts of the brain that are related to creativity, connection, pleasure, and perhaps poetry. Nerve branches can run through and bundle up around different parts of a female pelvis, which might explain why some but not all women report the ability to have orgasms at their clitoris, vagina, cervix, rectum, and/or anus. Scientists have argued for decades about whether or not vaginal

---

164   Wolf, Naomi. *Vagina: A New Biography*. New York, Ecco (2013): 10.

orgasms exist, but the truth may simply be that they exist for women whose pelvic nerves branch there and they don't exist for women whose pelvic nerves don't. Wolf explains, "Among the many incredible things about your incredible pelvic nerve and its lovely multiple branches is that [...] *it is completely unique for every individual woman on earth—no two women are alike.*"[165]

So whatever ideas we may have in our heads about what's supposed to work for all women, it's worth getting to know your own body and communicating with any individual woman, if any, who you're trying to please. Some people with vaginas love deep, cervix-poking thrusts; others find that painful. Some love anal play, and for some it genuinely does nothing. Many can orgasm with lots of clitoral stimulation, but others find they are too sensitive for direct contact there. Insisting that *all* women can have cervical orgasms, for example, or that *no* women can just isn't true: probably some of them can and some of them can't, simply depending on where their pelvic nerves are.

Though penises may be more similarly structured to each other, no two men have exactly the same kind of sexual response, either. I'll admit to having known a few men in my day in the Biblical sense, and no single move or technique works the same way for any given two of them. Some guys love blow jobs, some genuinely don't. Some of them can only come from fast, hard, shallow penetration, some come from slow, deep thrusts. Some only come from oral sex. Some of them like teeth. Others hate that. It's anyone's guess what's going to happen when you get your pants off (or keep them on, do your thing). When we allow ourselves to be present with what we're actually experiencing rather than what we've been told we should experience, whole worlds can open up.

As beautiful as our unique orgasms are, we must also consider the afterglow (or aftermath) of deep, pleasurable, connected sex. Journalist Jonathan Margolis explains in his book on the topic that an orgasm releases a bunch of feel-good chemicals, including endorphins, that have been shown to have pain-relieving properties. Orgasms are especially good, apparently, for headaches and period cramps—so take those off your list of excuses not to have sex. The moment after orgasm, however, is another thing altogether. The feel-good high plummets, and sometimes there's a moment of sadness. Margolis writes that the "slight (yet slightly gratifying) feeling of loss, of emptiness and sadness—or of a minor death to the dramatically inclined—is for many people as much an integral part of the sexual climax as the preceding euphoric sensation."[166]

This is a common experience for me. I get struck by a sudden sense of loneliness or loss. Insecurity floods my brain after spending so much time in the uninhibited high of sex. Sometimes it feels like the gravity of everything that was stolen from me comes crashing down all in one moment. In her book *Women, Sex, and Addiction*, Charlotte Davis Kasl points out that the vulnerability of loving, connected sex can bring up almost intolerable grief. Kasl writes:

---

165   Ibid, 19.
166   Margolis, Jonathan. *O: The Intimate History of the Orgasm.* New York: Grove Press (2004): 72.

If a woman has a history of incest or sexual abuse, intimate sex may bring up the profound pain of that abuse, for intimate sex will give her the experience of being loved, as opposed to being used. This gives her a perspective on her past, and her rage and grief may come to the surface when the reality of the early betrayal is internally experienced in full force. This is, in part, why so many women who have been abused flee from potential partners who have a capacity to love them.[167]

It's not just that loving, connected sex might bring up memories of a painful past, it can also bring up feelings of loss for what *didn't* happen, for the love and connectedness that was stolen by the abuser. When this depressing moment comes up after sex, I have found that it helps a lot to let my partner hold me. I try to breathe. I use my mindfulness skills. The feeling pretty much always passes in a few minutes.

Men may be more vulnerable to this after-sex depression than women are, whether or not they have experienced abuse, but perhaps especially if they have a history of substance use disorders. Women don't have as intense of a refractory period after sex, which means many women can go ahead and have another orgasm within a few minutes of their first one. (The studies that I've read on this don't mention whether this is a quirk of anatomy or hormones, so I'm not sure how these gender differences would play out for a transgender person at different stages of their transition. There is some anecdotal evidence, however, that multiple orgasms are a function of hormones, not anatomy.[168]) Most men orgasm with ejaculation just once, and then the party is over. Dopamine is exhausted and prolactin is released, triggering his need to rest and sleep, while she's wide awake, wanting to talk or dance or take over the world. The sudden dip in dopamine can make men feel tired, grumpy, or depressed. Some men reach for a cigarette or a drink immediately after orgasm partly because their brains need an immediate hit of pleasure as their dopamine dips below their baseline.[169] This may hit men harder if they've had addictions, because addiction can affect the brain's ability to bounce back to baseline after a surge of pleasurable sensations.

In some Tantric worldviews, sexual energy is a kind of nectar called *ojas*. When a woman takes in her partner's semen, she takes in his *ojas*, his life force, as well. Women's *ojas*, on the other hand, is in their menstrual fluid, so a woman doesn't lose any of this energy when she orgasms. That's why one of the most famous techniques of Tantric sex is for a man to learn to orgasm without ejaculation, keeping his *ojas* to himself and letting him keep building his sexual energy with his partner, giving her as many orgasms as he can and keeping his own pleasure at a heightened plateau for a long time with no dip. This isn't scientific, of course, but it's intuitive to me and other women that I've spoken to who sleep with men that taking in a partner's ejaculation is incredibly energizing for us

167   Kasl, Charlotte Davis. *Women, Sex, and Addiction: A Search for Love and Power.* New York: Harper & Row Perennial Library (1990): 10.

168   Tourjée, Diana. "'I Was a Slave to Testosterone': How Sex Changes for Trans Women on Hormones." Broadly, Feb 18, 2016. https://broadly.vice.com/en_us/article/jpy7g7/i-was-a-slave-to-testosterone-how-sex-changes-for-trans-women-on-hormones

169   Thorpe, J.R. "What Happens To The Body After Orgasm? How Women & Men Experience Post-Coital Bliss Differently, According To Science." Bustle, August 25, 2015. https://www.bustle.com/articles/105437-what-happens-to-the-body-after-orgasm-how-women-men-experience-post-coital-bliss-differently-according

and completely depleting for the guys. The slight depression and exhaustion post-ejaculation for men is much more similar to how we feel at the end of our periods when we've bled out our eggs, and theoretically our energetic nectar with them. I had a yoga teacher once who pointed out that, just as a woman might need affection and gentle attention during her period, men need gentleness and as many hugs (or as few!) as they want right after ejaculation, when they are feeling their most vulnerable.

Everyone is different, of course, but, in a heterosexual coupling, it's good practice to focus on her orgasm first: one female orgasm doesn't have to end the game, and some women need more than one to feel fully satisfied. For him, though, it can be like a switch has been turned off after one orgasm: he is so done. Now's a good time for cuddling and rest—at least, if you like the person. Cuddling boosts oxytocin, the bonding chemical, for most human beings, and we're especially susceptible to oxytocin after orgasm.

Oxytocin is one of the great dangers of casual sex. The release of inhibitions and emotional vulnerability plus the ambient oxytocin makes us want to bond with our sexual partners even when we know we really shouldn't. Great sex is the *worst* for trying to keep someone at arm's length. It seems to activate a kind of chemical addiction response, no matter whether we actually like or respect the person we're sleeping with or not. Many of us have experienced that thing that happens when we try to break it off with a great lover who we know isn't right for us—we can't help going back for more. We get chemical benefits from hot sex with another human being that are really hard, if not impossible, to access on our own. Naomi Wolf argues that this phenomenon is a form of withdrawal: "If this is the person with the right touch to activate your unique neural network, *you will go into withdrawal* if he or she is not around to do this again, and ideally soon: actual, painful, real withdrawal."[170]

The good news about this, I think, is that it gives us at least one reason to stay connected with other human beings. These days, we need each other less and less for companionship, money, entertainment, security, or (lonely) orgasms. The Internet age can scratch almost any itch we can come up with. But sex with another human being is a unique opportunity to access sensations and emotions we can't get to alone. This is at least one reason to step away from the phone or computer and look into another human being's eyes once in a while.

DATING AFTER ASSAULT

Dating after assault is a bit of a mixed bag. It requires reading people quickly while managing the confusing messages coming from your own body and brain. Being with a new partner is always scary for me, but it sometimes helps if I talk to them about why. One good thing about all the news out there about sexual assault and violence against women is that it comes up in conversation all the time. I used to feel fearful or ashamed

170   Wolf, Naomi. *Vagina: A New Biography*. New York, Ecco (2013): 72.

to bring it up, like it was some sort of high-stress coming-out moment. Now, rather than anxiously 'fessing up and apologizing for my shameful existence, I can talk about what happened with what I've come to think of as survivor pride. It's not something I need to feel ashamed of having experienced, and I'm hardly alone in having gone through a sexual assault. At this point, I assume the person I'm talking to already knows several people who have been through it—whether they know it or not. When people ask Paul Gilmartin why he talks about his experience with covert incest so publicly on his podcast, he simply says that it is empowering for him, it helps other people, and pointedly, "It's not my shame to carry."[171]

When I tell a potential date that I've experienced sexual assault, their reaction generally tells me a lot. I learn about their compassion, their self-awareness, and how they engage with the news. Besides, I've been through something that has forced me to learn intimacy with my own body, to communicate more effectively, and to feel compassion and curiosity about whatever my partner might be feeling. I don't generally tell potential partners this at first, but a little secret perk is that all the hard work of recovery has made me a more present, more connected, and more consent-focused (read: better) lover.

In my experience, sex is also better with people who have been through their own experiences of recovery. My last partner had his own complicated history with sex, and he was the one that asked that we go slow at first. He kissed me very gently once on our third date and told me he wanted us to take our time. We waited months to have sex for the first time. It surprised me—not a lot of guys are like that in the Tinder age in my experience, and nothing could have charmed me more. It made me feel like he cared about who I was as a person. It allowed our experience of sex to be very emotional, very connected, and stabilized with an intention to communicate and invite trust.

A lot of us, especially men, are taught that women like to be pursued, chased at all costs. Especially if she's been assaulted, however, she might be more turned on by respect and listening. Space and communication are sexy, especially when there's a painful past involved. It's important that we be clear about our intentions, but pursuing someone can include respecting their space, listening to their words, and backing off when they say back off.

One night I was lying in bed with my lover, who was trying to initiate sex. I was exhausted and said I wasn't feeling up to it. He immediately stopped and threw his arm around me, and less than fifteen seconds later he was snoring. I was lying there worrying about whether it was okay that I had said no, while he was so content to switch gears he veered right into dreamland. That was one of those moments where I came to know I could trust him—it was pretty clear he didn't feel entitled to my body. While everyone wants to feel wanted and valued, it's very easy for the chase to feel predatory. If your date understands that you are listening and you will respect them if they say no, they are a thousand times likelier to want to have sex with you. Pressuring someone generally stresses them out, which will tend to hit their brakes. Don't do that.

---

171   *I Survivor.* "Covert Affairs." Wondery, Oct 9, 2018. https://wondery.com/shows/i-survivor/

For me, dating after assault requires something of a selection process. I want to get to know someone and build a little trust before I can have sex with them. To be clear, I'm not against casual sexual partners. They can be great, and there are times when maybe we do need to explore that question of whether or not we can get our power back by fucking the whole town and not caring what anyone has to say about it. Do you. But in my experience, a deeper sexual healing becomes possible with people with whom I can also create a loving, trusting bond. I don't think this necessarily has to fit into the standard model of a long-term monogamous romantic relationship, but I at least want to feel like I can talk to the person I'm having sex with. I want to make sure I can trust my partners to listen to my body language, back off when I push them away, laugh with me if something awkward happens, and hold me if I start to cry afterwards.

Then again, sometimes a one-night stand with a sweet guy who is leaving town the next day is the best kind of risk. Sometimes he gives you three orgasms, makes your bed in the morning, and leaves a bottle of wine at your house (true story). It's hard to tell right away who is going to be a devil and who is going to be an angel at these sexual crossroads.

RED, GREEN, AND YELLOW FLAGS

When you've been assaulted, especially by someone you trusted, it can be hard to listen to your intuition about potential partners. Intuition can be helpful, but it's important to remember that it generally comes from subconscious information gathered through experience. I think we often misunderstand intuition: we think it means we should go with what feels right and avoid what feels wrong. But what feels right is usually simply whatever is familiar, and what's familiar isn't always the best thing for us. If we always follow the most comfortable path, we will absolutely keep perpetuating whatever habits we're already in anyway.

Doing what feels right over and over can manifest in a lot of different ways. Maybe we seek out rescuers, people who will never hurt us and make us feel safe—but don't turn us on in the least. Maybe we're looking for people who will prove our belief that we'll always be rejected/abandoned/abused. Many of us get into relationships with completely unavailable people because it protects us from the unpredictability of genuine intimacy. Still others find any excuse to reject a potential partner and avoid intimacy altogether. If we are with someone who loves us and treats us with kindness, it can feel so unfamiliar it can make us want to run for the hills. It *feels* wrong.

Survivors usually have the added challenge of the occasional trauma trigger—something will happen in a relationship that reminds us of something horrible from our past, and we can feel as if we are right back in the traumatic experience. We're not able to tell the difference between a minor issue in the present and the major one from the past. I remember once asking a counselor how I was supposed to tell the difference between a useful intuition about the present moment and a triggered overreaction to the past. Her answer was something along the lines of "you just know." Let me tell you, that's a crap answer to the question. None of us "just know." No crystal balls in our guts, remember?

What has helped me with that question, though, is the concept of red, yellow, and green flags. Most of us are familiar with red flags—those moments when it becomes crystal clear to us (usually in hindsight) that a certain partner was wrong or unsafe for us. Usually our intuition will have piped up in that moment, trying to let us know something was wrong. Especially if we've been hurt by people we've trusted, however, we can get really confused about the signals we're getting. Little things that are no big deal can seem like major problems, while we can sail blindly right through huge, blinking red stop signs.

It's easier for me to know whether or not something is a red flag when I have a few green and yellow flags to compare it to. Yellow flags mean slow down: there's information coming in that I don't yet know how to interpret. For example, not too long ago, a partner snapped at me harshly out of nowhere. I was not able to divine whether this was just a symptom of pre-coffee morning crankiness or if he had some underlying violence within him that he was just waiting to unleash on me. Rather than panic and break up with him (or pretend it never happened), I filed it away to see if more moments like that would crop up or if I simply needed to learn to leave him alone until after he'd had his coffee. Yellow flags are signals that tell me to wait and gather more information (as long as I'm not physically in danger). I can also compare them with my green flags.

Green flags are moments when I feel safe with a partner. They are indications that I can trust this person, that they have compassion and care for me, that they are interested in meeting my needs. In previous relationships, I'd been so on guard for danger that I'd forget to notice the good things that were happening in the relationship. It's easy for me to see a partner, especially if he's male, as an enemy who is secretly trying to destroy me (hey, it's happened before). So in order to stay present with the actual human being in front of me, I need to pay attention to the good things that are happening while making sure I'm not blinding myself to the bad things.

In the process of writing this chapter, I thought I'd reach out to my community and ask around a little bit about other people's practices with red and green flags. Asking about red flags was interesting: the women I know who date men had plenty of examples to share from their experience. They mentioned everything from calling his ex-girlfriends crazy to "he has Nazi regalia at his house." Everyone's red flags are different, because they are often about shared values, but there were a few themes that came out for the women who date men. First, there was physical safety. If he acts aggressive or violent, if he gets mad if she tries to cancel, if he rushes through the date to try to get to the sex part (and then "asks to use the bathroom after he walks you home" in an attempt to get into her house), if he tries to isolate her from her friends and family, if he doesn't respect her boundaries, if "he has a tattoo of Red Riding Hood being eaten by the wolf": these are all things that make a gal worry she's going to get raped or murdered. A secondary theme was behaviors that indicate internalized misogyny or a lack of respect for women in general, such as talking over her, interrupting her, denigrating her interests, or feeling uncomfortable with her successes or work ambition ("He told me I'd be one of the prettiest girls in the coffee shop if I wasn't concentrating so hard on my work"). A few women warned against men who are passionate fans of misogynist artists like Charles Bukowski, Lars Von Trier, or Quentin Tarantino. There's nothing wrong with liking these artists, of course, but when their work portrays a massive amount of violence against women and the guy you're trying to date can't stop talking about how much he loves the stuff, it can send a little chill down your spine.

Men who date women had less to say on the matter. It seemed they hadn't thought about it as much as the women had. Heartbroken women are often told they pick the wrong guys, that they need to get better at somehow predicting who is going to hurt them. Women spend a lot of time analyzing what went wrong and how to protect themselves from going through it again. Men, on the other hand, seem to simply move on as quickly as they can and avoid processing the experience too much. I can't think of a single time I've heard someone say, "He needs to get better at choosing his girlfriends" when a man's heterosexual relationship falls apart. Women are trained to blame themselves for whatever goes wrong in our lives, and men are trained *not* to think too reflexively about anything that has to do with their feelings.

That being said, several people, including a few of the men, had some thoughtful responses about red flags that would apply to any gender or sexuality. Being late all the time is "a sign that they've accepted a selfish behavior as okay for them and are not motivated to trying to be a better version of themselves." Treating others as disposable, for example, by consistently ghosting others, was a red flag, as were racialized dating behaviors, especially white men who only date Asian women.

Asking what behaviors people took as green flags was its own interesting experiment. More than one person said, "I have no idea," and another, a little chagrined, suggested, "the absence of red flags?" One man named how the whole thing tends to go down for him: "When looking at my dating history, it's mostly Q: did we make out once? A: yes; let us now date for three or more years." Beyond that, people looked for kindness to wait staff, panhandlers, and/or animals to show that they had compassion and consideration for others. Lots of people agreed it was a good sign if someone has friends of varying genders and is on reasonably good terms with their exes. More than one woman said, "He asks questions about me!" which seems like kind of a low bar, really (though perhaps not as low as, "They own more than one pair of pants and work for a living"). In one of his red flags, my friend Ryan wrote, "They talk more about what they don't want than what they do want," which might be something we are all doing a little too much of, considering how much more weight we seem to give red flags than green.

Survivors tend to either overreact or underreact with our fear responses. It's so hard to understand the nuances of our gut intuitions that we often end up either doing what someone else wants us to do (including when we are on a date with that someone else) or else we override our desire to connect and fall back on self-isolation. Red, green, and yellow flags are one way that we can actively engage with our intuitive responses and try to make better choices for ourselves when selecting partners. No relationship is perfect, but some are better than others. Keeping our flags color coded can help keep us rational and conscious about what's going on rather than blissfully ignoring all the warning signs or pushing away perfectly good partners because we're too terrified to see anything *but* warning signs.

At the same time, though, perfectly color coding our flags isn't going to protect us from ever getting hurt again. When we date, when we open ourselves to new experiences, when we—god forbid—let ourselves be vulnerable, we are taking a risk. It takes a long time to get to know someone, and if we are abused or betrayed or brokenhearted at the end of any relationship, it isn't our fault—even if the way was paved with bright flashing red flags we really wish we'd noticed at the time. We can learn from our experiences and try to do better next time, of course, but sometimes people are just assholes, and trust can't be completely contained to a list of flags, no matter how nuanced their colors.

CODEPENDENCY

One of the reasons it's so difficult to decipher red flags when it comes to sex and relationships is because we've all been conditioned to use sex as a tool to get what we want rather than as a genuine expression of intimacy. In her book *Women, Sex, and Addiction*, Charlotte Davis Kasl explains that sex addiction usually arises when someone is using sex to meet some other need, like security, comfort, or power. She writes:

> *When sex is separated from love and care, it can become addictive. Rather than bringing us close to someone, it becomes a block to intimacy. [...] Addictive sex does not open up feelings but is carried out in an attempt to hide them.*[172]

For Kasl, codependency is the opposite side of the sex addiction coin. It means we create our sense of self from our relationships, define ourselves by our lovers, and overfocus on our lovers' or families' needs at the expense of our own. Codependency is a dysfunctional pattern in relationships where the codependent person is "someone whose core identity is undeveloped or unknown, and who maintains a false identity built from dependent attachments to external sources—a partner, a spouse, family, appearances, work, or rules."[173]

It's very common for people with addictions to partner with people who have codependent patterns. I'd never thought of myself as codependent until I read Kasl's book and noticed my own tendency to get into relationships with people who are struggling with mental health issues: they take up so much energy in the relationship I never have to deal with my own shit. I didn't realize I was avoiding myself by overfocusing on my partners. I'm not alone: for Kasl, codependency is "women's basic programming."[174] She argues that women are taught to relinquish our power by taking

---

172   Kasl, Charlotte Davis. *Women, Sex, and Addiction: A Search for Love and Power.* New York: Harper & Row Perennial Library (1990): 10.
173   Ibid, 31.
174   Ibid.

care of everyone but our own selves. Sex is one of the few places we can wrangle a little power, so we end up in dysfunctional power struggles with our romantic others that often play out in the bedroom. Kasl goes on to say:

> *Think of the stereotypical female and how people praise her: She never thinks of herself. She is a devoted mother. She'd do anything for you. She is a saint. She always puts her husband first. She is patient, kind, and never complains. What her admirers omit is that she probably acts like an angel out of fear: fear people won't like her; fear of financial insecurity; fear her partner will leave her, fear of a fight. Notice that no mention is made of what she feels like inside. That's because to fill this role, you aren't allowed to feel inside; you have to be nice all the time.*[175]

It's not possible to enter into a vulnerable, loving, intimate sexual connection with another human being when you're too busy being *nice*.

Codependency is terrible for our sex lives. It essentially means that we trade our deepest internal feelings—our erotic force—for security, safety, or power. We can't ask for what we want, set boundaries, or be fully present with our pleasure when we feel it might get us abandoned in the forest with a pack of tigers. Indeed, changing these patterns can be terrifying. Kasl writes:

> *If the woman embarks on a course of recovery, she initially experiences profound guilt and shame as the primary symptoms of withdrawal. She feels awful if she says no to sex with her partner or to listening to her mother complain on the phone for half an hour. She thinks she is selfish, whiny, and fussy if she starts asking for what she wants, sexually and otherwise. She has an immense fear of abandonment. She is afraid of rejection and retribution every time she says I want, I feel, or I think. She also starts to have fleeting moments when she feels a surge of power within her as she takes on an identity that belongs solely to her. Her fear abates and her body starts to relax as she discovers herself and lives more in tune with her inner truth.*[176]

Feeling feelings isn't just hard because it's kind of uncomfortable. It's because our culture has taught us to feel shame when our feelings don't match the personality we've been taught we should have. Our closest people resist change in us at the best of times, but they especially hate it if the person who usually takes care of everyone else suddenly decides to stand her ground and ask for what she wants. Recovering from our social conditioning isn't easy, but it's worthy labor. We must take responsibility for the ways we've let ourselves down and work on building a self that belongs only to us.

Building a secure sense of self ain't easy, so many of us try to seek safety in other ways. "Safe" can mean a lot of different things. Maybe we're trying to get safety by having horrible sex and faking orgasms so that our partner sticks around to help pay for the kids' braces. Maybe we're trying to get safety by committing to someone we don't

---

175   Ibid, 35.
176   Ibid, 37.

respect who never asks anything of us, so we never have to be vulnerable with them. Maybe we feel safe when we only fuck unavailable jerks who we know won't threaten us with a real relationship. These are false forms of safety that often end up hurting us much more than our own vulnerability would. The truth is, when it comes to sex and relationships, there's no possible true, unassailable way to be "safe." No one can promise you'll always be safe with them, and there are no truly, unvaryingly safe spaces. The good news is, though, we can learn to cultivate trust with one person: ourselves. We can work on learning who we are, what matters to us, how to stand up for our needs, and how to take care of ourselves when other people continue to be unpredictable assholes. These are all better ways to feel powerful than committing to a life of bad sex.

True connection requires that we let go of these false versions of safety. Desire feeds on feelings of uncertainty and mystery, and those things can only be sustained in a partnership where both individuals have a secure enough sense of self that they can tolerate a little unpredictability. When two people are so enmeshed in each others' lives that they have no separate identities, they've crushed any possible attractive force. Cultivating a self separate from your partner might be the most erotic thing you can do in a long-term relationship. If you want to want your partner, get the hell away from them from time to time. Space is sexy. Codependency is not.

DESIRE AND AFFAIRS

Sometimes, when people feel lost in a relationship, they rebel by having an affair. Codependency can feel like a trap where one's erotic self is suffocated in the mundane realities of making lunches and changing diapers, and affairs can represent an escape route. It's not just that an affair is exciting and novel, it's that an illicit lover can provide a glimpse of a self you used to be or could have been if your life had taken a different direction. In her book on infidelity called *The State of Affairs*, psychologist Esther Perel writes:

> *Sometimes when we seek the gaze of another, it isn't our partner we're turning away from, but the person we have become. We are not looking for another lover so much as another version of ourselves.*[177]

This is one type of infidelity, which Perel calls the affair of "self discovery."[178] I have a feeling some version of infidelity may be a very common (if life-exploding) experiment for those of us who have experienced sexual violation.

For one thing, we need to feel safe to heal and we need to feel safe to feel desire. Paradoxically, affairs, which are dangerous by nature, are a very specific kind of safe. In a culture that has generally taught women to be codependent, we are set up to surrender our bodies and everything else to our partnerships. We are surrounded by men who have been conditioned to feel entitled to women's bodies—especially if they

177   Perel, Esther. *The State of Affairs: Rethinking Infidelity.* New York: Harper (2017): 156.
178   Ibid, 155.

are in a romantic relationship with those women. Marital rape was only outlawed in all fifty states in the US in 1993. Monogamy is the cultural standard, and marriage is the institution that sanctions it (at least for heterosexual couples, though this is increasingly the case for everyone else as same-sex marriage has been legalized). Having an affair is a powerful way for a woman to reclaim ownership over a body that has been suppressed and repressed by her culture, her perpetrator, and the institution of marriage—even if her husband is a really good dude. Perel points out, "When a woman struggles to stay connected to herself, an affair is often a venue for self-reclamation. [...] When you have an affair, you know for a fact that you're not doing it to take care of anyone else."[179] This reminds me of how I feel when, once in a blue moon, I have a cigarette: literally no one wants me to light up, so if I'm doing it, I am 100 percent sure I'm making my own choice about my body. In a culture that's always telling me my body doesn't belong to me, having a cigarette feels like a middle finger to anyone who is trying to make my choices for me.

I doubt there are many studies out there on how frequently married or otherwise committed sexual assault survivors have affairs, and it would be hard to find concrete numbers on that since rape and assault (let alone affairs) are so infrequently reported. But I would hazard a guess that it is something a lot of survivors have in common, perhaps especially the women. One of the most important phases of our recovery is taking our power back. Marriage and monogamy are institutions that have been oppressing women for a very long time, so it makes sense to me that the quickest and most powerful way to reclaim that power is to make the choice to sleep with someone— anyone—other than the person who signed a paper implying they are entitled to your body.

In addition to the rebellious tone of an affair, it can be a way of grasping on to life when death threatens. Surviving abuse can make you feel dead inside for a very long time, and when desire flickers once again, it's like an irresistible invitation to come back to life. Perel quotes psychotherapist Dalma Heyn, who defines "erotic silence" as an "unexpected, inarticulable deadening of pleasure and vitality."[180] While this erotic silence can come up for plenty of reasons, it sounds a lot like going gray, the phenomenon I've seen in so many of my friends when they are in an unhappy relationship or are feeling powerless or disconnected in their lives. Heyn goes on to say:

> *Whereas before their affairs these women experienced their bodies as fragmented, their voices muted, some vital organ or aspect of their personality missing, during the affair and after it they became changed. They let go of those muffled feelings and entered a clear reality, one filled with color and vibrancy, in which they felt alive and awake and strong and focused.*[181]

This experience is common enough that Perel has begun to ask her clients dealing with infidelity whether they've experienced some tragedy or trauma recently. An affair

179   Ibid, 185.
180   Ibid, 184–185.
181   Ibid.

can be a powerful affirmation of life after someone has threatened you with (literal or metaphorical) death.

This is one of the ways the wound that we all carry from generations of unequal gender dynamics manifests in our ability to inflict pain on each other. As powerful and life-affirming as it can feel for a survivor to find her desire again and have joyful sex outside of the bounds of a relationship that feels oppressive, it's also incredibly painful for the partner left behind. Trauma is never an excuse to cause trauma, but that's often how it happens. It's a complicated thing: we must feel free in order to heal, but our freedom sometimes requires that we hurt the people who count on us. Our recovery is our priority, and we must stand up for our needs, but our loved ones sometimes end up as casualties of that recovery. Freedom and commitment aren't a natural pair.

For some people, forms of non-monogamy provide a solution to this paradox of freedom within commitment. In most forms of non-monogamy, two people have a primary relationship with each other but come to some mutual agreement about contact with others. This could mean that they have a threesome from time to time, that they can make out with other people but not have sex, that they can have full sexual relationships with other people as long as they don't do it in the house, and so on and so on. It could be anything, as long as the partners agree to the boundaries together and stick to them. Some of these relationship structures are emotionally monogamous, while others, the polyamorous relationships, are structures where more than two people can form emotional and sexual bonds with each other and in which there may or may not be a primary pair. The key with non-monogamous relationship structures is that everything that happens is consensual for everyone involved. Infidelity, on the other hand, is not consensual.

I've experimented with some forms of non-monogamy; when I first started, I found it quite intimidating. I thought I would be plagued with jealousy and fear. I was surprised to find that when my partner and I agreed to a rule where we could sleep with other people when one or the other of us was out of town, it actually sort of solved my jealousy. I realized that if he slept with someone else, it wouldn't change anything between us, and that was what I really feared. That first weekend that we tried it, neither of us acted on our newfound roaming abilities, but I loved knowing that I could. I felt more powerful in my own body and my own choices. It was exhilarating. I know several women who always practice non-monogamy, and for them, it is a manifestation of a feminism that insists on their right to choose how to express their sexuality. Non-monogamy and polyamory (theoretically, anyway) reject the idea that anyone is entitled to anyone else's sexual body.

Experimenting with non-monogamy taught me that there are many ways to have a relationship, and what matters is choice, consent, and communication. I usually choose monogamy anyway, not because I think any partner is entitled to my body, but because I want to direct my sexual and emotional energy only to them. It's my choice, not an unspoken assumption, and it feels like a more powerful choice because I've tried out other ways of doing it. I don't think love is necessarily limited, but time and energy are, and the kind of intimacy I believe in takes a fair amount of those two things. I do appreciate, however, that monogamy doesn't have to be a given in my relationships. I haven't committed to monogamy till death do us part. It's an ongoing conversation, and whatever I decide with my partners can always be renegotiated if we decide we want to do so. We're not doing things in a certain way just because it's what's been sold to us, but because we're choosing it mindfully.

As useful as these relationship structures may be, however, they do not protect us from the pain of infidelity. No matter how wide we stretch the boundaries of a relationship, relationships always have boundaries, and they can be broken. Freedom within commitment isn't the same as freedom all by itself. Desire can be selfish. No relationship structure will completely protect us from the pain of a broken heart, but I do think it's worth considering these alternatives as ways to negotiate the sticky disagreement between commitment and freedom, especially when freedom is so necessary for healing.

I've never been married, so I haven't had the chance to experience an extramarital affair from the inside, but I did fall in love with a married man once. Well, sort of. It was one of those overblown romantic illusions where we sent each other desperate lines of poetry purple with metaphors and secretly communicated via coded tweets (something I later learned the kids call "subtweeting"). It was mostly an affair of the mind; it was long distance, and there was little to no sexual contact between us (but no one ever needs to know how many subtweets). It went on for a very long time while he worked on his failing marriage and I shuffled through boyfriends, and we kept trying to quit each other but couldn't. Finally, his divorce went through, we had sex, and—drumroll please—it was terrible.

We had such inflated fantasies about who the other person was that we really hadn't stopped to get to know each other. By the time the divorce went through, I had encountered many of the endless humiliations of being the other woman—being texted constantly and then suddenly told to stop in case she sees, having him ghost me for months after his therapist insisted he cut me off, and being told we couldn't be in touch but still seeing those damn subtweets. When we finally saw each other again after all that, I had started to consider that I might want something more in my life. "Yes, the lover gets the lust without the laundry," Perel points out, "but she lives without legitimacy—a position that inevitably erodes self-esteem and confidence."[182] I felt confused and hurt and wanted him to acknowledge that a lot of this had been hard on me. He wanted a weekend of non-stop fucking. When I hedged and told him I wasn't sure if I wanted to do that, he whined and wheedled at me, complaining about how long we'd waited and telling me that, basically, I owed him. It sounded pretty familiar, but I did it anyway. And, predictably, it was bad—really awkward. He talked about his therapist right in the middle of everything. I don't want to talk about it.

I'm not proud of this. For years, we insisted we were on some sort of moral high ground because "nothing really happened." I've wondered more than once if we'd just gotten

---

182   Ibid, 245.

the bad sex out of the way that first night we met, maybe we wouldn't have needed to have a years-long half-real emotional affair. But an emotional affair is an affair all the same. We hurt people. We hurt each other and we hurt ourselves. I'm sorry for that.

I think the reason I held on to this affair was because of that misguided search for safety and power. I was still very much in the beginning of my healing process and was trying to understand a world where someone I trusted had assaulted me. A married man is a *great* person to fall in love with because he provides no true threat of intimacy—especially when most of the relationship takes place over email and Twitter. When sex was always off the table, it could never be something I owed him (at least until the divorce papers were signed, I guess). He could be my knight in shining armor. He was never going to let me down if it was never possible for us to be actually, intimately, getting-to-know-each-other's-guts close. He provided a shadowy third to my other relationships, allowing me to avoid what Esther Perel refers to as the "vulnerability of two."[183] He was my escape route, a comforting fantasy of a different kind of life. I can't speak for him, but I get the sense I represented something similar to him. I idolized him, while his wife had to live with his shit every day. Each in our own way, we provided each other with an analgesic to the pain of the lives we were living at the time. We were enraptured, not by each other, but by the image each of us saw of ourselves in the other's eyes.

The fantasy helped, in its twisted way, but it was hurting, too. It kept us dreaming of a better life without ever actually having to do any work to make that life a reality. It created a very real threat to the people he and I were otherwise involved with. It let me avoid being honestly present in my life. The affair kept me safe from something, but the danger wasn't really out there with all the other men who might assault me. The thing I was really protecting myself from was me.

I've gotten much more courageous since then about sitting with the emotions that arise when, for example, I have sex with a new person, when I'm starting to trust again, or when I'm sitting alone wondering if my eggs have already shriveled up and died. Assault, violation, manipulation, trauma, and heartbreak are all things that can make us more vulnerable to fantasies and, paradoxically, to dangerous safety-seeking behavior. The crappy things that happened to us in our lives are never excuses for treating other people poorly, but the truth is, that's often the way that goes.

It's appropriate and important that we feel guilt for our bad behavior, no matter how good our reasons might have been for being assholes at the time. What's not useful in these situations is shame. Shame makes us feel that we are bad people, so there's no point in trying to do any better. Esther Perel points out that "The shift from shame to guilt is crucial. Shame is a state of self-absorption, while guilt is an empathic relational response inspired by the hurt you have caused another."[184] When we've done something hurtful and we say, "I'm a horrible person, I don't deserve your forgiveness," we've made it about us, not about the other person's pain. We're trying to get the other person to tell us we're not horrible people, to absolve us without actually forgiving us. Shame can

---

183   Ibid, 115.
184   Ibid, 71.

be a funny way of bypassing the work that we need to do to atone for our mistakes. Guilt, on the other hand, is appropriate when we've taken advantage of someone or crossed a boundary. It allows us to see that we've made a mistake but also to still believe we can do better in the future. Guilt requires that we not only feel our own feelings but also empathize with the people we've hurt, and that can be much more painful than familiar old narcissistic shame. Guilt is certainly uncomfortable, but it can help us change.

I don't know, honestly, if my involvement with this married man was the worst thing I did while I was trying to survive. I also (unconsciously) used more than one partner as a kind of shield against the world without ever allowing myself to be genuinely present with them. I treated my own body like it didn't matter, trying to starve myself of food and feelings. I wouldn't be surprised if I hurt the people around me in ways I didn't even realize at the time. Healing can be messy—especially when we haven't yet clued in that we really need to handle our scandal.

If you've done some crappy stuff as a result of your trauma, heartbreak, violation, or a shitty childhood, welcome to the goddamn club. You probably did it because, on whatever unconscious level, you were trying to survive, to feel safe, to reclaim some power somewhere. There's no point in feeling shame about being a flawed human being. It's important to acknowledge that our assholery often comes from a place of pain but to take responsibility for it anyway. That's all we've got to work with. The good news is, that's a lot.

CONSENSUAL SEX IS HOT

So you've gotten a sense by now of my sad and sordid sex life up until this point. There was good, bad, and ugly, but there wasn't a whole lot of awareness of what I was doing and why—and not a ton of great sex, either. A few months shy of turning thirty, I looked at my colorless life and felt I'd had enough. I was *this close* to getting engaged to a partner I had been with for a couple of years (and rarely had sex with), but I decided instead to shut it down. I called a new therapist and stared down the barrel of being single in my thirties, not sure what the hell was going to come next but knowing I didn't want it to be like this anymore. (Spoiler alert—it wasn't. Everything in my life is way better than it ever was before I turned thirty.)

That year, I met the first lover I had ever been with who made consent explicit. He wasn't the first with an intuition for consent—some had asked me if I was okay, noticed when I flinched or tensed up, and got turned on by me being turned on, but I'm not sure they had a vocabulary for what they were doing. Plenty of others had whined, wheedled, manipulated, shamed, and shoved me into a dark room and locked the door. Those guys did not have a great intuition for consent.

I knew this guy was different when we were having sex one day and he noticed me checking out a little bit. I was going through the motions, but my mind was elsewhere, kind of waiting for it to be over. He picked up on it right away, stopped, and lectured me (I remember his finger literally wagging at me): "Don't you ever keep doing something with me that you don't want to be doing. If you don't like it, we stop. Never, ever pretend to be into this. Don't do that to me." No one had ever yelled at me before for trying to please them against my own interests. I later learned that he had been assaulted himself as a teen and that consent was non-negotiable for him. He wasn't just setting a boundary for my sake, but for his own as well, in honor of his own healing. In that moment, we made a contract that I think everyone should agree to from the get-go: if anyone is not into it, we're not doing it. There is to be no pretending, no playacting, no doing it just to get it over with. Consent is non-negotiable on all sides. From that point on, the sex was incredible, connected, and deeply pleasurable. I found my desire was activated and supported, and I wanted it *all the time*. I felt alive, like I had finally gotten my color back.

When this man left my life, I was disconsolate. This may have had something to do with Naomi Wolf's argument that fulfilling sex is biologically addictive, but it also felt like I had lost a really powerful avenue for my healing. I thought my color would never return. I didn't know what sex was supposed to look like out there with other people who might not understand consent in this way. It infuriated me that I was thirty years old before I met someone who really deeply understood and enacted consent with me. I felt I was being shoved back into the forest of tigers.

Poor little younger Julie. I feel for that past self. I remember feeling like I had stumbled into the darkest timeline and that nothing could be right again. I didn't understand then that everything I had learned about consent from my ex hadn't gone away when he left. He left me with some really good things I could keep (along with a little emotional damage I wish he'd kept to himself). I think here of writer bell hooks' comment in her book, *All About Love*, that "When one knows a true love, the transformative force of that love lasts even when we no longer have the company of the person with whom we experienced profound mutual care and growth."[185] It's important that we take something with us from every relationship, whether it lasted decades or a few minutes, and if there was good there (and even if there was bad, too), the good doesn't break when the heart does. I had to honor what I'd learned from this man and let him go. I had to trust that, like Dorothy remembering Oz when she returns home to the farm the consent had been within me all along!

Now that I had experienced really good consensual sex, I knew what it looked like. It wasn't in any way contained to that one relationship. My color had always been mine, and even if this man had helped me find it again, he didn't take it with him when he left. With or without him, I would no longer stand for any intimacy that wasn't intimate. I would no longer be willing to have sex and feel numb. I resolved to stop dating uninspiring people and kept myself open to meeting the right person. It's not always easy, but the people I date now are so much more interesting than the ones I used to end up in relationships with. They are brave, they've done their own work, and they

---

185   hooks, bell. *All About Love: New Visions*. New York, W. Morrow (2000): 187.

are able to meet my vulnerability with their own. We can find each other a little more easily now because we're doing that scary and sometimes painful thing where we're honest about who we are and what we want. People who don't want to do that work aren't interested in me, nor I in them, but the ones that do can see me as someone they can really connect to. It's amazing how useful it is to be honest about who you are in dating—it turns the wrong people right off and lets the right ones find you much more easily.

It's true what they tell you—that sex gets better as you get older. It's not about finding the right person, it's about learning to trust yourself. You give a lot fewer fucks about what people think about you, and you start to learn the difference between what feels good and what really doesn't. It's scary, but it's absolutely worth breaking the social contracts that require you to be numb and nice.

THREE RULES FOR MINDFUL SEX

Now that I've been through some things and I have an idea of what kind of sex I want (and don't want) in my life, I follow three general rules in my sex life. These three rules are based on the concept of mindfulness, which basically means paying attention to what's going on and being kind to whatever you find there. It's all the same stuff we've been talking about throughout this book, this time applied in the service of hot, fulfilling, consensual sex. If you've read this far, you already have the skills for an enlightened sex life. You're welcome!

The first rule is to be present. Being present means being in the body. So often with sex we slip into distraction, dissociation, fetishization, or obsession to avoid intimacy with our own bodies, let alone with our partners. When our minds are on what the other person is thinking of us, whether they can see our belly folds, or how good our performance is, we're spectatoring—keeping our critical judging minds online—and that kills our desire and pleasure. As we've learned, in order to orgasm, we need to surrender to a loss of self-consciousness and be fully present to the sensations of the body. Naomi Wolf explains that a certain wildness arises with orgasm as the brain regions that control behavioral regulation in a woman go quiet:

> *One could say that she actually becomes, biochemically, a wild woman or a maenad. She becomes so disinhibited and impervious to pain that it is as if she is in a state of altered consciousness. Women in "high" orgasm go more deeply into this trance state than at any other time. Judgment is suspended in this state, and women do not even feel pain in the same ways as in normal circumstances.*[186]

Wolf argues that this is a specific feature of the "female" brain, but as we've discussed, I'm not totally convinced that's a thing. All humans have brains, so it wouldn't surprise me if this one carries over, regardless of sex or gender. Allowing ourselves to be present

---

186   Wolf, Naomi. *Vagina: A New Biography.* New York, Ecco (2013): 26.

with the sensations of the body allows us to let those self-critical functions turn off and feel some pleasure for once in our goddamn lives.

The second rule for mindful sex is to let go of goals. Orgasm isn't easy for a lot of people even if they haven't been assaulted. When we only focus on the body sensations that signal orgasm, we're missing all kinds of good stuff that is worth paying attention to even though it's never going to get us to the big O. Mindfulness practices in daily life teach us to pay closer attention to small sensations and learn to relax within discomfort. When we apply this to our sex lives, we can much more thoroughly enjoy the feeling of a lover's fingers stroking our thigh, the warmth and texture of a kiss on our lips, or the smell of our partner's sweat. All the senses are involved in a sexual encounter, and noticing what's already happening instead of what's *supposed* to happen can make the whole thing a lot more fun.

Many women are unlikely to have an orgasm from penetrative sex alone, but that doesn't mean penetration isn't deeply pleasurable and enjoyable. There are many parts of the body that probably won't get you to orgasm but feel amazing when they are touched in the right ways. When orgasm isn't a big deal, it's far more likely to come to the party. It should be the cherry on top of an experience that's full of play, exploration, pleasure, and intimacy. If you get down on yourself for not having an orgasm or not having a very good orgasm, that only feeds into the judging mind, which—you guessed it—prevents you from having an orgasm. So don't focus just on the cherry, enjoy the entire sundae.

The third rule for mindful sex is to listen with the body. Listening with the body is not unlike the intuitive eating practice we talked about in our chapter on food. It means involving the entire body in the process of sexual contact and honoring how it makes us feel before, during, and after. It means honoring the preferences of our unique bodies and learning those preferences through experimentation. Junk food tastes awesome but generally makes us feel like crap later—junk sex is the same.

Listening with the body means both listening to our own physical signals and paying attention to our partner's body. Genitals have their own language. Sometimes a hard penis or a very lubricated vagina mean being turned on and sometimes they don't. What else is the body saying? What is the flush of the skin, the heartbeat, or the breath telling us? This comes back to the question of consent. How do we know whether or not our partner likes what we're doing? We listen—to their words, of course, but also to how their body responds. Deep breaths, panting, and moaning tend to be signs that things are going well, while if your partner goes silent and stops breathing all of a sudden, that means they are tensing up, which is generally not a good sign. Sex is a conversation between two bodies, and while verbal communication is useful, it doesn't tell the whole story. I'm one of those people who kind of loses my words in that context, and sometimes it's hard for me to vocalize what's going on. It's important for me that my partner is able to clue in if I'm tensing up or checking out. We have a responsibility to our bodies to learn how they speak, and to do our best to learn our partner's unique body language, too.

Sex can be beautiful, emotional, intense, intimate, and incredibly healing. When we allow ourselves to be fully present to the vulnerability of our bodies and what might show up when we let someone touch us, we are opening to a new phase of the healing process that comes with its own challenges. We can't always trust other people to do or say exactly the right thing all the time, but we can practice knowing our bodies, breathing, staying present, and communicating our needs. We can become more self-aware about when we're using sex as a trading chip for security, control, or even love, and we might be able to learn to stop doing that. We can seek out partners who can meet us in the space of actual intimacy, but we can't control what they do and there's no way to prevent being hurt ever again. We can, though, discover our own capacity for healing, feeling, and taking the risk of trusting all over again. We can only truly surrender to the vulnerability of sex when we feel powerful enough in who we already are.

LOVE

Love has kicked my ass many, many (many) times. I've had my heart broken by a baseball cap-wearing high school sweetheart who cheated on me, a soulful hippie who wanted to live on a ship made out of garbage that would take him to Mars when earth became unlivable, a brilliant poet with OCD and absolutely no respect for me, a handsome helicopter pilot whose military job required him to be away for nine months at a time, a mad professor type who was amazing in bed but neglected to clean his kitchen so long he'd get maggots in there, and a gorgeous, brooding ex-bartender who used to shoot fire out of his mouth. You can't say I haven't had a breadth of experience when it comes to love, and even though it certainly hasn't always worked, I've always *tried* to break my same old relationship patterns. I think I have, actually. Every new relationship brought fresh innovative ways to get my heart trampled on.

The cool thing about all those heartbreaks is that, miraculously, I keep healing. Every time I think I'll never fall in love again, I do. I'll think my capacity for romance has completely dried up until I meet some weirdo at an event for amateur ukulele players and I find my heart capable, all over again, of giving itself away, of being willing to take the risk to let itself be broken—even though I know from experience that sometimes romance turns violent. My heart shrinks but then expands again, insisting on its own reinvented naiveté. To paraphrase the pop star Ariana Grande in her ode to self-love and romantic recovery titled "Thank U, Next": that shit's amazing.

Despite their external differences, my romantic relationships tend to fit into one of two general patterns: a shot at gaining security or an attempt to subconsciously fix my dad. Those relationships are easy—the roles are well defined and super familiar. Either he adores me and I can barely tolerate anything that comes out of his mouth, or I'm desperately chasing him down, trying to make myself worthy of his impossible love, which he's usually already told me ain't on the menu. I spent a long time dating men who didn't really want me because I'd learned from experience that men who wanted me sometimes stole from me. Their desire for me was, apparently, a reason to push me around, grab me in public, or get me alone in order to assault me. People always wonder why women keep dating men who don't treat them very well and reject the "nice guys" who want to be with them. Well, it's probably because one of those "nice guys" liked her so much he took something she didn't want to give. I kept men at arm's length by making sure they always wanted me at arm's length, too.

Eventually I'd had enough of this, and on my birthday one year, I decided it was time for something better for my exhausted champ of a heart. I'd dated many and sundry, and it was all lots of fun (though sometimes really not), but there was a frontier I hadn't yet explored: love with someone who was actually emotionally available, who could love me for who I am and offer me the chance to grow and learn and change with them. I knew that what I really desired was genuine, authentic connection, and I wanted to believe that there was someone out there who could meet me there (and that unicorns are real, but we can dream, right?). At the very least, I wanted to get really good at being alone so that I didn't have to tolerate crappy relationships for the rest of my life. So I made a resolution: I would do my damnedest not to get into the wrong relationship.

I've had more than one person tell me that my track record of medium to bad relationships was because I had "low self-esteem." I take exception to this diagnosis for a couple of reasons. First, I have pretty good self-esteem. In my view, self-esteem means having a loving relationship with yourself through good and bad. It doesn't mean thinking you're perfect, but rather that you forgive yourself when you make mistakes and take pretty good care of yourself on a day-to-day level. I like myself a lot, actually. I'm proud of what I've accomplished in my life. I didn't enter into the world of romance thinking I "deserved" to be treated like crap. I didn't ask for it. It just started happening.

Second, it's an accomplishment to have any self-esteem at all in a culture that systematically teaches us that women are inferior objects. It's hard enough to have loving relationships in this culture when you *haven't* been sexually abused or violated. It's hard to know what a healthy relationship looks like when you've never seen it or experienced it, or when despite all your hope and good intentions people keep treating you like an old Kleenex anyway. That's not our fault. That is the fault of our perpetrators. Don't blame the victim for having low self-esteem when the problem is systemic violence.

Third, I'm not the one who is fucked up about relationships. That's our whole society. We don't do love very well in our emotionally underdeveloped world. It's extremely difficult to have healthy relationships in an unhealthy society. It's not because we have low self-esteem. Survivors especially have to rummage around in the many tools we've picked up in our recovery process to get brave, get smart, and insist on a better kind of love than anything we've seen or experienced before. I believe that we can learn self-esteem and that's it's possible to be healthier in an unhealthy society (and that unicorns are real). I also believe we can learn to love better. Step Eight in our path to recovery is Love.

BOOKS OF LOVE

We don't have a great definition for love in our culture. The word is used as a blanket term for how we feel about anything we have a generally positive response to. A lot of what we learn about love in our lives is implicit: we pick up information from our friends, what we see on TV, and, most importantly, our first caregivers. As children, we are careful observers, watching how our parents act with each other, with our siblings, with their lovers, and with us. We notice if our parents choose to stay together, break up, date, or stay alone. We notice if their hearts get broken. We notice if they treat their lovers with kindness or disdain. We see the emotional consequences of all the romantic choices our parents make with other adults. Our unconscious internalized definition of love is whatever we experienced at home when we were young. In an essay for *The New York Times*, philosopher Alain de Botton points out that this is one of many reasons we end up marrying the wrong people:

> *Though we believe ourselves to be seeking happiness in marriage, it isn't that simple. What we really seek is familiarity—which may well complicate any plans we might have had for happiness. We are looking to recreate, within our adult relationships, the feelings we knew so well in childhood. The love most of us will have tasted early on was often confused with other, more destructive dynamics: feelings of wanting to help an adult who was out of control, of being deprived of a parent's warmth or scared of his anger, of not feeling secure enough to communicate our wishes.*[187]

We tend to fall in love based on a feeling, a sense of "rightness" or "just knowing." We stay with people who treat us poorly, reject us, or withhold their attention because that's what we know, that's what matches our unconscious definition of love. We not only seek out dynamics that are familiar to us, we reject potentially healthy relationships simply because they are unfamiliar. They don't *feel* right. Botton continues:

> *How logical, then, that we should as grown-ups find ourselves rejecting certain candidates for marriage, not because they are wrong, but because they are too right—too balanced, mature, understanding, and reliable—given that in our hearts, such rightness feels foreign. We marry the wrong people because we don't associate being loved with feeling happy.*[188]

This is a common enough problem for the average person, but it gets even more complicated for those of us who have experienced sexual or relationship abuse—those funhouse mirror versions of love—especially in childhood. When love has been mixed up with pain, humiliation, fear, and domination, it's difficult to imagine what a healthier love might look like. That doesn't mean survivors of abuse are incapable of loving—not at all. Rather, I think, survivors are pushed through a healing process that generally makes us face the truth about the love dynamics we learned from our experiences. We are required to pull our unconscious definitions of love to the surface in a way that others never have a reason to do. That might make survivors uniquely capable of making new, more mindful definitions of love in our adult lives.

Whether or not we've been abused, we live in a society that does tend to intertwine love with power, domination, transactionality, and money. Without many good models of love between equals out there, many of us confuse love with power. It's a relatively new concept in our society that people marry because they consensually agree to tie

---

187   de Botton, Alain. "Why You Will Marry the Wrong Person." The New York Times, May 28, 2016. https://www.nytimes.com/2016/05/29/opinion/sunday/why-you-will-marry-the-wrong-person.html
188   Ibid.

the knot. For most of our history, marriage was based on things like who owned and controlled the land and who would make the most babies to keep the family farm going. Centuries of witch-hunting in Europe and North America heralded the rise of capitalism and patriarchal control over the labor force. Women were prevented from working and were instead conscripted into the role of "motherwives" who could make more laborers for the new capitalist Christian patriarchal system that was coming into power at the time. Marriage is an institution that until pretty recently has been a legal way to own a woman.

Even now, as women are becoming more powerful at work than they have been in many generations, heterosexual marriage can still hold them back. In her book *All the Single Ladies*, Rebecca Traister points out that "a college educated woman who delays marriage until her thirties will earn eighteen thousand dollars more per year than an equivalently educated woman who married in her twenties."[189] Based on wage data between 1979 and 2006, Traister writes, "On average, men saw a six percent increase in earnings after becoming fathers; in contrast, women's wages decreased four percent for every child."[190] Marrying and having children in heterosexual pairs is still a boon for men that comes at a huge cost for women (at least in terms of economics).

More and more women are opting out of this institutional structure that keeps them oppressed. Traister found that while just 22 percent of high-income women tended to be unmarried in the 1970s, by 2011, that number had nearly doubled to 40 percent.[191] The upshot of all this is that marriage and motherhood affect the wage gap. "Nationally," Traister explains, "childless, unmarried women earn nearly ninety-six cents for every male dollar, compared to seventy-six cents to the dollar earned by married mothers."[192] As much as we like to think of love as simply a rainbows-and-flowers kind of *feeling*, it can have material costs, at least for women, if you put a ring on it (and a baby in it).

LOVE IN THE TIME OF PATRIARCHY

These economics of love form part of the reason we so often skip out on genuine intimacy and trade sex for security instead. Living in a capitalist patriarchal (Christian, white supremacist, colonialist, heteronormative) society affects the way we make our most intimate choices. "Reviewing the literature on love," writes feminist cultural critic bell hooks, "I noticed how few writers, male or female, talk about the impact of patriarchy, the way in which male domination of women and children stands in the way of love."[193] Even as women and other genders become more powerful and more financially independent in our society, we are still struggling within a gendered power dynamic. Regardless of our gender expression, sexual orientation, desire to marry, or

189   Traister, Rebecca. *All the Single Ladies*. New York, Simon & Schuster (2016): 175
190   Ibid, 176.
191   Ibid, 175.
192   Ibid, 177.
193   hooks, bell. *All About Love: New Visions*. New York, W. Morrow (2000): xxiv.

interest in having children, many of us still intuit that we need to please men in order to survive.

Beyond this need to please, a different kind of love might indeed exist. There may be a way to connect with other human beings that is not defined by power, control, hierarchy, gender dynamics, or economics. This version of love could be a place to heal from the wounds of living in a culture that does not see us as individual human beings worthy of love and respect.

In her book *All About Love,* bell hooks points out that our society is lacking in this revolutionary, visionary type of love. Without any examples for this more powerful kind of loving, we settle for merely caring, or what Freud has called cathexis. hooks writes:

> **Most of us learn early on to think of love as a feeling. When we feel deeply drawn to someone, we cathect with them; that is, we invest feelings or emotion in them. That process of investment wherein a loved one becomes important to us is called "cathexis."[194]**

We can cathect with our others when we care what happens to them and wish them well, but that's not the same thing as true, vulnerable, connected love between equals.

hooks turns to psychologist M. Scott Peck for a different definition of love. He writes that love is "the will to extend one's self for the purpose of nurturing one's own or another's spiritual growth."[195] Here, love is an act of will—a choice, not an instinctual experience of being swept away by romance. This choice is in the service of growth, notably either for another person or for one's own self. Self-love and other-love, then, involve a willingness to be with the discomfort of unfamiliarity and change. It is a mindful, intentional act, not simply a feeling that comes and goes. We can't control our feelings, after all, but we can choose where to put our attention. We can choose to put energy, intention, and action into cultivating space within a relationship for fun, connection, communication, and intimacy. That is a commitment we can make to another human being. It's impossible to commit to how we're going to *feel* forever.

It's interesting to me that the word "spiritual" exists in this definition. Neither Peck nor hooks seem to mean it in a religious sense, but it's worth defining a term that can mean such different things to different people. Some people find a lot of solace in a religious tradition and a concept of a god, and that's fair enough. For me, though, the idea that the world is organized according to justice, or that some all-powerful being out there was randomly taking the night off from looking out for me while I was being assaulted, only makes me feel worse. I do have a spirituality, and it lives in my yoga and mindfulness practices and certainly in my experience of love, but it doesn't match up with the concept of any specific god. The word *spirit* comes from the Latin *spiritus*, which can mean soul, animus, courage, energy, or breath, informing the word *inspirare*, which means "to breathe in." In a sense, we can understand spirit as life force, which we've been exploring throughout this book as the erotic energy that allows us to access

---

194   Ibid, 5.
195   Ibid.

our deepest feelings. Then we can define love as *an act of will that supports the growth of one's own or another's erotic force.* Loving ourselves means supporting that energy that underlies our ability to contact our deepest feelings, to be honest with ourselves, and to discern the difference between our momentary cravings and our deeper desires for connection and passion. Loving another means showing up with them, giving them the space to change and grow, listening to them fully, supporting them in contacting their deepest feelings, and encouraging them to follow their passions and trust their desires. Sometimes loving another means holding them accountable. Sometimes it means separating from them. So much of our healing work, then, is the work of self-love, of giving ourselves the space to feel and encourage our own possibilities for growth. Finding this with another human being can be incredibly healing and powerful, if admittedly rare.

Love lives in our choices. What we feel certainly draws us toward those choices, but when the first flush of hormones dies off, love is a commitment to keep showing up (especially when our lovers are driving us crazy). It insists on being honest about who we are, who we've been, and who we could be without getting too attached to any of those identities. It allows us to see our loved ones as their own shifting selves, giving them the space to move and adjust and change their minds. It means seeing another person as a whole, flawed human being, and allowing ourselves to be with them as whole, flawed human beings ourselves.

If you love yourself in this way, that's amazing. If you also love and feel loved by another in this way, you should take a moment to close this book, take a deep breath, and acknowledge how lucky you are. It is not common to love in the service of growth. Most of us love in the service of convenience, familiarity, and the roles we are given to play. We never saw love in the service of growth in our families, and we never learned it from the world around us. That's no one's fault, and there is nothing wrong with you if you don't currently feel loved in this way—you're in the majority. Love is a choice, an act of will, and even if there are no other human beings in our lives who we currently want to offer this work to, we can practice turning this love toward ourselves and, with time, toward other human beings, too. We can move deeper than cathexis in our existing relationships if we are committed to that choice, and we can search for others who are willing to join us in the project of true love. We can practice. We can get better at loving ourselves and we can get better at loving each other.

TRUE LOVE

In this chapter, I want to focus on a specific subset of this type of full-hearted loving. This type of love, which I'll call true love, is a commitment to encouraging one's own and another's spiritual growth, yes, but it is also a commitment to equality, vulnerability, and creating a space for each lover's erotic energy. It's not necessarily about sex, though sex can be a part of that commitment. It's about deep communication, but it also gives each lover the space to be their own version of themselves, to be sovereign over their bodies, and to change if they want to change. True love is *a commitment to the growth of one's own and another's erotic force along with a commitment to equality between you.* This love practice tends to come with plenty of stumbles and reversions to old patterns, and that's okay—committing to something doesn't mean you always get it right. Equality isn't always easy to find or even to feel when you have it. It's an honest attempt to work on yourself and to allow your other to work on themselves while forgiving the many inevitable moments when the relationship doesn't look like that. It's not something you simply *have*, it's something you work towards.

This kind of love can only exist between consenting adults. It is a love that strives for equality and resists power dynamics in an unequal world that is fueled by domination. There are powerful forms of love between a parent and child or a person and a pet, and these can certainly be acts of will in the service of another's spiritual growth. When there is caretaking and/or dependence, however, there is a power imbalance, which chokes off this radical commitment to equality and genuine vulnerability. Caretaking and dependence can be aspects of codependency, and codependency is not true love. You cannot be responsible for another being while also remaining committed to equality between you.

True love demands an unrelenting commitment to our own personal growth, to taking responsibility for our own flaws and nonsense, so that we can come to a loving relationship without a need to be rescued. It cannot exist when we are using another person to feel bigger, stronger, smarter, or safer or when we simply want to have the security of a ring on our finger. It cannot exist when there is abuse, domination, manipulation, or violation. This type of love can only happen between people who feel powerful enough within themselves to love each other truly, authentically, and with vulnerability. It is, indeed, a practice—it goes far beyond that "in love" feeling, which inevitably comes and goes. It means choosing to commit to doing our own work, which is in the service of our relationship with our other. True love means being responsible for yourself and allowing your lover to be responsible for themself, too.

Now, does this mean every love relationship I have is completely free of power dynamics and a shining example of blissful kindness and mutual respect? Hell no. This version of love is aspirational. I work toward it and do my best to choose partners who are willing to work on it with me, but I'm not always good at it. It is not easy to feel powerful enough within oneself to be vulnerable with another in this society. It is a practice and a commitment, and not everyone wants to do it with me. Sometimes I've found that if the relationship is somehow preventing my own or my other's growth, truly loving someone means ending the relationship. There are many forms of love that are based on caretaking or cathexis or mutually agreed upon power dynamics that work just fine and don't ask anyone to change, and that's okay. Plenty of people don't actually want to touch the dangerous possibility of true love, because true love *does* ask for change. It encourages spiritual growth. It asks for something more than the anemic version of love we've all been taught to settle for.

LOVING BOUNDARIES

Our culture glorifies codependency: we want our heroes to rescue our heroines. We want our heroines to swoon and surrender. We want two to become one, to paraphrase the immortal lyrics of the Spice Girls. We think love means breaking every boundary between us, telling every secret, forgiving every indiscretion. We don't want to hold our lovers accountable for their bullshit. We think love means being *nice* all the time.

I recently watched the 2018 film *A Star is Born*, in which Bradley Cooper's character Jackson struggles with addiction. In one scene, he tries to apologize to his love, Ally, played by Lady Gaga, for completely ruining the moment when he, drunk and high, peed onstage beside her as she tried to accept a Grammy award. He sits across from her in a treatment center, sober now, hanging his head in shame. He tries to tell her how sorry he is while struggling to hold back tears. She strokes him and interrupts, saying, "It's okay, it's okay." This is a natural reaction. She knows he is struggling, she has empathy, and she doesn't want him to be in pain anymore, so she tries to erase the mistake. This is not, however, a true love reaction. Her refusal to acknowledge the seriousness of what happened and the sincerity of his apology robs him of an opportunity to take on appropriate guilt, acknowledge his wrongdoing, and make a commitment to do better. He doesn't get that moment where she sees him for who he is, including his flaws, and loves him anyway, trusting him to do better in the future. She is so uncomfortable with his expression of pain that she simply tries to tell him "it's okay" instead of holding space for his suffering and offering him the love that comes with honoring our messed-up-ness.

We often think of and experience love as idolization—seeing our other as our perfect one—but it's not that. It's loving *after* seeing someone's worst aspects. Psychotherapist John Welwood has described a loving relationship as a sort of sacred space:

> *When we reveal ourselves to our partner and find that this brings healing rather than harm, we make an important discovery—that intimate relationship can provide a sanctuary from the world of facades, a sacred space where we can be ourselves, as we are.[196]*

This moment between Jackson and Ally is a moment of caretaking, of soothing pain. Ally wants Jackson to stop crying and keep being the husband she expects him to be. It's not that she doesn't love or care about him, she absolutely does. She falters in this moment because she can't tolerate the discomfort of letting him contact his deepest feelings. It's too painful to allow him to express his shame, be seen, heard, appropriately forgiven, and genuinely loved. It takes a lot of courage to love honestly in a moment of deep pain.

If someone gets drunk and high and pees on stage beside you while you are trying to accept a Grammy, that's an appropriate time to set a boundary. No matter how much

---

196   Ibid, 30.

empathy we feel for Jackson, he fucked up. That doesn't make him a bad person or unworthy of love, it just means he made a mistake. Ally had every right to be angry. She deserved that apology. Telling him everything is okay before he can even finish saying he is sorry is an example of Robert Augustus Masters' blind compassion, a tendency to want to forgive and let go without actually processing what went wrong, which "keeps love too meek, sentenced to wearing a kind face."[197] Love isn't always kind. Sometimes love is fierce.

It can be hard to imagine that we can love someone as well as hold them accountable, say no to them, or set a boundary with them, especially if we have codependent patterns. Sometimes the most loving thing we can do for someone is look them in the eyes and tell them, "No, that wasn't okay. You fucked up. You need to take responsibility for your mistakes. And I love you."

I learned a little something about loving boundaries during a period when I was stuck in a breakup that just wouldn't end. I was separated from my ex, but we still communicated in a way that did not allow me to move on. He had moved away to another country and we were (well, I was) haunted by this "maybe one day" caveat that we had about breaking up. Maybe he'd move back. Maybe I could move there. Maybe we could make it work. He didn't want to commit to me, but he wouldn't quite commit to the breakup, either. I was suffering.

This is not the first time I've struggled to get over someone. When I love, I tend to love hard, and I don't let go easily. I can't tell you how many times I've heard the words "just get over it" when stuck in a breakup that has long since gone stale. As I'm writing this chapter on love, I should disclose that while I am certainly not an expert on beautiful, perfect, long-term relationships I am something of an expert on breakups. I've had a lot of them. One thing I can tell you with some authority is that "just getting over it" is not a tactic that works.

This time, though, I tried a different strategy: asking for what I needed. I had been socialized to trade time, attention, and sex for security like all the rest of us, and my tactic of offering him anything he wanted and silently hoping he'd commit in exchange wasn't working super well. I was doing this thing where if I never actually asked for what I needed, the possibility could stay open that he *might just* give it to me. If I spoke up and asked and he said no, then the "maybe" window would have to close forever. My therapist suggested that I figure out what, exactly, I wanted from my interactions with him and ask him for it. So I did. I called him up, terrified, palms sweating, and laid out a few requests. I asked him to do a couple of things to help him decide what he really wanted so we could either move forward together or actually end things before we saw each other again, which we'd planned to do in six weeks. He agreed. This went against everyone else's advice to cut off contact and somehow magically stop thinking about it. All my attempts to do that were getting me nowhere. Rather than bury my feelings and shut up about it, which is what our culture usually advises us to do when we're in

197   Masters, Robert Augustus. Spiritual Bypassing: When Spirituality Disconnects Us from What Really Matters. Berkeley, North Atlantic Books (2010): 21–22.

pain, my therapist was helping me confront the problem, demystify it, and advocate for myself. She was encouraging my spiritual growth.

When my ex and I met again at the agreed upon date, sure enough, he hadn't done any of what I'd asked. He was no closer to making a choice and was clearly comfortable keeping me on the hook with no obligation on his part to make a decision. He was continuing on doing whatever the hell he wanted and leaving me to deal with the consequences—which had been a pattern when we were together, too. My strategy of giving him whatever I had and quietly hoping he'd commit to me in return was not only ineffective, it was manipulative. It wasn't loving. When I finally said out loud what I wanted and saw with my own two eyes that he couldn't follow through, I finally really, actually got it: he wasn't going to give me what I wanted. Ever.

The spell was completely broken. This man, who I had previously thought was the love of my life, suddenly seemed sort of pathetic and annoying to me. I wasn't angry, exactly, but it was like the rose-colored glasses of my codependent devotion had shattered. He was just a person. He was someone I had loved, sure, but he had lost his power over me completely. I never looked back. I had to process that breakup and relationship like any other, of course, but I stopped missing him; I never again wished we were still together. Advocating for myself, setting a boundary, and asking for what I needed made me feel powerful. I didn't "just" get over it. I spoke up for myself, saw that my needs were never going to get met, and *then* I got over it. I've been using this strategy in my relationships ever since, and it seems to be the key for me to break my codependent patterns. I no longer silently wait for a relationship to magically be what I want it to be. I lay out needs and boundaries, and I am willing to let go of people who can't meet me there. It's been an excellent way to avoid getting into the wrong relationship.

I thought of this empowering breakup moment when I watched the 2014 Australian horror film *The Babadook*. Amelia is a single mother who is being terrorized by the eponymous poltergeist-like monster. She is a sweet and lonely mother who helps everyone and never asks for anything for herself. You can tell the movie was written by a woman (Jennifer Kent): the true horror of the film is not so much the monster but the sometimes isolating and frustrating experience of mothering a difficult child alone (oh—and getting cockroaches. Horrifying). Near the end of the film, after weeks of being terrorized by the Babadook, who mostly seems to make Amelia feel anxious, exhausted, and sometimes murderous toward her child (which are all occasional side effects of motherhood, or so I've heard), Amelia has one final confrontation with the monster. She clutches her child to her, screaming, "This is my house! You are trespassing in my house!" and then, "If you touch my son again, I'll fucking kill you!" The Babadook literally falls out of the sky and then runs into the basement to hide. He is never a threat again. All Amelia needed to do was stand up for herself for once in her goddamn life. She gets her color back, her child relaxes, and her friends start coming over again. Single motherhood becomes much less terrifying. Amelia and I both confronted our demons and exorcised them from our hearts and houses. A little boundary setting goes a long way.

Breaking the Relationship Pattern

If you feel unable to get over someone, unable to leave when you know you should, or unable to stop fighting with someone you love, you are stuck in a toxic relationship pattern. You may be able to break it by clarifying your needs. As we discussed in our chapter on Rage, our anger is the key to letting us know we need to speak up. If you find yourself consistently angry within a relationship, it might be time to make an effort to change the pattern. Here are some tips on how:

⊕ First, identify what need is not being met or what boundary is being crossed. We all make compromises for the ones we love, and no relationship is perfect, but a need is a need—if it doesn't get met, it's not going to work. A preference is a whole other story.

⊕ What concrete actions and changes would allow you to be willing to go forward with this person? What would you need to see or hear from them to know that they are willing to change with you? What behaviors would you need to change within yourself? How long will you wait to see if these changes are happening? Don't fall back on feeling—remember that we tend to go for people who "feel" right simply because they are familiarly terrible for us. Look for concrete, measurable changes you can name.

⊕ Find a way to support yourself in setting a boundary before you have a conversation with your other. Remember that if the person cannot meet your needs or stop breaking your boundaries, you may have to find a way to separate yourself from them. That can be painful. What is your plan to commit to your own boundary? What are the consequences if the person does not change in the necessary ways?

⊕ Figure out how to name these concrete requests out loud to your person. Phrase the ask as "I need," and "This is what I want to see going forward," and "Would you be willing to try this?" Stick with "I" statements and questions. Don't tell the person what to do—they have a choice whether or not to meet you where you're asking them to go, and they are under no obligation to do it. It's not a command, it's a request.

⊕ Be honest with yourself about what happens next. Give the person a chance to show you they are trying to meet your request. Sometimes it takes a little time, effort, and practice to get it right. If they're unable to work with you or don't even try, refer back to your commitment to maintaining your boundary.

⊕ Sometimes this results in a standoff between two people that can last a little while. Set your intention to commit to your need and boundary no matter how uncomfortable it makes you feel and how much the other person wants to be in your life—despite their inability or unwillingness to meet your needs. Teach the other person that you care enough about yourself to uphold your boundary and that, if they want to be in your life, they have to meet you there. Teach yourself that you care enough about yourself to respect your own boundaries.

⊕ You may find that you can't live without this other person even though they won't meet your needs. You may discover that your need was a preference after all. You're allowed to change your mind. Perhaps you can find a way to meet your needs on your own and renegotiate your boundaries with the other person so that you are getting enough of your needs met to feel good about it. We want to get out of a pattern of being angry at someone for not being who we want them to be. People are who they are.

⊕ You may go back a few times before you can really stick to your boundary. That's okay—this is a practice like everything else. The more you work at it, the better you'll get. Keep trying.

LOVE AND COURAGE

Dating the wrong person is a common thing in our society at the best of times. Every time I've had my heart broken, I've thought about it, analyzed it, gone to therapy about it, and tried to prevent it from happening again—and every time, it happens again. I can't control other people or prevent myself from getting hurt if I keep insisting on having relationships. What I can do, however, is learn how to love who I am and stand up for myself. When I started to apply that in my romantic relationships, I became better able to weed out the people who didn't really respect me or see me as a human being. For me, loving in romantic partnerships has been less about falling into some irrational spell and more about loving myself enough to be honest about what I want and need.

A lot of people think good love is about luck, simply finding the "right person." In this society, we are indeed lucky to find human beings capable of seeing us as human beings, but it takes a lot of conscious work to sift through all the others who see us only for what we can give them (and to clearly perceive and transform our own tendency to do that to them). We are trained to objectify each other in this society, and it's not always obvious how to love each other truly.

When I resolved to stop getting into the wrong relationships, I was making a commitment to be in a relationship because I was choosing that journey mindfully. I refused to settle for someone who merely seemed safe or relatively unlikely to rape me. I wanted to know I could love myself fiercely and truly so that if I chose to love another, it would be because they could love me like that, too.

This promise was a manifestation of the erotic energy that we keep returning to again and again in this book. When she writes about this energy, Audre Lorde does not pretend it's easy to tap into it, and certainly the experience might make plenty of people run screaming. Lorde writes:

*Our erotic knowledge empowers us, becomes a lens through which we scrutinize
all aspects of our existence, forcing us to evaluate those aspects honestly in
terms of their relative meaning within our lives. And this is a grave responsibility,
projected from within each of us, not to settle for the convenient, the shoddy, the
conventionally expected, nor the merely safe.*[198]

When we start to tap into this energy, we don't have time for the bullshit we've always
been sold. We don't need it, either, because we feel powerful enough within ourselves to
access our own erotic energy. bell hooks agrees that not everyone will want to take this
journey down the path of true love. Many of us would much prefer to keep playing out
the same old dynamics we learned from our first families and never let anyone truly see
us. She writes:

*Our hearts connect with lots of folks in a lifetime, but most of us will go to our
graves with no experience of true love. This is in no way tragic, as most of us run
the other way when true love comes near. Since true love sheds light on these
aspects of ourselves we may wish to deny or hide, enabling us to see ourselves
clearly and without shame, it is not surprising that so many individuals who say
they want to know love turn away when such love beckons.*[199]

Fair enough. It's okay that not everyone wants to love in this way. It is hard and it is
uncomfortable. It's easier to believe in a world where we will somehow magically fall in
love without having to do any work for our part. To "fall in love" is itself a phrase that
implies the lack of responsibility most of us feel about our love relationships. hooks
points out, "If you do not know what you feel, then it is difficult to choose love; it is
better to fall. Then you do not have to be responsible for your actions."[200]

I believe that it is survivors who are most capable of finding the courage to empower
themselves and show up to their relationships with the uncompromising commitment of
true love. We have had to go through a lot of shit to recover from what happened to us,
and along the way we had to collect enough bravery to face ourselves. We are figuring
out how to trust our instincts, how to connect with our bodies, how to read people, how
to tell if someone is trying to use or manipulate us, and how to bounce back when that
happens anyway. We have had to learn to care for ourselves with a kindness we may
never have known as children, and accepting this kindness from others can feel deeply
uncomfortable, at least at first. It's messy and difficult, and we never really stop learning
these lessons, but these are the skills that make us capable of loving fiercely and truly,
with a commitment to seeing each other as equals. This is a kind love that can help us
heal, and that, when we can offer it to others, might help them heal, too. This is the kind
of love that might just change the world.

---

198   Lorde, Audre. *Sister Outsider: Essays and Speeches.* Berkeley, Crossing Press (2007): 57.
199   hooks, bell. *All About Love: New Visions.* New York, W. Morrow (2000): 186.
200   Ibid, 171.

THE WAR OF THE SEXES

Sexual assault is definitely not something that is only done to women by men. Women can assault, too, and any gender can certainly experience assault. Still, it is significant that women are more often than not the targets of sexual violence. We tend to think of sexual violence as a women's issue, but considering that, according to a National Intimate Partner and Sexual Violence survey, 90 percent of women and 93 percent of men report that their abusers were male, why don't we ever think of sexual violence as a men's problem?[201] Why are all these men acting out with violence and aggression? What's going on with men?

In his fascinating study *Love and War*, Tom Digby argues that there is an antagonistic battle between the sexes partly because North America is generally a culture based on militarism: like many other cultures in the world, it owes its success to fighting in wars. The country's economic and colonial success, along with its population's survival, have depended on fighting for resources and winning. In a culture that survives on war, heterosexuality is necessary and a gender binary is required. Digby explains,

> *If a lot of men get killed, the population can still be replenished fairly efficiently, but not so if a lot of women get killed. So members of the comparatively more expendable sex, men, get assigned the role of combat, while the women get assigned the role of breeding and nurturing.*[202]

This leads to several consequences, one of which is that men must be trained by the culture to be warrior-like and women must be trained to be mother-like. Everyone must perform their respective genders explicitly and unambiguously in order to keep these roles intact and keep the military structure running. The desired outcome of this system, Digby reports, is "maximum babies."[203] Women who do not wish to be mothers, men who show fear or compassion and thus a resistance to becoming a soldier, and anyone who rejects procreation by daring to love someone of the same sex must be shamed and punished mercilessly.

In order to be a "real man" in such a culture, a man must display the qualities of a warrior. The most crucial of these qualities, Digby writes, is that "he must be able to manage the capacity to care about the suffering of others, as well as his own suffering."[204] If these boys are going to become men able to witness the atrocities of war and even kill people in the name of it, they'd better get a handle on their compassion. The price of this quality is nothing less than an "emotional disability" according to Digby.[205] The heartlessness men sometimes display in our culture, especially toward women, is not a

201   Black, Michele C. et al. "The National Intimate Partner and Sexual Violence Survey: 2010 Summary Report." National Center for Injury Prevention and Control Centers for Disease Control and Prevention. November 2011. https://www.cdc.gov/violenceprevention/pdf/nisvs_report2010-a.pdf
202   Digby, Tom. *Love and War: How Militarism Shapes Sexuality and Romance.* New York, Columbia University Press (2014): 14.
203   Ibid, 20.
204   Ibid, 33.
205   Ibid, 103.

natural meanness men are born with. It is something a man has to be trained to do. It starts with the toy guns he is given as a child and evolves when his parents, peers, and coaches tell him to "man up" and that crying makes him, pointedly, a "pussy."

Men are taught that they must always be prepared to fight the enemy. That enemy is not necessarily other men invading from another warring nation, but women. In a culture that uses the phrase "opposite sex" to describe a strict gender binary, men must define their masculinity as being not-women. The absolute worst thing you can say to insult a man is to call him a woman: *pussy* and *bitch* are common enough, but as we saw with Chandler on the show *Friends*, who admonishes himself by saying, "Why am I such a *girl*?" after he dares to feel upset that someone tricked him into having sex, even simply using a direct word for a female person is an insult. Digby explains:

> *To be deemed a girl or a woman is not only a sign of failure as a man, it is a sign of having fallen to a status that is implicitly understood to be profoundly inferior. To be female is to have a status that is deeply despised—and feared—by boys and men. That is why misogyny is such an effective means of culturally policing their lives. Misogyny is at the emotional core of the gender binary as it is experienced by boys and men in militaristic societies.*[206]

In order to ensure that, even if we are not actively at war, our society is ready to defend our borders (or to steal oil or diamonds or whatever we want from other cultures), we must be replete with expendable warriors and baby tanks who know how to nurture. We must be expressly taught these roles precisely because they do not come naturally to every human being. Humans have a huge range of ways they would like to exist in the world, and they don't all fit into these narrow gender definitions.

In order to convince men to go through with their warrior training, to teach them to unlearn their natural compassion for others and reasonable fear for their own safety, the culture punishes them for behaving outside masculine warrior norms. They learn to fear showing emotion and compassion (especially for women), and, ironically, they must fear ever revealing that fear. I've felt many times that it takes an immense amount of courage for a man in this culture to admit confusion, vulnerability, or emotional pain. It takes a lot of bravery to do the work of unlearning the lessons patriarchy has taught them. Digby agrees:

> *Those men who ally themselves with women against misogynistic terrorism— against discrimination and sexual harassment, against sexist jokes, against overblown claims of false rape accusations, against slut shaming, against all the other cultural mechanisms that are used to disempower women—those allies of women are the courageous men.*[207]

It is smart for men to resist this social conditioning to see women as the enemy. That's not only because women are not the enemy, but because the "opposite sexes" are set up

---

206   Ibid, 62–63.
207   Ibid, 149.

as enemies in order to keep *men* disempowered. Misogyny is bad for women, obviously, but it's also bad for men, because it is the tool the culture uses to train men to be compassionless warriors.

Men perpetrate violence against women, absolutely, but they also perpetrate violence against each other. The percentage of violent crimes in general perpetrated by men is high: 85 percent. But the victims of those crimes are also overwhelmingly men: 85 percent of them.[208] Having effectively instilled the fear of being anything other than a "real man," the culture must then teach men to hate and subordinate women while also promising them access to women's bodies. Then, of course, it teaches them that if they don't get access to a woman's body, they are performing their gender badly.

This is the patriarchal promise that I believe made my perpetrator both want me and hate me at the same time. Men unconsciously swallow this promise, act like warriors, and expect women to appear and offer themselves up. They suffer through the performance of their masculinity in order to get access to women's bodies. The rage that men feel when their soul-sacrifice does not come with the reward of all-access pussy is not directed at the patriarchal system that lied to them, but rather at the women this system has taught them to hate. For some perpetrators, there is a desire for sexual gratification by the acts of rape, harassment, or assault, but for others, it's way beyond that. Some perpetrators simply want revenge on the women who block their access. They want to see women humiliated, degraded, and in pain. It's not even remotely about sexual desire for these perpetrators.

While most porn is meant to be an aid for masturbation and a tool for pleasure, there are a few subgenres of porn that men tend to use in this revenge-oriented way. Gonzo porn, which is essentially sexual torture and humiliation of women, is tellingly not usually watched by individual men by themselves, but rather by groups of men who perform their masculinity to each other by laughing at the humiliated women on the screen. Michael Kimmel writes in *Guyland*:

> **The sexual fantasies of many young men become more revenge fantasies than erotic ones—revenge for the fact that most of them don't feel they get as much sex as they think they are supposed to get—or as they think everyone else is getting.**[209]

Plenty of porn is fun and pleasurable, and there's nothing inherently wrong with using an aid for pleasure. But these violent forms of porn reach out to a wounded place in men, a place that has been cultivated by patriarchal culture and filled with rage and anger against women. It is a form of what Digby calls "gender terrorism."[210] Can we be surprised any longer at the prevalence of rape in a culture that teaches us to behave like this?

---

208   Ibid, 142–143.
209   Ibid, 118.
210   Ibid, 137.

SUBJECTIFICATION

We have to be taught to objectify each other in our society precisely because it is not what comes naturally to us. Naturally, we see each other as allies in the human community, but in order to conquer, colonize, and dominate, we have to learn how to dehumanize each other. Racial and gendered slurs teach us to see each other as parts of an enemy group, rather than as individuals just like us. This has been seen in wars and genocidal campaigns over and over—the epithets "rats" and "cockroaches" were used to refer to both the Jews in Nazi Germany and the Tutsis during the Rwandan genocide.[211] It is massively depressing to think about the ways we shove ourselves and each other into narrow categories in order to serve some violent end we never even agreed to, but we don't do this because it's in our nature but because we've been conditioned to do it.

Objectification is a word that's thrown around a lot, but it's really important that we understand what it is and how it affects our everyday life experiences. Hollywood has taken on the Me Too movement in a major way, and recent years have seen more and more movies and TV shows led by women and people of color. This might seem like a frivolous gain, but it's not. Entertainment is the vehicle through which we teach people how to be people. Mass media is the mechanism of what Digby calls "cultural programming," by which he means:

> *the manifold ways in which a culture effectively programs habits of belief, desire, preference, and behavior into its members. Sources of cultural programming include parenting, education, religion, peer pressure, movies, books, television, online videos, music, and social media. […] Although cultural programming works in a much less precise way than computer programming, it does result in a lot of automatic behavior.*[212]

There aren't any masterminds sitting on gold thrones in Hollywood writing scripts about how to make people feel bad about themselves—there don't need to be. When we create art, we tend to create what we know, what we've already learned from our parents, peer groups, and the media we have thus far consumed. Unless we have done a lot of work to unlearn our cultural lessons and explicitly intend to create feminist/anti-racist art (which is happening more and more), whatever comes out will tend to support the status quo.

So many of our most popular cultural narratives are about shaming and punishing people who behave outside of the bounds of approved norms. In her study on single women, Anthea Taylor points to popular movies from the late 1980s and early 1990s, which was an era when women were gaining power, so we needed a few films to teach us what happens when a woman dares to be single, sexy, and—god forbid—powerful:

211   Livingstone Smith, David. "'Less Than Human': The Psychology of Cruelty." NPR, March 29, 2011. https://www.npr.org/2011/03/29/134956180/criminals-see-their-victims-as-less-than-human
212   Digby, *Love and War: How Militarism Shapes Sexuality and Romance.* New York, Columbia University Press (2014): 77.

> **Hollywood films such as *Basic Instinct* (1992), with a highly eroticized, ice pick wielding Sharon Stone, or *Disclosure* (1994), featuring Demi Moore as sexual harasser, as well as *Fatal Attraction* (1987), all mobilize the trope of the castrating, often sexually voracious, woman in a position of power.**[213]

Taylor focuses on *Fatal Attraction*, a film in which the main character, a successful single editor named Alex Forrest, becomes obsessed with her married lover and behaves in more and more psychopathic ways throughout the film. Alex (played by Glenn Close) terrorizes the married man's family, and, having threatened his wife and child, meets a violent end: her lover nearly drowns her, and his wife shoots her in the heart. Taylor writes, "*Fatal Attraction* is, unsurprisingly, routinely seen as a cautionary tale against women's single subjectivity; not only is it unviable, it is punishable by death (and an especially gruesome and brutal one at that)."[214]

Thirty years later, Glenn Close has now spoken out about the problems in the film, noting that the story is not told from Alex's perspective. In retrospect, it seems clear that Alex has a mental illness and probably abuse in her past, but, as Close points out, "There's no way for the audience to know what her past was."[215] Originally, the film was supposed to end with Alex taking her own life and framing her lover for her murder, but according to former Paramount executive Ned Tanen, that wasn't going to be enough: test audiences "want[ed] us to terminate the bitch with extreme prejudice."[216] Even the filmmakers wanted a (slightly) kinder ending for Alex Forrest that left her with some agency, but the people demanded the status quo: this threat to the modern family must be destroyed and humiliated, completely stripped of her power.

Horror films are particularly interesting as forms of cautionary entertainment. They are filled with tropes and common storylines that (at least for a time) usually involved the black guy getting killed first, then the sluts; only the innocent virgin could survive. Horror films channel our cultural anxieties, bringing up our fears, manifesting them in some monster, and then soothing us by violently destroying the monster. We like to see the virtuous people who appropriately uphold their romantic and gendered roles survive.

In a film like *Fatal Attraction*, Alex Forrest is the object of the film, the other. Her married lover is the person the audience mostly identifies with. For many generations, popular Hollywood films have been dominated by straight, white, male subjects, protagonists that we follow and root for throughout the film. The fact that movies that have female subjects as the main characters are derogatorily called "chick flicks" says enough about the truth of this patriarchal norm. From the time we started watching movies, we—not just men, but everyone else, too—learned to see men as subjects and women and people of color as objects, as plot devices.

213   Taylor, Anthea. *Single Women in Popular Culture: the Limits of Postfeminism.* London: Palgrave Macmillan (2012): 53.

214   Ibid, 54.

215   Desta, Yohana. "30 Years Later: Why Fatal Attraction Never Sat Right with Glenn Close." Vanity Fair, Sept 18, 2017. https://www.vanityfair.com/hollywood/2017/09/fatal-attraction-30-year-anniversary-glenn-close

216   Ibid.

A useful definition of objectification comes from philosopher Martha Nussbaum, who has stated that hallmarks of objectification include "denial of autonomy, denial of subjectivity. Not taking people's feelings into account, but also treating them as a mere instrument."[217] The object in question has no agency or ability, it can be possessed, damaged, or even destroyed with no moral consequences. Murdering the object Alex Forrest is seen as a heroic, moral act, even, an act of removing danger from the sacred family unit.

The good news, though, is that humans are really good at turning an object back into a subject. All it takes is a moment of identification, a glimpse from the perspective of the objectified person—or even the inanimate object. Spike Jonze once directed a fantastic commercial for Ikea that showed the life of a lamp, lit in a warm home in one scene, and then discarded in the rain, replaced by a shinier model, its lamp-face drooping in sadness on the street corner. The Ikea guy steps into frame and says, "Many of you feel bad for this lamp. That is because you crazy! It has no feelings! And the new one is much better!"[218] It's funny and effective because we really do feel bad for this lamp. Even rewatching it right now, I couldn't help but want to take that lamp home and care for it for the rest of its little lamp life!

Objectification can be easily broken when we have a chance to subjectify the object, to align with it and see it as an individual with feelings just like us. Children are especially adept at this, possibly in part because so many of their movies involve talking dolls and teacups and cars and all kinds of inanimate objects that they learn to see as having thoughts and feelings. Then, as we grow older, we watch different kinds of films in which we're gradually taught to align only with the white guys.

Subjectification is one of the reasons I got so excited when I saw the 2017 horror film *Get Out*. It's a classic trope in horror films for there to be one black character (if any) who gets the chop first. *Get Out* stars Daniel Kaluuya as the main character of the film, the protagonist with whom we consistently empathize throughout. It's not just that this is a mainstream Hollywood film starring a black main character, but that this film is about racism from the perspective of a black person. Kaluuya's character, Chris, goes to his white girlfriend Rose's family home (essentially a cabin in the woods), where at first microaggressions and offhand comments seem vaguely but not explicitly threatening. We feel with Chris, we look at the world through his eyes, and we completely understand why he feels so uncomfortable in an all-white environment. He wonders if he's being paranoid until he discovers that he is indeed in extreme danger, and yes, he is absolutely being targeted because of his race. In a piece I wrote on the film for *Feminist Current*, I wrote:

In the mild hypnotism of watching a movie, we enter the world of the protagonist.
We see what Chris sees (sometimes even through his camera). We know what Chris

217   Gras, Patricia and Rose Marie Salum. "The Objectification of Women with Martha Nussbaum." Literal Magazine, July 2012. http://literalmagazine.com/the-objectification-of-women-a-conversation-with-martha-nussbaum/

218   Ikea "Lamp" Commercial-Hi Res. Directed by Spike Jonze. Online video. Dec 20, 2007. YouTube. https://www.youtube.com/watch?v=dBqhIVyfsRg

knows, we feel what Chris feels. We don't need a treatise on microaggressions, we actually kind of experience them. Of course a movie can't entirely represent a person's or a group's experience, but stories can do something no explanation ever has: give a person someone else's perspective.[219]

It matters that more women and people of color are making movies now and writing scripts that let us into different kinds of experiences. These films, books, and TV shows are doing powerful work in the revolution of love: they are pushing against our tendency to objectify each other, put everyone in groups, and leave our compassion at home when it's convenient for us to use someone else for our own gain. Seeing things from someone else's perspective isn't always easy—especially when, say, they vote differently than you do. But watching a fun, pulpy horror movie or reading a book by someone whose perspective you wouldn't normally have access to can remind us of our compassion and teach us that we are still capable of feeling with someone different from us, no matter how much the culture has tried to push our empathy out of us.

How to Tell if Someone Is Being Objectified

There is a lot of objectification in porn and advertising. That doesn't mean, though, that there can't be beautiful, delightful, and titillating images out there that are also subjectifying. Knowing how to spot the difference can help you to see what's going on and to choose to consume more subjectifying media when you can. These tips are based on image-based art like film and photography. You can read a longer piece by me on this topic with some visual examples at:_https://www.elephantjournal.com/2013/08/subjectify-me-5-ways-to-tell-if-an-image-is-objectifying/

- ⊕ Faces: Humans are so good at recognizing faces we have a whole separate brain region for it. Look for faces that are showing expressions (and in porn ideally faces that seem to be having a great time).

- ⊕ Pieces: Cutting meat into pieces makes it easier for us to eat because we forget that it once was a being with feelings. Images can do this too. Look for bodies in context, not close-ups of disembodied parts.

- ⊕ Visual distance: What is the point of view of the camera? If it's looking through a mirror or window, or if it seems to be sneaking up on an unsuspecting object, it's objectifying. It's more subjectifying to be on the same side of the window as the subject, so the viewer is in the room with them. It's even more so if those depicted are engaging with the camera, clearly consenting to being seen.

- ⊕ Context: Objects don't have a personality. Subjects do. Can you get a sense of the photographed person's mood, personality, and likes and

---

219   Peters, Julie. "The real reasons Get Out was the most profitable film of 2017: White absolution and toxic masculinity." Feminist Current. August 30, 2017. https://www.feministcurrent.com/2017/08/30/real-reasons-get-profitable-film-2017-white-absolution-toxic-masculinity/

dislikes? What is the environment like in the image? Can you sense how
the person feels in that environment?

⌗ Agency and ability: Objects don't have power. Does the photographed
person seem in control, strong, and able to change anything about their
circumstances, or is something being done to them? Do they seem weak
and helpless or capable and powerful? Do they have choices?

MASCULINE ROMANCE

Our cultural insistence on strict gender roles, heterosexuality, and "maximum babies"
has dire consequences for the prospect of love. For one thing, it sets us up for
transactionality, not connection, in our relationships. Heterosexual love in this culture is
a deal: for a man, the subtext of a wedding vow might be, "I promise to be a protector,
a provider, and a sperm donor for you," while for a woman, it might be, "I promise to be
a nurturer, a baby-maker, and a dependent subordinate to you with an all-access pass
to my body." At a very basic level, men are socialized to trade money and power for
sex, and women to trade sex for money, protection, and security. Digby warns that this
pressures "both 'sides' in the relationship to strategize to get the most advantageous
exchange, to get the best deal possible, even to the extent of exploiting the partner."[220]
Books, magazines, and websites are full of advice for women on how to manipulate men
into staying with them, and men's media teach them how to trick women into going
to bed with them. These forms of light entertainment are "about how best to exploit a
partner in the context of a heterosexual relationship that is inherently transactional."[221]
We are set up to manipulate each other on the battlefield of love.

This is not the kind of love I want for us. I want more than gender norms and
"opposite sexes" that have to fight the "battle of the sexes." This is clearly an issue for
heterosexual couples, but the gender binary requirement plagues same-sex couples
too, at least from the outside: how many times have you heard a gay couple being
asked the insulting question, "Which one of you is the 'woman'?" I am not a gay man,
so I am obviously not intimate with the cultural nuances of this, but I have noticed
a certain type of language on TV shows and podcasts featuring gay men in which
everyone is required to identify as either a "top" or a "bottom." Not only do these
men have to publicly declare their private sexual preferences, those preferences are
supposed to define something about their personalities ("top" being powerful and
"manly" and "bottom" being submissive and "womanly"). Even worse, those preferences
are oriented around penetrative sex, which we've already discussed as a potentially
oppressive expectation in the bedroom that simply doesn't work for everyone. We can
get around queerness as long as it's not too queer: there is still marriage and babies (and
penetration), and everyone is still playing the roles we're familiar with. We sacrifice

---

220   Digby, Tom. *Love and War: How Militarism Shapes Sexuality and Romance.* New York, Columbia University
Press (2014): 37.
221   Ibid.

our humanness in exchange for this twisted performance. It takes work to look into someone's eyes and see them as they are when we've been trained to objectify each other and insist everyone fit into one of two strict gender categories.

Things, are, of course, changing in our society, and our experience of love is changing with the times. More and more people are challenging the gender binary by coming out as trans or gender non-conforming. As women begin to have more power, protection, and security that they can gain on their own, they are less and less willing to marry or stay with a compassionless man who treats them like shit. More women than men now attend college, at around 56 percent of women nationwide,[222] and it seems that, despite the stereotype that women want to settle down and men want to wander forever, lately, men are at least as interested in committed, long-term relationships as women are, if not more so. One survey found that in general, 70 percent of women and 73 percent of men said they wanted a long-term relationship.[223] A survey focusing on African Americans in particular found that 43 percent of single black men were interested in a long-term committed relationship while only 25 percent of black women wanted that same thing.[224]

I have started noticing this trend myself, particularly on my drive to work, when I indulge in my not-so-secret love for top forty pop music. The radio is filled with female singers talking about self-empowerment, partying at the club, and hanging out with their girlfriends while the men croon about falling in love and having five hundred babies. In one of her delightful songs, Meghan Trainor insists, "If I was you, I'd wanna be me too," and that "I can't help lovin' myself / And I don't need nobody else."[225] Hailee Steinfeld doesn't need any help from a man when she purrs, "I feel it deep inside without you, yeah, know how to satisfy [...] I'm gonna put my body first/ And love me so hard til it hurts."[226] These female singers are powerful, in control, and do not want to deal with the mess of misogynist men.

The male singers tell a completely different story about romance. Poor Drake lets a little insecurity slip on "One Dance" when he pleads, "as soon as you see the text reply me."[227] Young Charlie Puth keens, "'Cause even after all this time I still wonder/ Why I can't move on/ Just the way you did so easily."[228] James Arthur nostalgically remembers how "I held your hair back when / you were throwing up," and insists "I want to stay

222   Marcus, Jon. "Why Men Are the New College Minority." The Atlantic, Aug 8, 2017. https://www. theatlantic.com/education/archive/2017/08/why-men-are-the-new-college-minority/536103/
223   Bradshaw, Carolyn, Arnold S. Kahn, and Bryan K. Saville. "To Hook Up or Date: Which Gender Benefits?" Sex Roles, Volume 62, Issue 9–10 (2010): 661–669.
224   "African Americans' Lives Today." NPR, Robert Wood Johnson Foundation, and the Harvard School of Public Health. June 2013. https://www.rwjf.org/content/dam/farm/reports/surveys_and_polls/2013/rwjf406076
225   Trainor, Meghan. "Me Too." 2016, Thank You, Sony/ATV Music Publishing, Universal Music Publishing Group, Kobalt Music Publishing Ltd.
226   Steinfeld, Hailee. "Love Myself." 2015, Jem and the Holograms soundtrack, Warner/Chappell Music, Inc, Universal Music Publishing Group.
227   Drake. "One Dance." 2016, Views, Sony/ATV Music Publishing LLC, Kobalt Music Publishing Ltd., BMG Rights Management, Sentric Music.
228   Puth, Charlie. "We Don't Talk Anymore (Feat. Selena Gomez)." 2016, Nine Track Mind, Warner/ Chappell Music, Inc, Universal Music Publishing Group, Kobalt Music Publishing Ltd.

with you until we're gray and old."[229] Arthur's grand romantic fantasy is making his lover breakfast in bed and then taking the kids off to school.

These men would have no luck with Marshmello and Anne Marie, who are not interested in any romantic gestures, especially anything that looks like that ol' boom-box-in-the-rain cliché. In the song "FRIENDS," they sing:

> *Have you got no shame?*
> *You looking insane*
> *Turning up at my door*
> *It's two in the morning, the rain is pouring*
> *Haven't we been here before?*[230]

Romance seems to be dead, at least for the ladies.

There was a time when I wanted to be swept away into a whirlwind romance, but I've since learned that if a guy wants to get really committed really fast, it's a red flag for me. It's what my friend Emilee calls an emotional boner: he gets really excited because you look just like the fantasy of what he thinks he wants, but the second you show yourself to be a human being with skin, the illusion crashes down. Or, worse, he's trying to manipulate you into an abusive relationship, which is sometimes what's happening with guys who move too fast. Wanting to "lock it down" indicates a certain possessiveness and an entitlement to your attention and commitment. There's a desperation there that women have started to catch on to. Digby calls this "masculine romanticism,"[231] suggesting that men

> **may be trending toward taking romantic love *seriously* and seeing their happiness as dependent on it. Of course, what that really means, though, is that they are more likely to feel dependent on achieving an entirely unrealistic fantasy that entitles them to the possession of a woman.**[232]

No wonder women are less interested in romance like this: it's a lazy way to possess someone. No matter how many roses and serenades it might come with, many of us are hoping for something more than a soulless transactional romance. More and more women are choosing the single life, having babies on our own, and living self-sufficiently without the threat of relationships with men. That could be a good thing, but there's a downside: many women have gotten so used to distrusting men and their intentions that we reject any man who seems to like us. It's not always easy to tell the difference between a genuine expression of romantic like and the masculine romanticism that is trying to use, abuse, and possess us—especially if that's happened before.

229   Arthur, James. "Say You Won't Let Go." 2016, *Back From the Edge*, Ultra Tunes, Sony/ATV Music Publishing LLC, Kobalt Music Publishing Ltd.
230   Marshmello and Anne Marie, "FRIENDS." 2018, *Speak Your Mind*, Sony/ATV Music Publishing LLC
231   Digby, Tom. *Love and War: How Militarism Shapes Sexuality and Romance*. New York, Columbia University Press (2014): 90.
232   Ibid, 94.

LOVE AND SPINSTERS

As women gain more power and get wise to the raw deal heterosexual romance has thus far offered us, many of us are opting out. As Rebecca Traister found in her study of single women, singleness is on the rise in the US: "There were 3.9 million more single adult women in 2014 than there were in 2010."[233] The age of first marriage for women held steady at between age twenty and twenty-two from 1890 to 1980, but today, it has jumped up to age twenty-seven, and even higher than that in some urban areas.[234] We are in an age of spinsters, perhaps, but that may not be a problem—at least not for women.

In her book *Singled Out,* Bella DePaulo busts some of our many cultural myths about the benefits of marriage. In a study on happiness over time, DePaulo looked at single, married, and divorced populations to see if, as the culture insists, marriage really does make us happier. She found that, in general, people's happiness tended to stay pretty much the same whether they got married, stayed single, or got divorced. For the marrieds, DePaulo writes, there was

> *a tiny blip in happiness. On average, they were about a quarter of a scale point happier around the time of their wedding than they had been about five years before. Notice also, though, that within a few years that small puff of happiness disappeared; the continuously married people were then, on average, no happier than when they were single.*[235]

She does note, however, that men do tend to benefit from marriage in terms of health. Getting married is better for men at first, and widowhood is bad for men at first, but things tend to equalize within a few years. She writes, "In all findings, was there any evidence to support a claim that marriage makes people healthier? Yes, for men—when they first married. But they got over it."[236] There is also some evidence that men who are married tend to live longer. For women, though, there is no health benefit:

> *As for the women, the stability of their health was rather remarkable. Basically, nothing fazed them. Regardless of whether they got married, got unmarried, stayed married, or stayed single, women (on average) noticed no real changes in their health.*[237]

So women don't benefit physically or economically from getting married, while men essentially get a pay raise and enough support at home to boost their wellbeing at least a little bit. Oh, and by the way, DePaulo adds:

233   Traister, Rebecca. *All the Single Ladies.* New York, Simon & Schuster (2016): 8.
234   Ibid, 5.
235   DePaulo. Bella. *Singled Out: How Singles are Stereotyped, Stigmatized, and Ignored, and Still Live Happily Ever After.* New York, St. Martin's Press (2006): 36.
236   Ibid, 48.
237   Ibid.

Violence against women is primarily intimate partner violence: 64.0 percent
of the women who reported being raped, physically assaulted, and/or stalked
since age 18 were victimized by a current or former husband, cohabiting partner,
boyfriend, or a date.[238]

Romance, for women, is looking paler and paler next to a good job, a safe apartment and a sense of independence, along with maybe a cat or three.

The rise of spinsterism sounds like a women's problem because of the negative connotations of the word "spinster" (for which men have no equivalent). But single women are doing just fine without oppressive romance narratives controlling their lives. The lonely, frustrated (and sometimes violent) men who are left out are the ones with the problem. The negative spin on spinsterism is another example of cultural marketing that is trying to teach us that men are dominant over women in a world where patriarchy and militarism prevail. Tom Digby points out that these patterns

> *point our attention to an extremely important meta-pattern in militaristic*
> *cultures: the tendency to assume that all the items in that list are not men's*
> *issues, but rather women's issues, or, even more narrowly, feminist issues.[239]*

The problem of violence against women in our culture is not a "women's issue" or a "feminist issue." It's an everyone issue, and a big source of the problem is men's suffering and rage in a culture that wants them to be soldiers, not human beings. Women don't want to be reduced to just being womb tanks, either, but when we are forced into a subordinate role in a society that is swimming with semiconscious hatred for us, it's pretty tough to feel like we can do anything to change this reality. Feminist work is incredibly powerful and important, and I'm not saying we shouldn't keep fighting for women's rights. We should. But if things are really going to change in our society in the long term, *men* are going to need to change.

I absolutely identify as a feminist, and one of the things that means to me is working to create a world where we all get to see each other as human beings worthy of love and respect. We live in a system that oppresses women and insists on domination by men, but, ironically, this system functions by dominating men at the same time. Men suffer under patriarchy, and maybe a little compassion and support for men might help them stop raping us all the time. As bell hooks insists:

> *To truly address male pain and male crisis, we must as a nation be willing to*
> *expose the harsh reality that patriarchy has damaged men in the past and*
> *continues to damage them in the present. If patriarchy were truly rewarding to*
> *men, the violence and addiction in family life that is so all-pervasive would not*
> *exist.[240]*

---

238   Ibid, 164.
239   Digby, Tom. *Love and War: How Militarism Shapes Sexuality and Romance.* New York, Columbia University Press (2014): 73–74.
240   hooks, bell. *The Will to Change: Men, Masculinity, and Love.* New York, Washington Square Press (2004): 31.

It's not any individual woman's job to help a man who wants to change. Women have enough emotional labor to do in our lives without having to drop everything to emotionally support a man who is struggling. That's not our job. One of the damaging tendencies we have in this culture is to blame a man's female partner when he acts like a jerk, and it's really not her fault. When Ariana Grande's ex-boyfriend Mac Miller died of a drug overdose shortly after they broke up, Grande was harassed so harshly on Twitter and Instagram by fans blaming her for his death that she had to go dark for a little while—quite a statement for a pop star with most of her fans on social media. When she came back online, she pointed out, "I am not a babysitter or a mother, and no woman should feel that they need to be. I have cared for him and tried to support his sobriety and prayed for his balance for years (and always will, of course), but shaming/blaming women for a man's inability to keep his shit together is a very major problem."[241]

Still, men do need support to change, and it's natural for men to lean on the women in their lives for emotional support: men have been socialized to fear showing emotion to other men, and women have been socialized to take care of men. I don't think men should *never* talk to women about what they are going through, but perhaps part of their work could be figuring out ways to support each other rather than expecting the women in their lives to drop everything and fix them. I'll reply to your text when I damn well feel like it, Drake.

It's vital that we understand that we *all* participate in a culture that dehumanizes everyone, in part by insisting that we fit into the narrow gender binary of "women" and "men." As we work toward equal rights for LGBTQ+ people, power for women at work, and compassion for men at home, we are fighting back against this violent militaristic battle of the sexes. We are fighting to live in a culture of love, not war. Refusing to fit into these narrow categories along gendered lines is a step toward making it okay for us to be human beings worthy of love, respect, and equality.

LOVING MEN

Men aren't the only ones who can be violent; in this culture that tries to strip us of our empathy, of course, anyone can be. Our suffering creates rage and pain, and when we don't know how to channel that pain, we can end up lashing out and hurting each other. One of the first times I was ever touched nonconsensually was by a woman—well, a girl—at church camp (Yep. At church camp). We were treading water in a lake, and she kept putting her hands on my body, touching me everywhere, including my child breasts and thighs. I kept trying to tell her to stop, that I didn't like it and it was creeping me out, and she wouldn't stop. Church camp is certainly a place where a young lesbian might feel confused enough to touch another girl under the water, and I don't really blame her. When our identities are frozen in an "other" place that we can't talk about (in

---

241   Weisenstein, Kara. "Ariana Grande, Mac Miller, and Why We Blame Women for Male Substance Abuse." Vice, Sept 19, 2018. https://www.vice.com/en_ca/article/a38g5k/ariana-grande-mac-miller-and-why-we-blame-women-for-male-substance-abuse

front of God!), it can lead us to some bewildering places. A few months later she sent me a postcard with a picture of a cathedral on it wishing me the best from Jesus. I do hope that girl was able to come out eventually and learn a few things about consent in her adult life.

Mothers, the eternal martyrs of our patriarchal stranglehold, can sometimes be the worst perpetrators of patriarchal violence against their children. They want their boy children to be good warriors and their girl children to be good mothers, just like the culture always taught them. hooks writes:

> **No wonder then that male rage is often most directed at women in intimate relationships. Such relationships clearly trigger for many males the anger and rage they felt in childhood when their mothers did not protect them or ruthlessly severed emotional bonds in the name of patriarchy.**[242]

Women have been just as indoctrinated into this system as men have been. In order to be good nurturers, we've been encouraged to learn the language of emotion, to express our feelings, to ask for help when we need it, to care for others, and to put up with men who are unable to fully love us. When our men start to rebel against their own emotional disability and tell us honestly about their pain, we don't always like it. If he starts to change the way he plays his role, our role (as the "opposite sex") may have to change, too. The terror of losing our own identity, along with all our patriarchal good-girl points, arises. We fear that if our men show vulnerability, they may not be able to protect us— something we've always been taught we need. hooks tells a story of her feelings when her male partner started to show some vulnerability and woundedness: "I did not want to hear the pain of my male partner because hearing it required that I surrender my investment in the patriarchal ideal of the male as protector of the wounded. If he was wounded, then how could he protect me?"[243]

Changing the way our culture indoctrinates us will not be a project of castigating individual men who are violent toward women. We must all look deeply within ourselves and admit the ways we've been trained to think that there are only two genders and that they must play very specific roles. There's work for all of us to do here, not just the men.

Many women are very strongly identified with our role as relationship people—the people who keep everyone together, who manage feelings, who perform the emotional labor. We think this makes us better at loving, but it doesn't. We are trained to be better at managing emotions and organizing the home life, but we aren't necessarily any better equipped to see other human beings as human beings. In order for men to change, they are going to have to feel their pain, and men don't currently have much support for feeling their feelings, certainly not from other men and not necessarily from women (and, again, that's no one's obligation). hooks writes, "Many women cannot hear male pain about love because it sounds like an indictment of female failure. Since sexist

---

242   hooks, bell. *The Will to Change: Men, Masculinity, and Love*. New York, Washington Square Press (2004): 61.
243   Ibid, 143.

norms have taught us that loving is our task, whether in our role as mothers or lovers or friends, if men say they are not loved, then we are at fault; we are to blame."[244]

We are not to blame, of course, not at all. It is not women's project to fix men, which is one reason violence against women should not be understood solely as a feminist issue. The fear, rage, and aggression that underlies that violence is a men's issue, but we women have our issues, too. The transformative work of insisting on a better world that is not so reliant on these gender roles is quite a project, and we need each other to get through it. As we do, we must offer compassion to men (along with appropriate consequences), but we must also offer compassion to ourselves for all the ways we haven't figured this out yet. We have to find ways to work on ourselves and love each other without taking responsibility for everyone else's problems. Trying to change our conditioning is a little like deciding you're a freshwater fish in the middle of the salty ocean. It's hard to even imagine what that freshwater world would look like—but it's worth gathering a few other fishes around to try to find out.

As a woman who usually dates men, my most intimate choices are defined by these cultural realities whether I like it or not. With the awareness I have thus far cultivated, I must protect myself from further violence by being able to clearly see what is happening when a man is trying to get close to me and creating strategies for getting away if I need to. Love is sometimes quite literally a battlefield. I must conserve my energy for my work and self-care and avoid getting into too many fights about feminism with people who are not interested in hearing what I have to say. But I am also doing my best to continue to choose love and compassion, not only in my intimate relationships, but also with the men I know who struggle to remain human while performing their cultural roles. I try to support men who are brave enough to show their vulnerability, whatever that looks like. And sometimes I work with David Hatfield, a facilitator here in Vancouver who runs a men's group called Manology that meets every Monday to talk about modern masculinity.

The first time I went to an all-gender meeting of the Manology group, I encountered men (and myself) in a completely new and honestly quite shocking way. Sitting in a circle with the men who had been coming to this group for months along with several others of different genders, I listened to their stories. I'll never forget one man who explained that he had started coming to the group after he hit his wife. He had realized that he had all this anger and no way to express it other than through violence. He felt horrible about it and wanted to find a way to change, so he started seeking resources that could help him understand his feelings and find other ways to express them. Up until that point, I had always felt that the moment a man showed any sign of violence, I would head for the hills. This is a good survival strategy (and I'm sticking to it), but I didn't realize how much I was dehumanizing men in the process. It hadn't occurred to me that a man might be violent because it was the only way he'd learned to express his feelings, and that he might be willing to do the work it takes to change. I hadn't confronted the ways I had objectified men—the ways I feared them and saw them as

---

244   Ibid, 7.

other. Hearing this man's story and those of many others in the room, I saw the male heart, possibly for the first time in my life. I saw their vulnerability and humanness and how much they were just like me. I hadn't even realized I was looking at the world that way. It was incredibly powerful simply to hear these men's stories. It gave me hope in a way I had never felt before.

The point I'm trying to make here is not that everyone should be forgiven or that we should all sit down and listen to men more. Rather, I think we need to be honest with ourselves and acknowledge that no one escapes cultural conditioning. We're not bad people because we play the gender roles we've been given. But once we become aware of how this system works, we can start trying to change it, both within ourselves and within our intimate relationships. We don't all need to be activists or go into politics (but if you want to, go for it, and thank you for your service!), but there are many ways that we can participate in making the world kinder and more compassionate. bell hooks argues that we need a revolution in order to change the toxicity of patriarchy and militarism in our culture, and with it, end the epidemic of male violence. "That revolution," she argues,

> *will necessarily be based on a love ethic. To create loving men, we must love males. Loving maleness is different from praising and rewarding males for living up to sexist-defined notions of male identity. Caring about men because of what they do for us is not the same as loving males for simply being. When we love maleness, we extend our love whether males are performing or not.*[245]

Working on seeing each other truly and with love is powerful and radical in a culture that wants us to perform our roles precisely and make maximum babies. We can find power in transformative love, which often begins in figuring out how to love ourselves first.

Loving Men

Whatever our gender or sexual orientation, there are usually at least a few men in our lives we could work on loving better. The gender dynamics in our culture can make it hard to relate to men, let alone support them in changing. Here are some things to consider:

- ⊕ Check yourself. What is your pattern of emotional connection to men? Consider how you talk to men and how you listen.

- ⊕ Show up. If you're a man, acknowledge that you can potentially be a powerful influencer of change among other men. Modeling emotional maturity in front of other men can be a game-changer.

- ⊕ Take care of yourself. Women have been socialized to take care of men and try to fix all their problems. For a woman, sometimes the best way to

245   Ibid, 11.

support a man is to take care of yourself instead. Let him be emotionally strong on his own.

⊕ Open up. Men have been socialized to expect women to take care of them and to avoid emotional conversation with each other. If you are a man, consider ways that you might create some space to open up those conversations. Often the best way is to start with sharing your own feelings with another man.

⊕ Model self-care. Whatever your gender, getting help for yourself (therapy, groups, whatever works for you) means you're changing the culture from the inside out. Talking about the benefits with men might help encourage them to do it too.

⊕ Listen. Sometimes it feels like men get all the airtime already. But are we really listening to them? Are we seeing them for who they really are, or just expecting them to fulfill a role in our lives? What would it be like to listen more deeply, to really hear what he's saying? Showing men compassion can help encourage their compassion.

⊕ Speak. Sometimes women and other genders protect men by avoiding telling their stories. I know plenty of men who didn't realize there was a problem in their society until they got close to someone who had experienced the actual effects of living in a patriarchal/militaristic culture. If you feel comfortable, tell a man some of your stories.

⊕ Bring it up. There are plenty of moments in our lives where we might notice something misogynistic in a commercial or in a movie. If you feel comfortable, point it out to the man you're watching with. Not everyone is open to this; sometimes it's helpful to ask first if he's interested. Make sure you're willing to have the conversation, too. Ask him what he thinks. Give him a chance to think about it, and listen to what he says. This isn't about starting an argument, it's just about bringing up the conversation.

⊕ Be a good bystander. If you are in a group and someone starts making misogynistic jokes or belittling a man for having feelings, say something (as long as you feel safe to do so). Let him know you don't think it's funny. This can be incredibly powerful for changing the culture around you, especially if you are a man in that culture.

⊕ Be a joiner (or a leader). If you're a man, join a men's group where men can feel safe enough to talk about their feelings. If there isn't one in your area, create one. This is especially important for male survivors of sexual assault, as they tend to have access to fewer of these kinds of resources than women do.

SELF-LOVE AND OTHER-LOVE

At the end of every episode of the drag queen reality TV show *RuPaul's Drag Race*, the great RuPaul Charles calls out, "If you can't love yourself, then how the hell are you gonna love somebody else? Can I get an amen up in here?" And all the drag queens on the stage respond, "Amen!"

It's true—well, sort of true. The practice of love must be happening within ourselves in order for us to live in a loving way. So much of this book is about practices of self-love: prioritizing pleasure, eating mindfully, and caring for our bodies are all concrete actions in the service of self. It's important that we understand that self-love isn't a given—at least for most of us. Even if we had a really nice family and have never been traumatized in any way, our culture makes it tough for us to love ourselves as we are. Loving ourselves is a radical act in a society that wants us to perform our given roles, sacrificing our authenticity and emotional connectedness along the way. Letting ourselves feel is a profound practice of self-love in and of itself, but sharing that vulnerability with another person is a key aspect of that practice.

RuPaul is absolutely right in that having a healthy relationship with ourselves is the foundation for everything else. But it is not a prerequisite for us to love others or for other people to love us. Our self-love is bolstered by a supportive community, and sometimes other people can help teach us how to love ourselves. We don't necessarily get any examples of the kind of love that supports our growth in our first families, and RuPaul's drag queens know that story firsthand. Many of them have families that rejected them, excommunicated them, or forced them to try to pray the gay away. They were not seen and loved for who they were at first, because they were not performing their gender roles the way our war-reliant society requires in order to make soldiers, breeders, and maximum babies. But one of my absolute favorite things about that show is that the queens find love in their lives in other ways. They find love in their communities, they make new families, and they let other people support them and build them up while they try to recover from their past traumas—sometimes even on camera while they are putting their makeup on. Even though it's a competition, *RuPaul's Drag Race* is also a community of people who support each other's art, and the art is at its best when it's authentic, vulnerable, and creative—connected to that erotic force that manifests in our connection to ourselves, our passions, and, sure, that perfect runway look.

We must find our chosen families when our first families don't teach us how to love, and our friends and community can help us learn those new ways of loving. In her book *Trauma and Recovery*, Judith Herman writes, "The core experiences of psychological trauma are disempowerment and disconnection from others. Recovery, therefore, is based upon the empowerment of the survivor and the creation of new connections.

Recovery can take place only in the context of relationships; it cannot occur in isolation."[246]

Yes, loving ourselves matters, and doing our own personal work is deeply important. We have to establish physical and emotional safety first, which can mean certain types of isolation. We have to build up our courage to deal with other human beings and their unpredictable ways. Others are not necessarily trustworthy. We can't control whether someone says the wrong thing or hurts our feelings or accidentally triggers something about our experience of trauma. Establishing some safety within the self is vital because it helps us find courage in the face of unpredictable love. It's not that we learn to love ourselves and then somehow magically we know how to love other people. Loving others is a whole other skill set that takes its own kind of practice. When we're ready for that, others can help us heal in ways that were impossible alone. That's why the last stage in this book is Love.

This is one of the reasons I think groups can be really helpful for survivors. When I first started to directly face what had happened to me and get some help, I wanted one-on-one therapy, which was the model I was used to. But what was affordable at the time was a group at the Women Against Violence Against Women center and a course on cognitive behavioral therapy at the Mood Disorders Association of BC. The one-on-one therapy I eventually got was helpful, for sure, but in a different way from what I experienced in the groups. It wasn't a replacement for therapy, but rather a different kind of healing. Being in a room full of other people who had gone through something similar or who struggled in similar ways was incredibly healing for me. Trauma is always isolating. It always makes us feel that we are facing this singular shame meant for us alone. While every traumatic experience is unique and everyone responds in different ways, the fact of having been through something is hardly rare in our society. There are many of us here. We need the right contexts and good facilitators to help us connect with each other in appropriate ways, but these are the communities that can help us get started on the project of intimacy after pain.

Many survivors are lonely. We feel isolated and like no one understands us. We feel there is something deeply rotten inside of us and that if we let anyone see who we really are, we'll inevitably be rejected. Sure enough, sometimes people do reject us, that's a thing that happens. People have no obligation to like us, and most people are not trained to be able to hold our painful stories well.

I've had an interesting journey trying to figure out what to say when people ask me what the book I've been working on is about. When I didn't want to talk about it, I'd say something neutral like, "Oh, it's about mindfulness for healing," which is true but kind of vague, and no one ever had any follow-up questions. If I felt like opening a can of worms, I'd tell them it's about recovering from sexual assault. Then people would kind of nod and smile and seem interested, but then they'd get stuck on what to say and quickly change the subject (I'm terrible at cocktail parties). I don't think they dodged because

246   Herman, Judith. *Trauma and Recovery: The Aftermath of Violence—from Domestic Abuse to Political Terror.* New York: Basic Books (1997): 133.

they didn't want to hear about it or because they think there's something wrong with me for having experienced assault. I think it's because it's a big topic that is usually so hidden and silenced that they just had no idea what to say. Or maybe they had been through something themselves that they didn't know how to talk about because they've always been encouraged to keep their silence. Sure enough, just bringing up the topic can be triggering and upsetting for people even if you don't share any details, but I think that's because we are taught to feel so much shame about these experiences. This is probably an unpopular opinion, but I think we should bring it up a bit more often, talk about it the way we talk about car accidents or, I don't know, shingles—things that aren't great but happen to enough of us that it's not weird to talk about good strategies for prevention and healing in mixed company. Anyway, if we did maybe I'd seem less awkward at cocktail parties.

Romance can be a terrifying prospect for survivors of sexual assault or intimate partner violence. Some of us want to engage in it one day but it feels impossible from where we stand. Some of us have decided to let that aspect of life fall away, and some of us are in committed partnerships with people we want to connect to but feel we can't after what happened to us. Whatever the situation, any practice of intimacy feeds every other practice of intimacy. We do not need romantic partnerships to have intimacy and connection in our lives. We need friends and community relationships whether or not we have partners, despite the cultural messaging that a spouse should be one's absolutely-everything. It's important that we honor and acknowledge the ways we already cultivate intimacy in our lives and keep working to create more, whether that's in a romantic context or not. If romantic connection is a goal, we have to keep in mind that those other intimacy practices with our friends and community members can support our capacity to love others on any level.

LONELINESS

Besides, loneliness isn't such a bad thing. In fact, loneliness is a powerful form of desire. It's an expression of the erotic force that is asking for *more*. It's is a call for deeper connection, for being with people who can really see us for who we are.

Loneliness isn't the same thing as alone-ness. I've felt desperately lonely at a party full of people in my own house. I've felt it in many of my romantic relationships where I had a committed partner, but I didn't feel seen or heard. I love the way the philosopher Osho has phrased it: "Loneliness is the absence of other. Aloneness is the presence of oneself."[247] Loneliness has an object, even if it's an imaginary person or community. It lets us know that we don't feel connected and pushes us toward that connection, possibly even past our fear of putting ourselves out there. Aloneness can be a delight, an indulgence even. It's a space for us to feel internally connected, held in the relationship we cultivate within our own selves.

---

247   Osho. "Loneliness is the absence of the other. Aloneness is the presence of the self." Oshoworld newsletter, Sept 2008. http://www.oshoworld.com/newsletter/sept08/pdf/14_loneliness_is_absence_of_the.pdf

Loving in the model our culture currently gives us, which requires us not to connect but to play out certain roles, is an incredibly lonely form of relationship. It's not true love. It's a hollow performance. Feeling lonely means you're not satisfied with that arrangement and want something deeper.

Sometimes loneliness actually wants us to be alone. It can be a call to end a shallow love relationship or get away from people who do not support our spiritual growth. It can feel lonely to choose something the culture around us doesn't want us to choose. But the alternative—to keep performing, never change, and never allow anyone to truly see us— is a raw deal. Our loneliness knows it is, even if we don't realize it consciously.

In a poem called "My Eyes So Soft" (translated by Daniel Ladinsky), the fourteenth century Persian poet Hafiz wrote:

> *Don't surrender your loneliness so quickly.*
> *Let it cut more deep.*
> *Let it ferment and season you*
> *As few human or even divine ingredients can.*
> *Something missing in my heart tonight*
> *Has made my eyes so soft,*
> *My voice so tender,*
> *My need of God*
> *Absolutely*
> *Clear.*[248]

In this poem, the speaker is called to intimacy with the energy he calls "God." For me, this energy *is* love, true intimacy, that mysterious experience that can exist between people. Loneliness calls us to true love. Loving ourselves is deeply important, but loving other people is a vital part of our healing practice that supports that self-love, too. Self-love and other-love are part of a cycle, they don't have to go in any particular order. Loving fully can be scary. It doesn't always work out, and it can break our hearts. But when we are bolstered by our connections with ourselves and with our communities, we know heartbreak is a pain that we can tolerate. We are supported, so we can be brave. Our loneliness shows us the way.

LONELINESS PRACTICE

For me, meditation is a practice of self-love. It's often an unstructured experience of sitting with whatever's on my mind, hanging out with myself, and just being with whoever I happen to be that day. Sometimes, however, it's very powerful to meditate directly with our emotions, and loneliness is a beautiful one to work with.

---

248   Hafiz, Trans. Daniel Ladinsky. *The Gift: Poems by Hafiz, the Great Sufi Master.* New York: Penguin Compass (1999): 277.

- Find a comfortable position to meditate in. It doesn't have to be anything formal, a chair is fine or even lying down if that works better for you. Stay awake, though!

- Take a few deep breaths and check in with how you are feeling.

- Call in the emotion of loneliness. Say its name in your mind. There might be a particular reason you're feeling lonely right now; you can bring that in, too.

- Try to find the particular place in your body where you feel your loneliness. I usually feel it around my heart. Place your hands on or near that place and breathe into the sensation. Relax into what you feel and try to stay with the feeling of loneliness.

- Silently to yourself, say the phrase "Hello, loneliness. Thank you for talking to me. I'm listening." Then leave some space to really listen (and by *listen*, I mean *feel*). Thoughts will come and go. Your mind will wander. Keep calling your loneliness back and breathing into it.

- Be curious about your loneliness. Don't try to fix or change it, and do your best not to judge yourself for it. Keep breathing and let yourself feel the discomfort of the emotion.

- Sit with your loneliness until the timer goes off. Pay attention to how it feels, if it moves, what other thoughts and feelings may arise. You may discover grief or anger hanging out at the corners of your loneliness; that's fine, they are invited too.

- When you are finished with your meditation, take a couple of deep breaths. Optionally, take a few minutes to journal about what you noticed.

THE PRACTICE OF INTIMACY

The yoga teacher, Buddhist meditation teacher, and psychotherapist Michael Stone has defined the word yoga to mean "intimacy." For Stone, intimacy means understanding our interconnectedness with all things. It means seeing every choice we make as having consequences on some level. It means *practicing* relationships. In his book *Awake in the World,* Stone writes, "Intimacy does not simply refer to sex. I translate the word yoga as 'intimacy' to connote the fact that everything is inherently contingent on everything else, from the basic molecules and strings that hold the world together all the way to the familial bonds that give rise to families and character."[249] For Stone, intimacy is the practice of being close to reality as it is, moment to moment. It means allowing ourselves to fully feel our pain, our loneliness, our desires, and our joy and letting them be present as they change. He goes on to say:

---

249   Stone, Michael. *Awake in the World: Teachings from Yoga and Buddhism for Living an Engaged Life.* Boston, Shambhala (2011): 12.

When we see that interconnectedness runs through each and every thing that we encounter, we begin to see that entering our lives fully is the deepest kind of intimacy we can ever encounter. In fact, in order to heal, we need to find an intimate connection to whatever it is that ails us. To be intimate with pain, sadness, or even loneliness is to enter that state of mind fully. This doesn't mean becoming completely absorbed, obsessed, or wallowing. It means riding the lively wave of anxiety or joy until it disperses and becomes something else.[250]

For Stone, nonattachment is the practice of intimacy. We often think of the concept of nonattachment to mean that we shouldn't get too attached to anything because everything dies. For Stone, the opposite is true: precisely because everything is impermanent, we should get as close to each moment as we possibly can, understanding that it's never going to be quite like this ever again.

For hooks and Digby, the problem of love is a problem of living in a social system that requires us to perform certain roles according to patriarchal or militaristic requirements. Stone believes that we manifest this problem by getting stuck in our narratives of who we think our others should be instead of seeing them for who they really are. We have all kinds of stories about what our relationships are supposed to look like. The problem of attachment isn't that we love too fiercely, it's that we're so attached to the story of our other that we're not truly present with the living, dying person in front of us.

There's nothing wrong with having narratives about the world and our others; in fact, they can be quite useful to us. Narratives are essentially a set of expectations, and it would be pretty hard to live in a world completely free of expectations. Alice didn't want to live in Wonderland *forever*. The problem is that we can become addicted to these narratives. We start to *need* things to go according to our expectations. Those expectations can blind us to the possibility of any other story that could also be there. "I really think that addiction at bottom is an addiction to a narrative," Stone has said, and also that "One sign that there's addiction to a narrative is that your imagination isn't there."[251] We are in pain because we believe we're not acting out our story the way we think we're supposed to, and we're plagued with narratives like "I'm never going to be good enough" and "I'm a failure." This can close us down to hope, to the possibility of any other self that we might possibly be. When we insist everyone act in exactly the ways we expect them to and never change, we can't begin to imagine the world being anything other than exactly what we expect it to be.

Loving imaginatively, then, means showing up for your others and listening to what they have to say. It means feeling with them and giving them a chance to change. We get very uncomfortable when our loved ones threaten to change something about themselves. They take up a new hobby or make a new friend or (god forbid) start asking for what they need, and it terrifies us. We're afraid not so much of losing the person as of losing the narrative we have about who they are and who we are with them—of losing

---

250   Ibid.
251   Stone, Michael. "Mindfulness & Social Action: Towards a Secular Spirituality." Lecture, Semperviva Yoga Studio, Vancouver, Jan 2015.

the role they play in our lives. When a close person threatens to change, we think it must force us to also change. When we are unimaginative about what that might look like, it's pretty terrifying. So yes, part of loving fully means loving ourselves enough to know that whatever another person does won't change who we are or what we are trying to be. It means getting curious about the other, seeing who they are from day to day. "In fact," Stone writes, "we can define healthy relationships as the ability to take in someone or something without superimposing our biases and expectations on them."[252]

For couples therapist Esther Perel, this tendency to see the story of our lover instead of seeing who they actually are is one of the ways passion dies within a long-term relationship. "Many of the couples who come to therapy imagine that they know everything there is to know about their mate," Perel writes.[253] She urges them "to recover their curiosity and catch a glimpse behind the walls that barricade the other."[254] When there is no mystery left in the relationship, Perel argues, there can be no spark, no passion, no interest or curiosity in getting to know the other's internal world. There is no space for desire when everything is already known—especially when what is known is the same boring old story it's been for decades.

The idea that there's nothing left to know about our lover isn't true, however. It's that we don't really want to know more. It's not just that we are unable to imagine our lover is anything other than what we're used to, but that we feel safer when our partner remains predictable. Perel goes on to say:

> *Our need for constancy limits how much we are willing to know the person who's next to us. We are invested in having him or her conform to an image that is often a creation of our own imagination, based on our own set of needs. [...] We see what we want to see, what we can tolerate seeing, and our partner does the same. Neutralizing each other's complexity affords us a kind of manageable otherness. We narrow down our partner, ignoring or rejecting essential parts when they threaten the established order of our coupledom.*[255]

This does a disservice to our partners, of course, but it also does a disservice to us. When our partner must remain the same at all times, we are locked in a choreography that must simply repeat itself, never allowing either partner to access their creativity, their individual selfhood, their capacity to change, or their passion. When we reduce our others in this way, Perel warns, "we also reduce ourselves, jettisoning large chunks of our personalities in the name of love."[256]

One of the reasons it's so difficult for us to love each other fully is because it's intensely vulnerable. Love feels good, but it can also be very painful. There is always the awareness of loss on the other side of love, as well as the anxiety of uncertainty. If we let ourselves

---

252   Stone, Michael. *Yoga for a World Out of Balance: Teachings on Ethics and Social Action.* Boston, Shambhala (2009): 30.
253   Perel, Esther. *Mating in Captivity: Unlocking Erotic Intelligence.* New York, Harper (2006): 13.
254   Ibid.
255   Ibid.
256   Ibid.

fully feel the love we feel, we are also letting in the possibility of loss. Grief is, after all, a form of love. There can't be grief if there wasn't love.

The film and television director Norman Buckley survived the deaths of two of his intimate partners—the first, Timothy Scott, in the AIDS crisis in the 1980s, and the second, Davyd Whaley, after ten years of marriage when Davyd died by suicide in 2014. Buckley wrote a beautiful piece on grief in a blog post after the loss of Davyd, in which he thinks about the incredible pain that wraps around him daily:

> *And then I realize that the pain has always been there. I felt this sweet agony every time I looked at Davyd during our ten years together, knowing subconsciously that one or the other of us would die first. The more you feel for another person, the more you are aware of loss. And all of us live with loss every single day, whether we admit it or not.[257]*

Loving is dangerous. Letting another person see us for who we are and creating a space of intimacy with them is incredibly precious and rare. It can feel far too scary to let that sort of intimacy in, especially if we're doing just fine on our own. Buckley warns us against rejecting the vulnerability of loving:

> *The building of the wall against it I think is a big mistake. And I think that's the culture we live in, it's that, "well, I just want to be happy all the time." To really feel a loss of a loved one is an absolutely crucial phase. And recognizing how much you loved them. If you detach from the experience, then you're detaching from the love.[258]*

No one wants to feel the grief that comes with losing a loved one, but if we truly let ourselves be present with the ones who are in our lives now, we might have to feel a little touch of that grief every time we see them. This is one of the reasons I think survivors might be so much more capable of choosing this radical, dangerous love: we've already dealt with grief. We've already faced the worst of ourselves and some of the shadows of the toxicity of the culture we were socialized in. We've learned (or we're learning) to sit with uncomfortable emotions and to choose presence anyway, to choose survival. I think we are capable of choosing love, too.

Whether we are working on these patterns of love and intimacy in our romantic relationships or in other ways, we do need to practice love. Loving ourselves, loving other people, and letting others love us are three separate but interconnected practices. We must learn how to be intimate with our world, our community, and our closest people if we want to be able to access joy, connection, and a healthier relationship with the world we occupy. "You can't get happy by yourself," Stone has said, "It's an

257   Buckley, Norman. "Davyd Whaley's Birthday 2014." normanbuckley.com, Dec 6, 2014. http://normanbuckley.com/blog/davyd-whaley/davyd-whaleys-birthday-2014/
258   I, Survivor. "Life After Death." I Heart Radio, Oct 2, 2018. https://www.iheart.com/podcast/272-i-survivor-29655305/episode/life-after-death-29931005/

oxymoron. The path toward joy, the path toward freedom, has to include other people."[259] We have to be brave to let them in.

LOVE AS A RADICAL ACT

Mindful, honest, vulnerable, deeply connected true love is radical. It rejects our social conditioning to objectify each other and insists on seeing other human beings as human beings, whole, flawed, and capable of changing. Loving ourselves in this way makes us more powerful, and thus less susceptible to the messages about what we need to buy to shove down the loneliness and despair that come with being forced to perform social roles we never agreed were right for us.

Choosing a different path for love might be difficult, but when we find others who are willing to be vulnerable with us, we feel that thing we've always been looking for: connection. We get to enter into that special place John Welwood describes as "a sanctuary from the world of facades, a sacred space where we can be ourselves, as we are."[260] True love works to reject dynamics of power and domination, even though it may never be able to completely eradicate them. It aims to subjectify the human beings in front of us despite having been taught nothing but how to objectify. True love is powerful enough to hold our darkness and our pain with kindness. True love gives us the chance to change and grow, to connect to the erotic power that lives with our deepest feelings. As we choose this form of love in our intimate lives, we are pushing against the status quo of performance, domination, dehumanization, and objectification.

This type of loving is a practice that involves daily action, and it is not always easy. But I believe that we, the survivors, may be uniquely equipped to choose this courageous form of love because of what we've gained in the crucible of recovery. We've seen the true face of what we've been sold, and it's a flimsy form of love. Our loneliness calls us to something better, so we learn to love ourselves, we let others love us, and we practice loving them. We learn to access true love as a source of power within us—as an expression of our erotic force that resists our oppression. We don't need to dominate others when we see ourselves as enough. We can change this place from a battlefield to a field of love simply by showing up and loving more. All we have to do is practice. As the American poet Rod Smith has written:

> *We work too hard*
> *We're too tired*
> *to fall in love.*
> *Therefore we must*
> *overthrow the government.*

259   Stone, Michael. "Mindfulness & Social Action: Towards a Secular Spirituality." Lecture, Semperviva Yoga Studio, Vancouver, Jan 2015.
260   In hooks, bell. *All About Love: New Visions.* New York, W. Morrow (2000): 30.

We work too hard
We're too tired
to overthrow the government.
Therefore we must
fall in love.[261]

---

261   Stone, Michael. "Mindfulness & Social Action: Towards a Secular Spirituality." Lecture, Semperviva Yoga Studio, Vancouver, Jan 2015.

ACKNOWLEDGMENTS

First of all, thank you for reading this book. Writing it was strange and hard and amazing. For months I felt so vulnerable, like all my nerve endings were coming out of my skin, every emotion, no matter how fleeting, bright and fully visible on my face. I stared into space a lot. I had at least three giggle fits. I sang off-key to pop songs in my car. I screamed at a lot of drivers who didn't signal their goddamn lane changes. I lost my filter for a while and had a few awkward conversations at parties when I got just a little too excited about the science of healing from trauma, or what happens in your intestines when you're on a first date, or how penises and vaginas *really* work. I cried at a lot of credit card commercials. I wrote from the gut, from the butterflies in my vagina, sheets of words coming straight from my tender organs. One day after a flurry of writing, I looked up at my lover, sitting on the couch reading a book nearby, and said, "Man. I got some shit to say." He laughed pretty heartily at that.

In those first drafts, I set aside any fear of what anyone was going to think of my story and what I had to say so that I could *say it*. I needed time to be in the vulnerability of simply getting the story out. Editing was a different process. I edited with you in the room with me, my reader. I tried to hold your heart and your uniqueness and everything I don't understand about you and your experience tenderly in my hands. I tried to shape a narrative that could offer hope and sweetness and everything I've learned that I thought might help. But that whole time, you were the one helping me. The thought that someone might read my story, care, and even get something out of it kept me willing to keep my nerves all a-jangle while I remembered and analyzed and researched and thought and asked questions and got feedback and worried about what my parents would think and obsessed about the fantastic, harrowing, and often beautiful process of recovering desire after sexual assault. For me, writing this book was Step Nine. I'm sure there will be many more steps to go from here as I encounter new phases in my life, but I feel incredibly fortunate to have the opportunity to take what happened to me and turn it into something that might possibly be helpful to you. I really hope it is. Thank you for being a part of my healing journey. I hope I can be a part of yours.

Thank you to my agent, Robert Lecker, who has believed in me for a long time and pushed me to keep going deeper, to stop hiding from this story, and to find out what was at the heart of what I really wanted to say. I feel incredibly lucky to trust Robert to push me to be brave but also to let me know in no uncertain terms when I can do better. That support is invaluable. Thank you.

Deep thanks to Erin Kirsh, a brilliant writer and fantastic editor who knows just how to ride that fine line between being supportive and encouraging while also being honest about what needs some work. You held a tender story in your hands, and you made it so much better. Thank you.

Thank you to Brenda Knight and the entire team at Mango for the huge amount of support and your belief in the need for a story like this.

Thank you, Kaelyn Elfert, Emilee Nimetz, Nicole Marcia, Megan Laven, Neil Griffith, Ryan Cho, Chris White, Jeremy Radin, and Rahel Claman for your perspectives, the many deep conversations, and your willingness to listen to me bumble through my ideas with you. Thank you to David Hatfield and all the men I've had the privilege to encounter at Manology. Thank you to Jess Owen and Katrina Topping for your invaluable emotional support. Thank you to my parents, Jane and Mike, for your absolutely unconditional support. Thank you, Rena Graham, Matt Loeb, Kelsey Savage, Alex Roth, Zack Peters, Ann Robson, and Tanille Geib for your willingness to show up and offer support in all kinds of ways.

RESOURCES

ORGANIZATIONS

1. RAINN, the Rape, Abuse, & Incest National Network, has a web page at rainn.org and runs a toll-free national US hotline at 800.656.HOPE. Their website also has an extensive list of resources here: www.rainn.org/national-resources-sexual-assault-survivors-and-their-loved-ones

2. Forge Forward supports transgender individuals in particular: forge-forward.org

3. Women Against Violence Against Women Rape Crisis Center in British Columbia has many resources: www.wavaw.ca

4. 1in6 ('One in Six') supports male survivors of sexual violence: 1in6.org

FURTHER READING

1. Brotto, Lori. *Better Sex Through Mindfulness.* Vancouver, Greystone Books (2018).

2. DePaulo, Bella. *Singled Out: How Singles are Stereotyped, Stigmatized, and Ignored, and Still Live Happily Ever After.* New York, St. Martin's Press (2006).

3. Digby, Tom. *Love and War: How Militarism Shapes Sexuality and Romance.* New York, Columbia University Press (2014).

4. Herman, Judith. *Trauma and Recovery: The Aftermath of Violence—from Domestic Abuse to Political Terror.* New York, Basic Books (1997).

5. hooks, bell. *All About Love: New Visions.* New York, W. Morrow (2000).

6. hooks, bell. *The Will to Change: Men, Masculinity, and Love.* New York, Washington Square Press (2004).

7. Kasl, Charlotte Davis. *Women, Sex, and Addiction: A Search for Love and Power.* New York, Harper & Row Perennial Library (1990).

8. Lerner, Harriet. *The Dance of Anger: A Woman's Guide to Changing the Patterns of Intimate Relationships.* New York, HarperCollins (2005).

9. Lorde, Audre. *Sister Outsider: Essays and Speeches.* Berkeley, Crossing Press (2007).

10. Nagoski, Emily. *Come as You Are: The Surprising New Science That Will Transform Your Sex Life.* New York, Simon and Schuster (2015).

11. Perel, Esther. *Mating in Captivity: Unlocking Erotic Intelligence.* New York, Harper (2007).

12. Perel, Esther. *The State of Affairs: Rethinking Infidelity.* New York, Harper (2017).

13. Real, Terrence. *I Don't Want to Talk About It: Overcoming the Secret Legacy of Male Depression.* New York, Scribner Paperback, Simon and Schuster (1997).

14. Taylor, Shelley E. *The Tending Instinct: Women, Men, and the Biology of Our Relationships.* New York, Holt Paperbacks (2003).

15. Wolf, Naomi. *Vagina: A New Biography.* New York, Ecco (2013).

ABOUT THE AUTHOR

Julie Peters is a writer and yoga teacher in Vancouver, BC, where she runs Ocean and Crow Yoga Studio with her mom, Jane. She has a biweekly column for *Spirituality and Health Magazine* and has published articles on feminist film critique and other topics on various websites and magazines. Julie's first book, *Secrets of the Eternal Moon Phase Goddesses: Meditations on Desire, Relationships, and the Art of Being Broken,* was published by SkyLight Paths in 2016. This is her second book.

CPSIA information can be obtained
at www.ICGtesting.com
Printed in the USA
LVHW021025271021
701641LV00003B/3

9 781633 539648